Radiation Therapy for Skin Cancer

Armand B. Cognetta Jr. • William M. Mendenhall
Editors

Radiation Therapy for Skin Cancer

Springer

Editors
Armand B. Cognetta Jr.
Dermatology Associates of Tallahassee
Chief, Division of Dermatology
Florida State University College of Medicine
Tallahassee, FL, USA

William M. Mendenhall
Department of Radiation Oncology
College of Medicine
University of Florida
Gainesville, FL, USA

ISBN 978-1-4939-4258-9 ISBN 978-1-4614-6986-5 (eBook)
DOI 10.1007/978-1-4614-6986-5
Springer New York Heidelberg Dordrecht London

Softcover reprint of the hardcover 1st edition 2013

Printed on acid-free paper

Springer is part of Springer Science+Business Media (www.springer.com)

This book is dedicated to all present and previous editors and contributors, to our trusted colleagues and coworkers, to all of our families, and specifically to our wives Nancy and Suzanne who continue to inspire us.

Preface

In reading the preface of *Radiation Treatment and Radiation Reactions in Dermatology* by Renato Pannizon M.D. and Jay Cooper M.D. (Springer 2004), we are reminded that we are following a great work which has been the standard text book for radiation therapy of skin neoplasms for the last 10 years. It is a very succinct work with renowned contributors and expert editing which, through its various reprints, has guided dermatologists around the world for the last decade.

When asked to become editors of this 2013 edition of *Radiation Therapy for Skin Cancer* we knew it would be a hard task to equal their success. We decided that this text would continue to serve as a primer on the physics, radiobiology, and practical aspects of radiation therapy as it applies to appropriate treatment planning for patients with select tumors. We expanded the chapters on patient selection and fractionation to include flexible guidelines for calculating, and if necessary, adjusting the TDF (Time Dose and Fractionation) as well as other practical additions. In addition, we greatly expanded the chapters dealing with high risk tumors and their management by radiation oncologists. It is hoped that the specific chapters on high risk squamous cell carcinoma, Merkel cell carcinoma, angiosarcoma, lymphomas, and adjuvant radiation for melanoma will be a useful reference for all cutaneous oncologists.

The list of those to thank for their assistance and support is too long for this preface. The overall goal of this book is to aid practitioners in the safe, effective, and judicious use of this time-honored treatment method. We also believe that the continued collaboration of radiation oncologists and dermatologists will result in further knowledge and refinements of the radiobiology and physics of radiation and its broad spectrum and untapped potential. We hope this will result in this modality being more recognized and utilized by knowledgeable practitioners in both of our specialties for our increasingly aging and frail patients.

Tallahassee, FL, USA — Armand B. Cognetta Jr.
Gainesville, FL, USA — William M. Mendenhalll

Contents

Contributors

Murad Alam Department of Dermatology, Northwestern University Feinberg School of Medicine, Chicago, IL, USA

Jeffrey Bennett Department of Radiology, University of Florida, Gainesville, FL, USA

Armand B. Cognetta Jr. Dermatology Associates of Tallahassee, Chief, Division of Dermatology, Florida State University College of Medicine, Tallahassee, FL, USA

Michele N. Edison Florida State University, Tallahassee, FL, USA

Jeremy L. Edwards Dermatology Associates of Tallahassee, Tallahassee, FL, USA

Kerry M.W. Fike Dermatology Associates of Tallahassee, Tallahassee, FL, USA

W. Harris Green Division of Dermatology, Florida State University College of Medicine, Tallahassee, FL, USA

Bradford S. Hoppe Department of Radiation Oncology, University of Florida Proton Therapy Institute, University of Florida, Jacksonville, FL, USA

Carolyn M. Johns Smilow Cancer Hospital Care Center, Guilford, CT, USA

David E. Kent Dermatologic Surgery Specialists, PC, Macon, GA, USA

Jeffrey M. Long Pearlman Comprehensive Cancer Center, South Georgia Medical Center, Valdosta, GA, USA

Nancy P. Mendenhall Department of Radiation Oncology, University of Florida Proton Therapy Institute, University of Florida, Jacksonville, FL, USA

William M. Mendenhall Department of Radiation Oncology, College of Medicine, University of Florida, Gainesville, FL, USA

Kenneth F. Morse Clinical Applications, Sensus Healthcare, Boca Raton, FL, USA

Rosalind Sandell Loyola University Chicago Stritch School of Medicine, Maywood, IL, USA

Thomas Shakar Dermatology Associates of Tallahassee, Tallahassee, FL, USA

Christopher M. Wolfe Lake Erie College of Osteopathic Medicine, Erie, PA, USA

History of Radiation Therapy in Dermatology

W. Harris Green and Thomas Shakar

On November 8, 1895, a German physicist and professor named Wilhelm Roentgen conducted some experiments with a cathode ray tube that led him to discover "eine neue Art von Strahlen"—"a new kind of rays" [1]. He chose the term X-*strahlen*—"X-rays" as the type of rays because the frequency and characteristics of these rays were unknown. He had made the discovery when observing that the invisible cathode rays caused a fluorescent effect on a small cardboard screen painted with barium platinocyanide. The intensity of the fluorescence was diminished proportionally by distances and by certain filter materials of various thicknesses. Roentgen was later awarded the first Nobel Prize for physics in 1901 for his efforts and a bustling new era of applied physical science was spawned from the discovery and development of the X-rays.

The discovery of X-rays also generated interest in natural sources of radiation such as the study of visibly fluorescent compounds. In 1896 Becquerel discovered that radiation was naturally occurring in all uranium compounds. After an initially unsuccessful attempt to induce fluorescence, Becquerel placed the uranium salts and the photographic plates used in his experiments in a drawer with plans to recommence the experiment at a later date. Months later when he developed the photographic plate, he discovered a darkened area which could only be explained by something intrinsic to the uranium salts. Maria Curie furthered this research by testing various materials and discovered that compounds containing thorium also exhibited radioactive properties. Pierre Curie and his brother Paul-Jacques Curie subsequently created a device known as the piezoelectrometer which allowed study

W.H. Green (✉)
Division of Dermatology, Florida State University College of Medicine, 1707 Riggins Road, Tallahassee, FL 32308, USA
e-mail: DATresearch@gmail.com

T. Shakar
Dermatology Associates of Tallahassee, 1707 Riggins Road, Tallahassee, FL 32308, USA

A.B. Cognetta and W.M. Mendenhall (eds.), *Radiation Therapy for Skin Cancer*,
DOI 10.1007/978-1-4614-6986-5_1,

of the intensity of radioactive emissions. While studying the substance, pitchblende, Marie and her husband Pierre Curie discovered emissions that were too intense to be explained by the amount of known uranium in the substance. Through careful experimentation, they isolated a new element polonium (after Maria's home country) and soon after came the discovery of radium. The Nobel Prize for physics was later awarded to Becquerel, Maria, and Pierre [2].

The similarity of radium's effect on the skin to that of the X-ray was noted in 1901 by Pierre Curie and Becquerel following the work of German scientists Giesel and Walkoff which ultimately gave rise to Brachytherapy (from the Greek word brachys, meaning "short"). Brachytherapy involves the placement of the radiation source inside or in short proximity to the lesion or skin condition to be treated. A more detailed history of Brachytherapy can be found at the beginning of Chap. 13.

Less than a year after the discovery, X-rays began to be used in the treatment of skin disease. The first reported use of X-rays for the treatment of a disease of the skin was done by Leopold Fruend of Vienna in 1896 on a nevus pigmentosus piliferus located on the back of a 5-year-old girl. Multiple reports surfaced describing the efficacy of X-rays in the treatment of skin cancers, including J.W. Pugh's article in 1902 entitled, "Four Cases of Rodent Ulcer Treated by X Rays," in which before- and after-photographs were displayed [3] (Fig. 1). A year later in 1903, a British dermatologist named Sequeira reported similar success in treating a longstanding, biopsy-proven BCC of the right ala of a 31-year-old female with before- and after-photographs [4] (Fig. 2). With multiple early reports of success treating skin cancers with X-rays and a tremendous enthusiasm for its potential, Pusey, an American dermatologist attempted to formulate an appropriate therapeutic window for this new, powerful, and potentially dangerous modality in his lecture entitled "Rationale of and the Indications for Therapeutic Use of Rontgen Rays," given at the 27th Annual Meeting of the American Dermatology Association in Washington on May 13th and 14th, 1903. This new treatment modality proved to be a tremendous dermatologic breakthrough affording success in treating numerous previously recalcitrant skin cancers and diseases.

Although the initial cathode ray tubes were somewhat erratic and unreliable in regard to the quality and intensity of their beams, new innovations in technology allowed for greater control of X-ray delivery via cathode ray tubes. In 1913 Coolidge introduced a modification of the cathode ray tube by increasing the vacuum and using a tungsten anode. These improvements allowed for a more reliable machine that could operate at higher voltages (150 kV) for longer periods of time. This led to the eventual development of a 200 kV machine in 1922 which enabled physicians to treat deeper tumors [4]. With the advent of these more reliable tubes, dermatologists such as George Miller MacKee served as pioneers in the field of radiation therapy for skin cancers and provided a benchmark textbook in 1921 entitled "X-Rays and Radium in the Treatment of Skin Disease" which, along with the subsequent editions, proved to be the gold standard for decades to come.

Before the discovery and widespread use of systemic and topical steroids, superficial radiation and Grenz ray therapy were both successfully utilized by dermatologists and non-dermatologists alike in the treatment of several benign yet recalcitrant

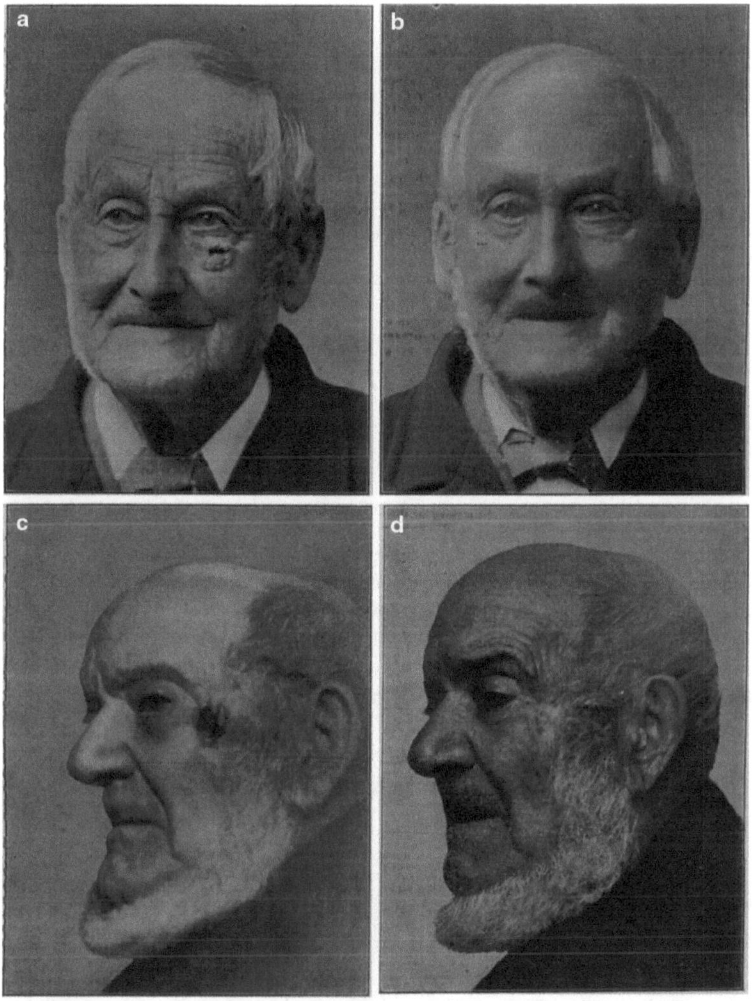

Fig. 1 Representative cases from Pugh's original study from 1902 of a 93-year-old man with a rodent ulcer on his *left* upper cheek before (**a**) and 2 years after (**b**) radiation therapy and in an 83-year-old man with a rodent ulcer on his *left* temple before (**c**) and after (**d**) 34 "sittings" of radiation therapy (reproduced from Br Med J, Pugh J.W., Four Cases of Rodent Ulcer Treated by X Rays, vol. 2154, pp. 882–88, © 1902 with permission from BMJ Publishing Group Ltd.)

skin conditions such as chronic inflammatory diseases, acne, and hirsutism [5–7]. With time, however, numerous reports of radiation dermatitis, atrophy, wrinkling, telangiectasias, ulceration, and secondary malignancies in these larger treatment site applications followed. Non-dermatologists and beauticians began using X-rays in the treatment of hirsutism and removal of superfluous hair via the "Tricho System and the "X-Ray Razor" yielding thousands of cases of unwanted radiation-induced sequelae [8] (Fig. 3). This prompted the American Medical Association's Bureau of

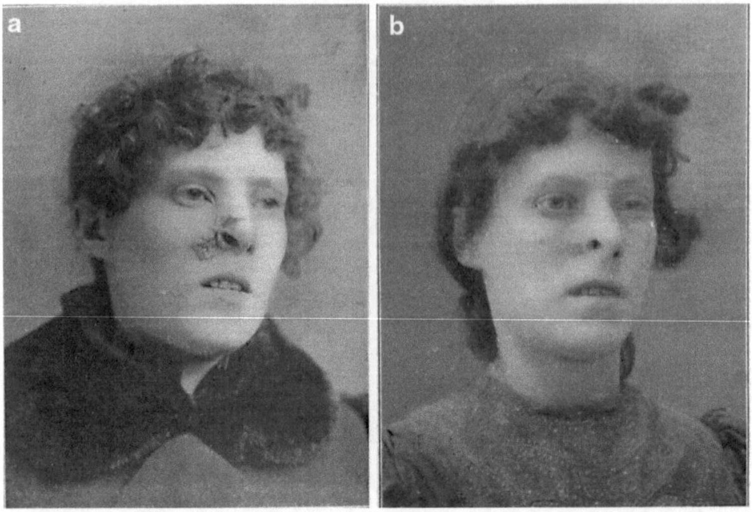

Fig. 2 Representative case from James H. Sequeira's report from 1903 showing a rodent ulcer on a 31-year-old woman before (**a**) and approximately 1 year after (**b**) X-ray therapy (reproduced from Br Med J, Sequeira J.H., Further observations upon the treatment of rodent ulcer by the X rays, vol. 2214, pp. 1307–1310, © 1903 with permission from BMJ Publishing Group Ltd.)

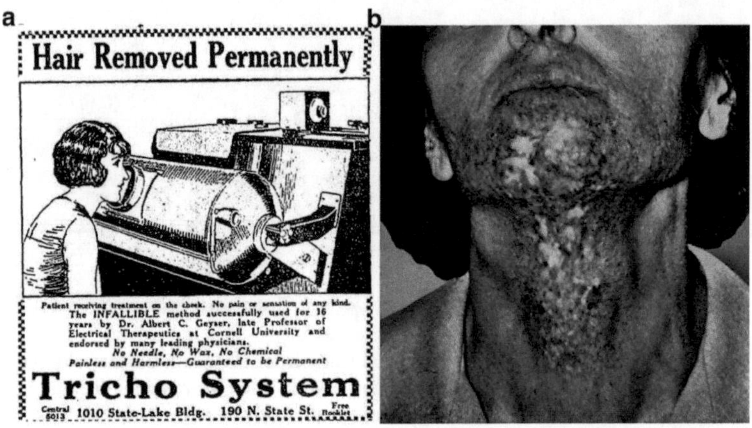

Fig. 3 An advertisement for the Tricho System unit for the removal of excess hair via X-ray (**a**) and long term sequelae including radiodermatitis and scarring in treated areas 35 years later (**b**) (**a**, from the March 7th, 1926 *Chicago Tribune* Classifieds section; **b**, from Cipollaro and Crossland 5th edition text: X-rays and Radium in the Treatment of Diseases of the Skin, Figure 20–13, pg 377)

Investigation to get involved via investigations and public warnings in the 1930s. George Miller MacKee's quote in the preface of his 1921 first edition textbook entitled "X-Rays and Radium in the Treatment of Skin Disease" proved to be a prescient charge for dermatologists and the medical community: "Unfortunately they [x rays and radium] are dangerous agents in unskilled hands. Every physician who employs x rays and radium should have a thorough training and should possess modern knowledge and equipment."

In addition to superficial X-ray therapy and radium therapy, a lower energy therapy with similar effects was also advanced. In 1923, Bucky described what became known as the Bucky ray, or Grenz ray. Grenz is German for "border" as the rays were on the border of ionizing radiation as they had a wavelength longer than that of X-rays, but shorter than that of the ultraviolet region. During the time of its discovery, the Grenz ray was produced at a peak kilovoltage (kVp) at around 8–12. With the development of the beryllium-window tube, the scientists were able to increase the kVp to roughly 14–15. Because the claims made by Bucky of the Grenz ray having no radiation sequelae proved to be inconsistent and because of the differences between Grenz and Soft X-rays being somewhat unclear at the time, there was disagreement over its uses and limitations of its popularity. In 1931 at the Council on Physical Medicine of the American Medical Association, MacKee stated, "In general, it is doubtful whether any skin disease… can be cured with Grenz rays that cannot be cured with X-rays- of short wavelengths of with beta rays of radium." It seems that the important aspect of the Grenz ray, which lies in its increased margin of safety compared to X-rays, was lost to many dermatologists [9]. Grenz rays did however continue to be used successfully by some dermatologists in the treatment of lentigo maligna and benign skin diseases such as psoriasis and refractory hand and foot eczema. A fuller history and discussion of Grenz ray therapy can be found in Chap. 11.

Topical and systemic steroids began to be used with success in the 1950s for inflammatory conditions establishing a radiation-sparing alternative. Although Grenz ray therapy for inflammatory conditions declined in lieu of topical steroids, superficial X-ray treatment regimens for cutaneous malignancies became more established, refined, and predictable and with far fewer side effects as more systematic reviews of treatment thresholds were performed. In 1944, Strandqvist presented the isoeffect curve where the total accumulated dose for each of the 280 cases of carcinoma of the skin treated by X-ray, which was followed for at least 5 years, was plotted on a log scale against overall treatment time [10]. In the 1960s and early 1970s, the initial Strandqvist isoeffect curve of 1944 was further modified with the efforts of Orton and Ellis, who, in addition to time and dose, incorporated the number of fractions, the interval between fractions, and decay factor into applied dosimetry and planning [11, 12]. The resulting time dose fractionation (TDF) reference tables that were instituted in the early 1970s provided a standardization of treatment and fractionation schemes. The ensuing treatment parameters allowed dermatologists greater consistency and confidence in delivering non-recoverable injurious effects on radiosensitive, mutagenically altered tumor cells while imparting recoverable and nonlethal injuries to healthy surrounding cells, providing greater efficacy rates and cosmesis outcomes. On the shoulders of early pioneers such as George MacKee and Anthony Cipollaro, newer generation dermatologists such as Herbert Goldschmidt and Renato Panizzon continued to contribute to the collective understanding of radiation therapy in dermatology through their studies and definitive textbooks which became an intrinsic part of dermatology residency training programs. Despite the significant progress made in the field of radiation therapy for skin cancers by such dermatologists in the 1960s and 1970s, its overall reported use continued to decline. According to a large survey amidst dermatologists by Goldschmidt in 1974, 55.5 % of dermatology offices used radiation as a treatment modality [13]. Fewer and fewer superficial X-ray machines were manufactured and the last Picker NR2 Zephyr Superficial X-ray machine was manufactured around 1965 and the last Universal Superficial X-ray machine around 1988. With the advent and increasing availability of Mohs surgery and its associated tumor clearance rates and relative absence of late side effects, the emphasis on superficial radiation therapy in dermatologic training centers gradually decreased. According to a survey conducted by Kingery in 1986, only 12 % of dermatologic training centers used superficial radiation [14]. Fewer and fewer machines became available and fewer dermatologists, upon the completion of residency training, continued this once widely utilized treatment modality. Similarly, the number of radiotherapy lectures at the American Academy of Dermatology (AAD) national meetings declined over the years.

Despite the waning of its usage amidst dermatologists, there have been recent signs of a persistence and possible resurgence in the dermatology community. New and modernized in-office machines are being built and sold among dermatologists and Mohs surgeons alike. These machines have new safety, calibration, and display features which greatly facilitate the treatment delivery process. Superficial X-ray therapy forums are surfacing once again at the AAD national meetings. Recently, Cognetta et al. reported 10-year results of SXRT of over 1,700 lesions in over 1,500 patients with 5-year cure rates around 95 % [15]. With an aging population and an increasing number of poor-surgical candidates, we may see a renaissance of this modality that may once again become an important and common tool in the dermatologist's armamentarium.

References

1. Roentgen WC. [On a new kind of ray (first report)]. Munch Med Wochenschr. 1959; 101:1237–9.
2. Mould RF. The discovery of radium in 1898 by Maria Sklodowska-Curie (1867–1934) and Pierre Curie (1859–1906) with commentary on their life and times. Br J Radiol. 1998;71(852): 1229–54.
3. Pugh JW. Four cases of rodent ulcer treated by X rays. Br Med J. 1902;1(2154):882–3.
4. Sequeira JH. Further observations upon the treatment of rodent ulcer by the X rays. Br Med J. 1903;1(2214):1307–10.
4. Buschke F. Radiation therapy: the past, the present, the future. Janeway Lecture, 1969. Am J Roentgenol Radium Ther Nuclear Med. 1970;108(2):236–46.
5. Scholefield RE. Treatment of lupus by the X rays. Br Med J. 1900;1(2053):1083–2,1081.
6. Semon HC. The X-ray treatment of acne vulgaris. Br Med J. 1920;1(3099):700–2.
7. Cleveland DE. The removal of superfluous hair by X-ray: The Marton Laboratories, Tricho System, etc. Can Med Assoc J. 1931;24(6):847–8.
8. Cipollaro AC, Einhorn MB. The use of X-rays for the treatment of hypertrichosis is dangerous. JAMA. 1947;135(6):349–53.
9. Hollander MB. Grenz rays. J Investig Dermatol. 1953;21(1):15–25.

10. Strandqvist M. Studien über die kumulative Wirkung der Röntgenstrahlen bei Fraktionierung. Erfahrungen aus dem Radiumhemmet an 280 Haut -und Lippenkarzinomen. Acta Radiol (Suppl). 1944;55:1–300.
11. Ellis F. Dose, time and fractionation: a clinical hypothesis. Clin Radiol. 1969;20(1):1–7.
12. Orton CG, Ellis F. A simplification in the use of the NSD concept in practical radiotherapy. Br J Radiol. 1973;46(547):529–37.
13. Goldschmidt H. Ionizing radiation therapy in dermatology. Current use in the United States and Canada. Arch Dermatol. 1975;111(11):1511–7.
14. Kingery FA. Radiation therapy in dermatologic training centers. J Am Acad Dermatol. 1986;14(6):1108–10.
15. Cognetta A, Howard B, Heaton H, Stoddard E, Hong G, Green WH. Superficial X-ray in the treatment of basal cell and squamous cell carcinoma: a viable option. American Academy of Dermatology, Annual Meeting. San Diego, CA; 2012.

Radiobiology

Kenneth F. Morse and Christopher M. Wolfe

Introduction

Radiobiology refers to the wide array of cellular effects of electromagnetic radiation to biologic systems. Electromagnetic radiation is radiant energy in motion that demonstrates both wave and particle characteristics. The effects of radiation depend on the type of radiation, quantity, and the biologic system affected and include cell killing, DNA damage, genetic mutation, neoplastic transformation, and cell cycle disturbances among others. Radiobiology as it relates to radiotherapy focuses on radiation that has the ability to cause ionization of atoms. In general, radiation energy above 10 eV is capable of producing ionizations. The most significant effect of radiation is cell killing as a result of the chemical bonds broken due to the ionization of atoms.

Interaction of Radiation with Matter

In superficial radiotherapy (low-voltage X-ray) electrons are accelerated towards a target such as tungsten to yield a resultant beam of photons when treating skin cancer. Radiation methods may be categorized based on kilovoltage. Photons (X-rays) with kinetic energies between 20 and 100 keV are referred to as superficial or soft X-rays, between 200 and 400 keV orthovoltage X-rays, 400–800 keV supervoltage X-rays, and those with kinetic energies above 1,000 keV are called megavoltage

K.F. Morse, CMD (✉)
Clinical Applications, Sensus Healthcare, 851 Broken Sound Parkway NW #215, Boca Raton, FL 33487, USA
e-mail: ken@sensushealthcare.com

C.M. Wolfe, BS, PA-C
Lake Erie College of Osteopathic Medicine, 1858 West Grandview Boulevard, Erie, PA 16509-1025, USA

A.B. Cognetta and W.M. Mendenhall (eds.), *Radiation Therapy for Skin Cancer*,
DOI 10.1007/978-1-4614-6986-5_2, © Springer Science+Business Media New York 2013

X-rays [1]. Other methods involve the use of linear accelerators to produce a continuous stream of electrons (electron beam radiotherapy), typically in the range of 6,000–9,000 keV to treat skin cancer, all of which are capable of producing ionizations in matter.

Interaction Types

Photon interactions: A photon can penetrate matter without interacting, it can be completely absorbed by depositing its energy, or it can be scattered (deflected) from its original direction and deposit part of its energy as follows:

1. Photon to electron interaction: a photon transfers all its energy to an electron located in one of the atomic shells, usually the outer shell. The electron is ejected from the atom and begins to pass through surrounding matter.
2. Compton interaction: only a portion of the energy is absorbed and a photon is produced with reduced energy. The photon that is produced leaves in a different direction than that of the original photon. This reaction is classified as a scattering process because of this change in direction.
3. Pair production: the photon interacts with the nucleus in such a way that its energy is converted to matter producing a pair of particles, an electron and a positively charged positron. This only occurs with photons with energies in excess of 1.02 MeV.

Electron interactions: Energized electrons transfer energy to surrounding tissues. These electrons are produced by the dislodging of an electron from an atom's outer shell by use of photons or by a direct stream of electrons produced by linear accelerators. Electrons immediately begin to transfer their energy to surrounding material, interacting with other electrons without touching them because they carry an electrical charge. As these energized electrons pass through material they push other electrons away, if the force is sufficient to remove another electron subsequent ionizations result. For example, in air a 50 keV photon undergoing a photon to electron interaction can eject an electron capable of ionizing over 1,000 additional atoms. The major biological effect of photons (X-ray) is due to electron interactions.

Within cells radiation may interact with DNA or water. The damage caused by these interactions is categorized as either direct (DNA is damaged directly) or indirect (cells are damaged indirectly via free radicals). Radiation is more likely to interact with water as it accounts for 70 % or more of the total cell mass [2] and DNA is present only as a tightly folded double strand within the nucleus. Therefore the majority of cell killing with radiation is through the indirect action of free radicals on the cells that are ionized. Direct damage to DNA, when it occurs, more often causes reproductive death; i.e., cells continue to undergo normal metabolic function but are unable to undergo cell division. When the radiation has enough energy it can eject an electron from the orbital shell of the hydrogen atom of water; it causes the water molecule to disassociate into hydrogen and a hydroxyl-free radical and is therefore ionizing. The highly reactive free radicals formed by radiolysis of water are capable of adding to the direct DNA damage of radiation by migrating to and damaging the DNA indirectly [3, 4].

$$\underset{(\text{XRT})}{\text{DNA}} \rightarrow \underset{(\text{ion pair})}{[\text{DNA}^{+} + \text{e}^{-}]} \rightarrow \underset{(\text{DNA-free radical})}{\text{DNA}}$$

$$\underset{(\text{XRT})}{\text{H}_2\text{O}} \rightarrow \underset{(\text{ion pair})}{[\text{H}_2\text{O}^{+} + \text{e}^{-}]} \rightarrow \underset{(\text{Hydroxyl-free radical; DNA-free radical; water})}{\text{OH} + \text{DNA} + \text{H}_2\text{O}}$$

Ionizing radiation deposits energy as it traverses an absorbing medium; when it does, it may produce interactions that occur along a path. Photons and displaced electrons deposit random and discrete packets of energy referred to as "spurs" (100 eV or less deposited), "blobs" (100–500 eV), or "short tracks" (500–5,000 eV). Discrete is the term used because the energy deposition is discontinuous and a relatively large amount of energy is deposited (on a microscopic scale) in a small volume of tissue. The average amount of energy deposited on a macroscopic scale, however, is minuscule. This is considered an efficient process for producing biologic damage. If the beam of energy used to treat a skin cancer were converted entirely to heat it would raise the temperature of the tissue by less than 0.01 °C [5]. This efficiency is demonstrated by another example, the total amount of energy deposited in a 70-kg human that will result in a 50 % probability of death is only about 70 cal, the same energy absorbed in one sip of hot coffee [4].

Dose/Units

There are several basic measurements that pertain to radiation. Within the realm of radiobiology only the absorbed dose is of primary concern. As stated previously radiation may pass through material totally unaffected, may be partially absorbed resulting in reduced energy, or it may be completely absorbed. The absorbed energy is considered biologically effective. In the past the absorbed dose of radiation was expressed in units called "rad" (radiation absorbed dose). A dose of 1 rad is equal to the absorption of 100 ergs of radiation energy per gram of absorbing material. The modern SI units used today are the gray (Gy). A dose of 1 Gy is equal to the absorption of 1 J of radiation energy per kilogram of absorbing material. For comparison, 1 Gy (100 centigrays) is equal to 100 rads, thus centigrays (cGy) and rads are equivalent.

Linear Energy Transfer

The total absorbed dose is, by itself, insufficient in determining the net biological effectiveness of different forms of radiation. Linear energy transfer (LET) is a measure of the energy transferred to a material as an ionizing particle traverses it, and is used to quantify the effects of ionizing radiation on biological systems. Different forms of radiation produce a different number of ionizations along a particle's track. In the microdosimetric pattern of energy deposition, the density or spacing of ionization events determines the biological effectiveness of that specific radiation. The closer the ionization events are to one another within a given length the more the energy will be deposited, and hence the more biologically effective per unit dose the type of radiation will be. It is a function of both the charge and mass of the ionizing particle and is measured in keV/μm. Heavier particles such as alpha particles will produce more events per unit length than photons which set in motion electrons with negligible mass. For example, a 250 keV X-ray (photon) has an average LET of 2.0 keV/μm, whereas alpha particle has an LET of 100–150 keV/μm. It is also important to note that for a given type of radiation, the LET increases with decreasing particle energy and the number of ionizations increases as a particle slows down [6].

Relative Biological Effectiveness

Relative biological effectiveness (RBE) is a number that expresses the relative amount of damage that a fixed amount of ionizing radiation of a given type can inflict on biological tissues. The International Committee on Radiological Protection (ICRP) uses the term "radiation weighting factor" to determine the equivalent biological effectiveness of different radiation types (Table 1) and went on to say "The RBE of one radiation compared with another is the inverse ratio of the absorbed doses producing the same effect." In light of the differences between high LET (alpha particles) and low LET (X-rays), it allows for comparison of two radiation beams of different LETs required to give the same biologic endpoint. Early on it was established that X-rays, gamma rays, and beta radiation were equivalent for all cell types in biologic effect, therefore X-rays (photons) at 250 keV energy were

Table 1 International Committee on Radiological Protection (ICRP) summary of the equivalent biological effectiveness of different radiation types

Radiation	Energy range	Radiation weighting factor/RBE
X-rays, gamma rays, electrons, positrons, muons		1
Neutrons	<10 keV	5
	10–100 keV	10
	100 keV–2 MeV	20
	2–20 MeV	10
	>20 MeV	5
Protons	>2 MeV	2
Alpha particles		20

Adapted with permission from 1990 Recommendations of the International Commission on Radiological Protection [7]

used as the standard and assigned an RBE of 1. This formula is applicable to all subsequent forms of radiation modalities (positrons, neutrons, alpha particles) and allows for useful comparison. Below is the formula for RBE:

RBE = Dose of reference radiation (low LET) / Dose of test radiation (high LET)

For example, if 40 Gy of X-rays (photons) kills 50 % of tumor cells and it takes 2 Gy of alpha particles to produce the same effect, the RBE would be 40/2 = 20 using X-rays as the reference radiation.

It is expected that research conducted in radiobiology to determine RBE values will state the exact experimental conditions, as it is highly variable and depends on several radiation parameters such as type of radiation, total dose, dose rate, fractionation schedule, and the biologic endpoint being measured. It is also important to note that there is a linear relationship between LET and RBE, with increasing RBE as the LET increases up to a maximum of 100 keV/μm, beyond this point the RBE begins to fall due to "over-kill effect." A given radiation type may have several RBEs depending on the biologic endpoint being measured. For example, the RBE for alpha particles whose measured biologic endpoint is tumor death is different from the RBE for the same alpha particles when the measured endpoint is radiodermatitis.

Cell Survival Curves

In radiotherapy for cancer, cell death is the biologic endpoint of greatest interest. Cell death to radiobiologists is somewhat different from the traditional definition of death, referring to a permanent cessation of vital functions. In the radiobiologic sense it refers to the loss of reproductive ability of a cell and is termed "clonogenic" or "reproductive" death. It follows that the cell may remain physically intact and metabolically active for some time after undergoing irradiation, with some cells even undergoing a few additional mitoses before dying in the traditional sense.

Cell survival curves are determined by an in vitro plating method. A known number of tumor cells are plated then irradiated. The numbers of surviving colonies are counted to determine the proportion of cells able to survive that dose of radiation. The fraction of surviving cells is plotted on a logarithmic scale against radiation dose on a linear scale. Initial survival curves were based on a single-hit, "all-or-nothing" inactivation of a single target, followed by survival curves based on target theory (multiple target or multiple hits to the same target). The single-hit, multi-target model has since been invalidated though its parameters are still used for comparative purposes today. In the 1970s the linear-quadratic or "alpha-beta" formula was introduced to reflect what was observed in practice, clinical studies, and mammalian cells at the low dose region of the survival curves and with fractionated doses [8]. The equation proved to fit survival data well and was based on the

Fig. 1 Alpha-beta formula representing the rate of cell kill from the interaction of two sublesions. α = the rate of cell kill by a single-hit process; β = the rate of cell kill by a two-hit mechanism

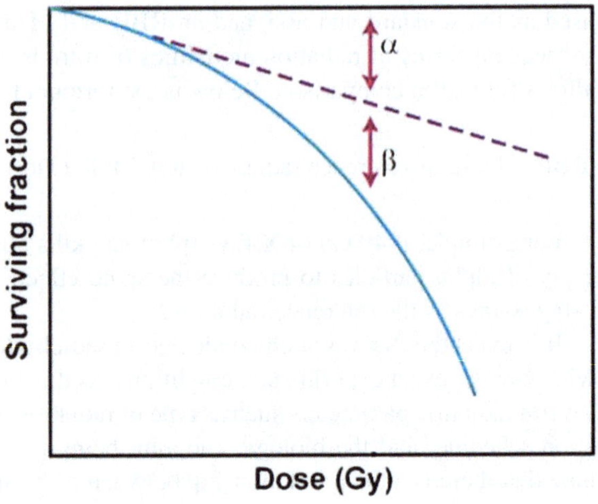

proposition that a radiation-induced lethal lesion resulted from the interaction of two sublesions or events [9]. Fig. 1 shows α which is the rate of cell kill by a single-hit process and β which is the rate of cell kill by a two-hit mechanism.

Powers of Ten

The goal of radiotherapy is to reduce the number of clonogenic cells. Tumor control is achieved when these cells are killed or inactivated. The probability of local tumor control is derived from Poisson statistics using the equation $P = e^{-n}$, where P is the tumor control probability and n is the average number of surviving clonogenic cells. The "powers of ten" describes the logarithmic relationship of tumor control based on exponential cell killing. The "powers of ten" terminology does not infer the percentage probability of cure relates by a factor of 10 to the number of clonogenic cells left after a course of radiotherapy but rather describes the logarithmic (10^x) numbers of clonogenic cells that must be eradicated to achieve a certain percentage of cure probability. For example, in most tumors if an average of two clonogenic cells exists at the end of radiotherapy the control rate would be 10 % (i.e., 9 out of 10 tumors of the same size and radio sensitivity will recur); at 0.1 clonogenic cells per tumor the control probability increases to 90 % and at 0.01 cells the control would be 99 % [6].

Oxygen Effect

Molecular oxygen is the best known chemical modifier of radiation action. The presence or absence of oxygen within a cell influences the biological effect of ionizing radiation. The larger the cell oxygenation, the larger the biological effect of radiation. This effect was observed first in the early 1900s whereby decreased radiation skin reactions were noticed when pressure was applied to skin decreasing the blood flow [10]. A simple model of the effect of oxygen holds, in that oxygen is required to create free radicals necessary to damage DNA following irradiation and it is believed that hypoxic cells are 3 times more resistant to radiation damage [4]. Furthermore, irradiation converts previously hypoxic cells to "Oxygenated" cells making them radiosensitive. Conceptually this may explain why anoxic tumor cells or tissues' locations with naturally lower oxygen levels, such as the lower extremities, have higher recurrence rates as well as longer periods of healing.

Cell Kinetics

Radio sensitivity of a cell depends on its phase within the cell cycle. The two well-defined periods of cell proliferation are M (mitosis) and S (DNA synthesis), with G_1 and G_2 occurring as apparent gaps of inactivity between the mitosis and the synthetic phase. In general, cells are the most sensitive to radiation in the M and G_2 phases and the most resistant in the late S phase. Ionizing radiation can cause perturbations of the cell cycle to influence radio responsiveness of tissues directly and indirectly. In tumors there is an asynchronous population of cells at various points in the cell cycle. Following radiation tumor cells are thought to be set in synchrony, and following redistribution (commencement of the cell cycle), the cell population as a whole becomes sensitized to subsequent doses of radiation [11].

Fractionation

Fractionation is the term used to describe the period of time over which a radiation dose is given (usually 2 weeks or more) rather than as a single dose. Its goal is to achieve an optimal therapeutic ratio, which is the destruction of tumor cells and the recovery and viability of normal tissue. Conclusions based on early research revealed that repair of sublethal damage occurred quickly within 6 hours of radiation, that cells become synchronized following a first dose of radiation, and that the sensitivity of a cell is dependent on the cell cycle phase [12]. Due to cell recovery between fractions, a larger total dose for a given biologic effect is needed than if given as a single dose. Healthy cells recover faster and more completely which allows for preferential killing of tumor cells and survival of healthy cells.

Strandquist [13] was the first to correlate dose with treatment time to produce an equivalent biological isoeffect. He utilized a 250 keV X-ray machine at a standard fractionation of 2 Gy/day at five treatments per week in his research of 280 skin carcinomas. He plotted a logarithm of dose versus log time for skin and connective tissue tolerance with a straight line separating the incidence of skin necrosis from that of recurrences. Later Ellis [14], using the isoeffect data for skin from Strandquist, attempted to correlate the number of fractions with the dose and total time over which the treatment was delivered. His introduction of the concept of nominal standard dose (NSD) allowed comparison of various treatment schemes or the changing of one scheme to another to gain equivalent biological effect. The formula which will be discussed in more depth in Chap. 9 is $D = \mathrm{NSD} \times T^{0.11} \times N^{0.24}$, where D is the total dose in rads, N is the number of fractions, and T is the overall time in days. Ellis' clinical observation was that fractionation was twice as important as time [15]. Time Dose Fractionation schedules are discussed further in the chapter on superficial radiotherapy treatment planning.

References

1. Goldschmidt H. Treatment planning: selection of physical factors and radiation techniques. In: Goldschmidt H, Panizzon RG, editors. Modern dermatologic radiation therapy. New York: Springer; 1991.
2. Cooper GM. The molecular composition of cells. The cell: a molecular approach. 2nd ed. Sunderland, MA: Sinauer; 2000.
3. Hutchinson F. Molecular basis for action of ionizing radiations. Science. 1961;134(3478): 533–8.
4. Hall EJ, Giaccia AJ. Radiobiology for the radiologist. 7th ed. Philadelphia: Lippincott Williams & Wilkins; 2011.
5. Goldschmidt H, Breneman JC, Breneman DL. Ionizing radiation therapy in dermatology. J Am Acad Dermatol. 1994;30(2 Pt 1):157–82; quiz 83–6.
6. Gunderson LL, Tepper JE. Clinical radiation oncology. 3rd ed. Philadelphia: Elsevier/ Saunders; 2012.
7. ICRP. 1990 Recommendations of the International Commission on Radiological Protection. Ann ICRP. 1991;21(1–3):1–201.
8. Obaturov GM. Kellerer-Rossi dual action theory. Radiobiologiia. 1977;17(5):764–71.
9. Alper T. Keynote address. Survival curve models. Radiation biology in cancer research. New York: Raven; 1980. p. 3–18.
10. Kaplan HS. Historic milestones in radiobiology and radiation therapy. Semin Oncol. 1979;6(4):479–89.
11. Withers HR. Cell cycle redistribution as a factor in multifraction irradiation. Radiology. 1975;114(1):199–202.
12. Elkind MM, Sutton H. X-ray damage and recovery in mammalian cells in culture. Nature. 1959;184:1293–5.
13. Strandquist M. A study of the cumulative effects of fractionated X-ray treatment based on the experience gained at radiumhemmet with the treatment of 280 cases of carcinoma of the skin and lip. Acta Radiol. 1944;55(Suppl):300–4.
14. Ellis F. Dose, time and fractionation: a clinical hypothesis. Clin Radiol. 1969;20(1):1–7.
15. Ellis F. Fractionation in radiotherapy. In: Deeley TJ, Wood CA, editors. Modern trends in radiotherapy. London: Butterworth; 1967. p. 34–51.

Physical Aspects of Dermatological Radiotherapy

Armand B. Cognetta Jr. and Kenneth F. Morse

Electromagnetic Spectrum

X-rays that are used in radiation therapy are easier to understand when reference is made to the electromagnetic spectrum. The electromagnetic spectrum is a continuum of all electromagnetic waves arranged according to frequency and wavelength (the distance between one wave crest to the next). An electromagnetic wave, although it carries no mass, does carry energy. We are exposed to electromagnetic waves daily from the sun, earth, and man-made devices. An electromagnetic wave transmits outwards from a source at the speed of light. These waves comprise an electric and magnetic fields which are at right angles to each other. The two fields oscillating perpendicular to each other as they travel away from the source. The E and B fields, along with being perpendicular to each other, are perpendicular to the direction the wave travels, meaning that an electromagnetic wave is a transverse wave. The energy of the wave is stored in the electric and magnetic fields (Fig. 1).

At one end of the spectrum are gamma rays, which have the shortest wavelengths and high frequencies. At the other end are radio waves, which have the longest wavelengths and low frequencies. Visible light is near the center of the spectrum. X-rays are just above the ultraviolet range of the spectrum. The X-ray wavelength is thousands of times shorter than that of ordinary light. The energy of electromagnetic waves is directly related to their frequency, X-rays are much more energetic and penetrating than light waves (Fig. 2).

A.B. Cognetta Jr. (✉)
Dermatology Associates of Tallahassee, Chief, Division of Dermatology,
Florida State University College of Medicine, 1707 Riggins Road, Tallahassee,
FL 32308, USA
e-mail: acognetta@gmail.com

K.F. Morse
Clinical Applications, Sensus Healthcare, 851 Broken Sound Parkway NW #215, Boca Raton,
FL 33487, USA

A.B. Cognetta and W.M. Mendenhall (eds.), *Radiation Therapy for Skin Cancer*,
DOI 10.1007/978-1-4614-6986-5_3, © Springer Science+Business Media New York 2013

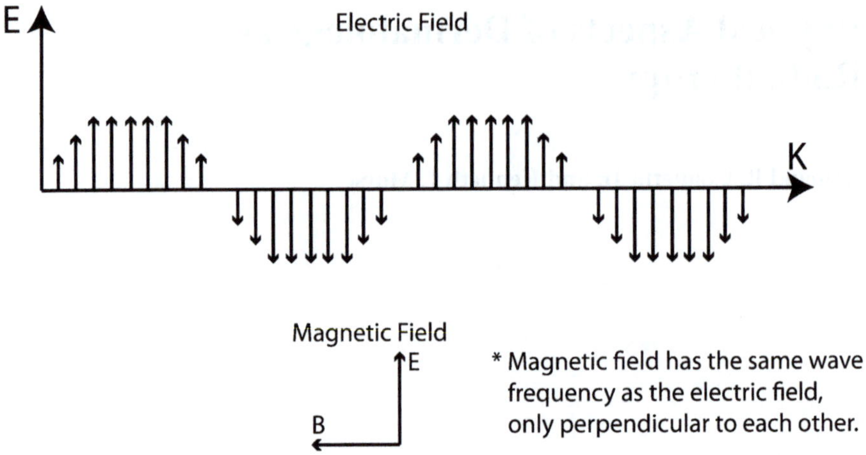

Fig. 1 This image shows a propagating transverse oscillating wave of electric (E) and magnetic fields (B), which are perpendicular to each other and have the same wave frequency. The direction of propagation is in the direction of K

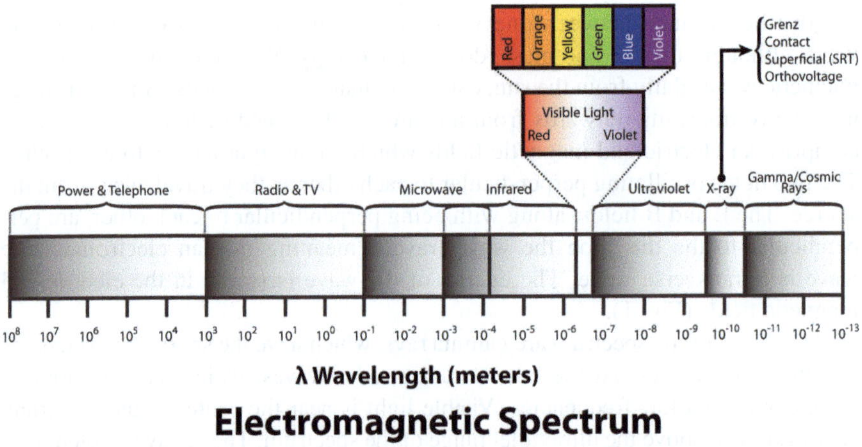

Fig. 2 The electromagnetic spectrum is a range of frequencies of electromagnetic radiation. The electromagnetic spectrum extends from low frequencies used for power and telephone to gamma/cosmic rays at the short-wavelength (high-frequency). X-rays fall between ultraviolet and gamma/cosmic rays and encompass Grenz, Contact, Superficial (SRT), and Orthovoltage energies

Nonionizing vs. Ionizing in Electromagnetic Spectrum

Nonionizing radiation refers to any type of electromagnetic radiation that does not carry enough energy to completely remove an electron from an atom or molecule, but causes excitation. In atoms, excitation transfers enough energy to an orbital electron to displace it further away from the nucleus. The absorption of nonionizing radiation in tissue creates local heating or a photochemical reaction. In a molecule, the energy is absorbed not only by the electrons but also by the whole molecule. The molecules will exhibit discrete modes of vibration and rotation [1].

X-rays are the start of ionizing section of the electromagnetic spectrum, just above ultraviolet. Ionizing radiation is any form of radiation that has enough energy to knock electrons out of atoms or molecules. The by-product of this reaction is ions. Each of the ionizations releases approximately 33 eV (eV) of energy [2]. Material surrounding the atom absorbs the energy and is electrically charged so that their properties are changed. X-ray radiation consists of packets of energy known as photons.

Two types of interactions occur with ionizing radiation, direct and indirect. When ionizing radiation directly acts on a cell, it can strike the DNA and macromolecules. When DNA or macromolecules sustain a direct hit, it can be fatal or alter the behavior of the cell. In direct action the radiation interacts directly with the critical target in the cell. Direct action is predominant with high LET radiation, especially particle ionizing radiation.

In indirect action the radiation interacts with other molecules and atoms (mainly water) within the cell to produce free radicals, which can damage the critical target within the cell. In interactions of radiation with water, short-lived reactive free radicals such as H_2O^+ (water ion) and $OH^\bullet$ (hydroxyl radical) are formed. The free radicals in turn can cause damage to the target within the cell. Indirect action is predominant with low LET radiation, X-ray, and gamma rays. The photon packets that are created are considered indirect radiation. When an ionizing photon interacts with material it sets free an electron. The electron that is set free constitutes ionization. Photons are not capable directly of producing the multiple ionization events that characterize the interactions of a charged particle. The energetic electron that is produced by the photon interaction goes on to produce multiple ionization events. The electron then interacts at a molecular level producing free radicals from fragmented water molecules. The main productions of ionizing events occur via the liberated electron and its subsequent interaction with tissue, which gives rise to the designation of photon X-ray as indirect radiation (Fig. 3).

X-ray Production

X-rays are produced in a vacuumed tube, which is composed of a cathode (filament) and an anode (target). The tube is vacuumed so the electrons used to produce X-rays will not interact with air molecules. The cathode is composed of a tungsten filament which is centered in a focusing cup. The focusing cup has a negative charge equal to the kV setting, like the electrons, and this repels and accelerates the electrons to the target. The electrons are produced by heating the filament, which in turn produces electrons by thermionic emission. Thermionic emission pertains to the heating of a metal to incandescence (glowing hot). Loosely bound valance electrons are given enough kinetic energy from the heating, to "boil off" and are accelerated towards the anode.

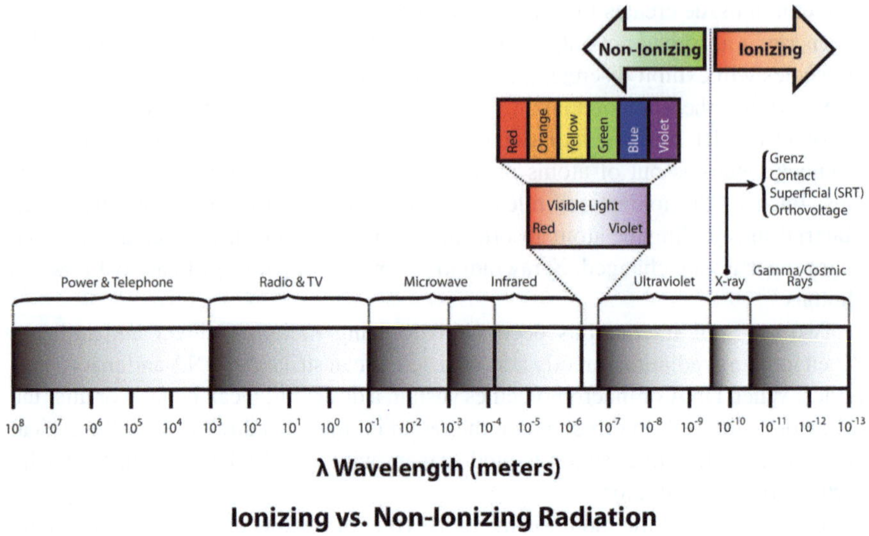

Fig. 3 Nonionizing wavelength energies occur when valance electron vibrates, but are not ejected from their orbitals, are energies up to realm of ultraviolet. The section of X-ray starts the ionization spectrum

The anode in the X-ray tube is composed of a tungsten target embedded in a copper stem. The copper helps to take some of the heat away from the anode. The anode (target) is the component in which the X-radiation is produced by electron bombardment. It is a relatively large piece of metal that connects to the positive side of the electrical circuit. The two primary functions of the anode are to convert electrons into X-rays and dissipate heat. When high potential difference measured in kV is applied across the tube, the result is a high negative charge to the cathode, and an equally high positive charge to the anode. The resulting electric field causes the electrons to be repelled by the cathode and pulled towards the anode at a very high speed. The electron stream represents the tube current measured in amps. When electrons from the filament hit the target, a lot of heat is produced. The anode is usually made of tungsten which has a unique ability to maintain its strength at high temperatures. The efficiency for X-ray production in the superficial energy range is on the order of 1 % or less. Most of the electron kinetic energy deposited in the X-ray target is transformed into heat and must be dissipated through a cooling system of circulating water, oil bath, or fan. X-ray production can be either through excitation or ionization. Excitation is where electrons acquire energy from a passing charged particle, but are not removed completely from their atom. Excited electrons may emit energy in the form of X-rays during this event before returning to a lower energy state. Ionization is the complete removal of an electron from an atom following the transfer of energy from a passing charged particle. The X-rays produced by the target are of two types, characteristic X-ray and bremsstrahlung X-ray. The majority of the X-rays produced by the anode are bremsstrahlung radiation (Fig. 4).

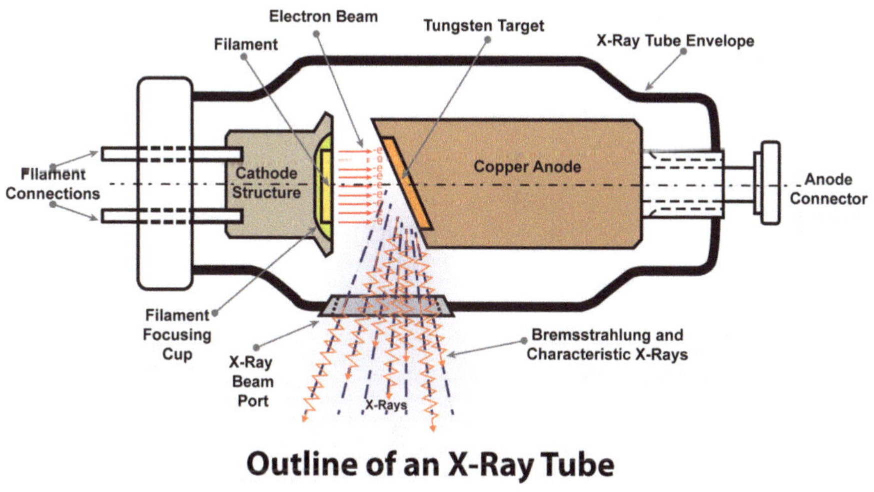

Fig. 4 A vacuum containing a cathode where the electrons are boiled off by thermionic emission and an anode were the electron beam collides with the tungsten target. The interaction of the electrons with the target produces X-rays in the form of Bremsstrahlung and characteristics

Characteristic X-rays

Characteristic X-rays are produced when a high-speed electron from the filament collides with an electron in one of the orbits of a target atom. The electron is knocked out of its orbit and creates space. This space is immediately filled by an electron from an outer orbit. When the electron drops into the open space, energy is released in the form of characteristic X-ray photons (Fig. 5). The energy of the high-speed electron must be higher than the binding energy of the target electron with which it interacts in order to achieve the ejection of the target electron; both electrons will then leave the atom. The amount of electronic energy that is converted into X-radiation depends on two factors: the atomic number (*Z*) of the anode material and the energy of the electrons. Although this process can take place in both low-*Z* and high-*Z* atoms, only for high-*Z* atoms are the binding energies sufficient to produce radiation in the X-ray portion of the electromagnetic spectrum [3]. All atoms will produce characteristic radiation but not all are visible in the X-ray portion of the electromagnetic spectrum. Elements with higher atomic numbers have their K, L, M, or N shells of sufficient energy to produce ionizing radiation. The X-ray energy is proportional to the atom's Z. Where the incident electrons have energies less than the electron binding energy, there will be no characteristic radiation emitted.

Bremsstrahlung X-rays

High-energy electrons interact directly with the electromagnetic field of a target nucleus. The electrons are deflected and lose a portion of their energy due to deceleration. The energy lost is then emitted in the form of radiation called

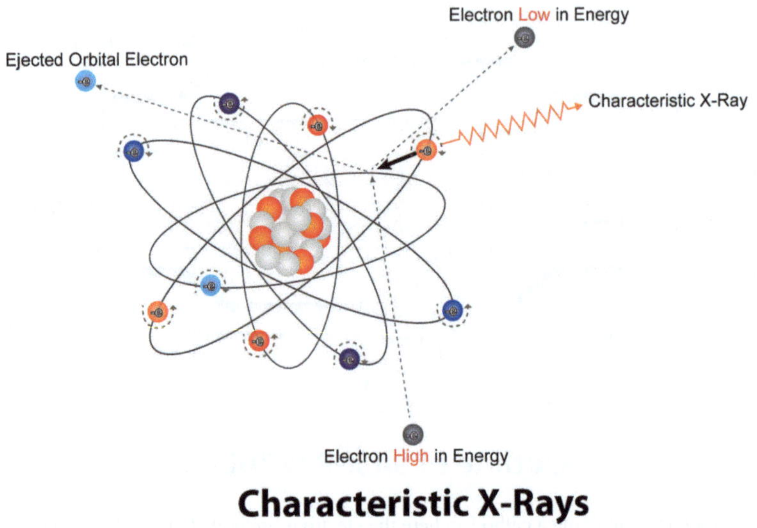

Fig. 5 A high energy electron strikes and ejects an orbital electron from a valance orbital. The high energy electron loses a portion of its energy and changes direction leaving the atom. An electron from an outer orbital drops down and fills the vacancy, the difference in the binding energy is released as a characteristic X-ray

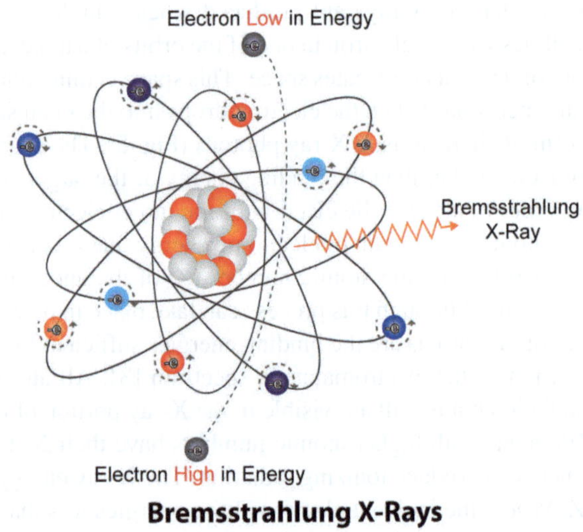

Fig. 6 A high energy electron comes in the vicinity of an atomic nucleus of the target material; its deflection by another charged particle gives of Bremsstrahlung X-ray

bremsstrahlung (braking radiation). The incident electron can lose any portion of its energy in this process. The variation in the loss of energy can produce bremsstrahlung X-rays from nearly zero to the full energy of the incident electron and up to the tubes kV (Fig. 6).

Spectrum of X-rays

The X-ray spectrum is a histogram showing the distribution of the various X-ray energies in the beam. The spectrum is a hump with several vertical spikes. The two different types of X-rays are forming the spectrum. The continuous hump represents the varying energies of bremsstrahlung X-rays. The vertical spikes are the characteristic X-rays. Together they form the X-ray spectrum unique to the tube and selected kV (Fig. 7).

X-ray Beam Quality and Filtration

The general term "quality" refers to an X-ray beam's penetrating ability. For X-ray beams that contain a spectrum of photon energies, the penetration is different for each of the energy. The overall penetration generally corresponds to the penetration of photon energy between the minimum and maximum energies of the spectrum. This energy is defined as the effective energy of the X-ray spectrum. X-ray machines produce a continuous spectrum of X-rays with energies ranging from near zero up to some maximum value, determined by the selected tube potential. The largest number of X-rays occurs at energy much lower than the maximum. This means that

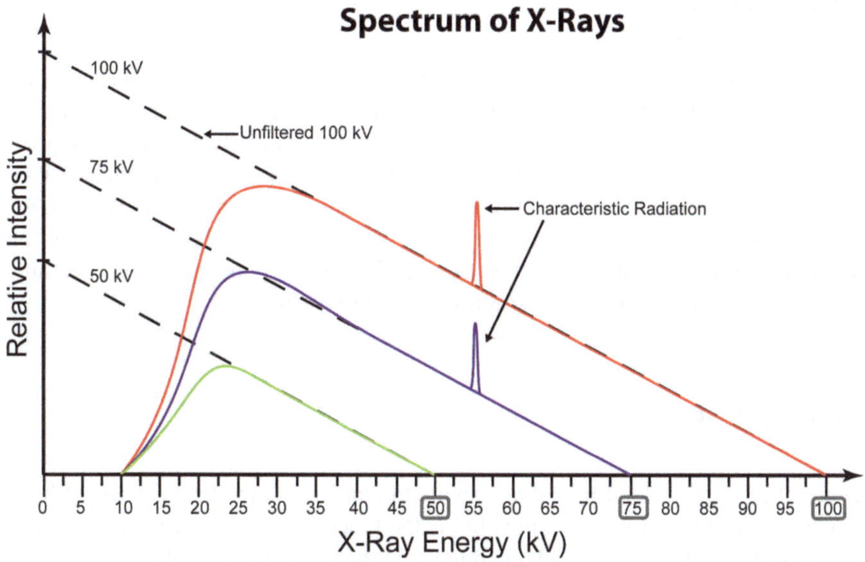

Fig. 7 An X-ray spectrum shows the distribution of various X-ray energies in the beam that is produced by an X-ray tube with a specific energy potential. This diagram shows three energy potentials of 50, 75, and 100 kV. Energy potentials above 68 kV start to produce characteristic radiation

the beam's physical properties are comparable to monoenergetic X-rays of that energy. A good estimate of the effective energy of an X-ray beam is approximately 1/3 of the maximum energy.

Filtration is achieved by placing a measured thickness of aluminum or copper between the window and the cone, this ultimately improves the quality of the X-ray beam. Filtration also reduces the intensity of the X-ray beam. The filtration minimizes the absorbed dose to the patient by eliminating the weaker portion of the spectrum. In determination of the amount of filtration required for a particular X-ray machine, Kilovolt Peak (kVp) and inherent filtration of the tube and its housing must be considered. Inherent filtration consists of the materials that X-ray photons encounter as they travel from the focal spot of the target to form the usable beam outside the tube enclosure. The total filtration of an X-ray tube is the sum of the inherent and the added filtration. The filtration provided by the X-ray tube housing assembly itself is termed the inherent filtration. The amount of inherent filtration by an X-ray tube is strongly dependent on the tube voltage, the maximum wavelength of the tube current, the choice of glass or beryllium window. Added filtration can be accomplished by placing a material in the path of the beam. The most common X-ray filtering media are tin, copper, and aluminum. For kilovoltage beams in the superficial region; aluminum is used to filter the beam. Aluminum has two significant applications in an X-ray system. It is used as a material to filter X-ray beam and also as a reference material for measuring the penetrating ability (HVL) of X-rays.

HVL Concept

HVL is that thickness of a specified material which will reduce the intensity of a beam of X-radiation to half its original value. For clinical beams, an indication of kV and HVL is recommended as a specification of beam quality. It is accepted practice to express beam quality in terms of the HVL, although most also include kVp and TSD. Increasing the penetrating ability of a radiation increases its HVL. HVL is related to, but not the same as, average photon range. The effective energy of an X-ray spectrum is the energy of a monoenergetic beam of photons that has the same penetrating ability (HVL) as the spectrum of photons (Fig. 8).

Kilovolt Peak

kVp is the peak accelerating voltage applied in an X-ray tube between the cathode and anode. The kVp (units of kilovolts) is the kinetic energy imparted to electrons boiled off the cathode and accelerated towards the anode by the voltage difference. A small fraction of the photons produced will have a kV equal to the kVp setting. The rest will have heterogeneous energies following a Gaussian distribution with the exception of characteristic X-ray vertical spikes, if the kVp exceeds the required kV

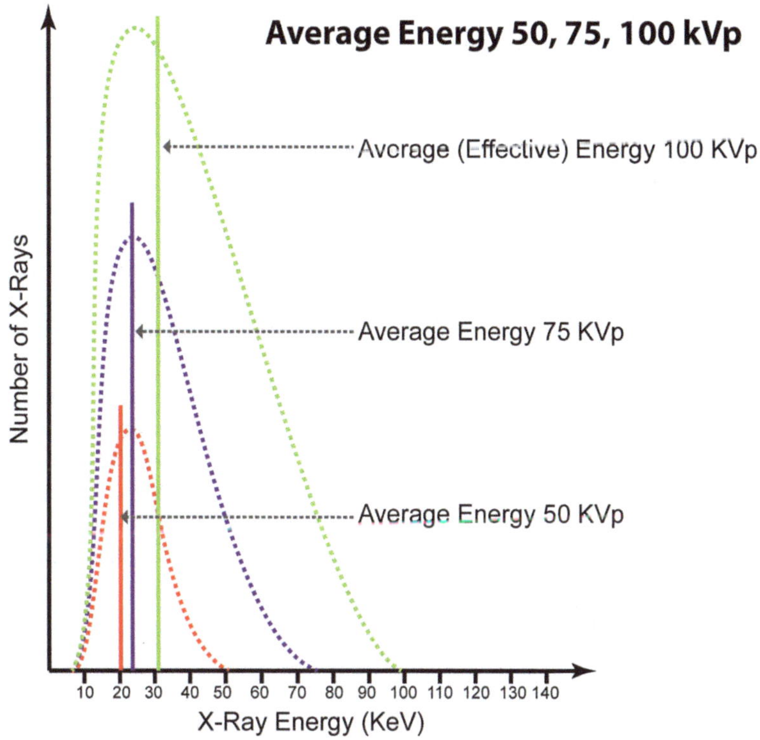

Fig. 8 Although each of the three energies has the potential of 50, 75, and 100 kV, the average therapeutic energy is much lower. The average can be anywhere around 2/3's to ½ the potential based upon the filtration which is used

of the anode material (in the case of tungsten 68 kV). The efficiency of X-ray production by bremsstrahlung increases with increasing kVp and resulting X-rays have a shorter and more penetrating wavelength [4]. Once again, if the kVp is higher than the binding energy of an electron shell of the X-ray tube target material, then characteristic radiation from that electron are produced in addition to bremsstrahlung.

Milliamperage (MA)

The measure of the electric current flowing through an X-ray tube between the cathode and anode is expressed in milliamperes. The number of X-ray photons produced depends on the number of electrons that boil off the filament. The X-ray tube current is proportional to the number of electrons per unit time arriving at the X-ray tube target. The number of electrons liberated depends on the temperature of the heating element which in turns depends on the current flowing through the filament.

The amount of current flowing through the filament is controlled by the mA setting. Therefore, for a given kVp the rate and amount of X-ray produced is directly proportional to the mA current.

Dosimetric Profiles

Dose homogeneity and the sparing of healthy tissues are the primary concerns in the management of superficial cancers. With this understanding the dose at the surface and deepest part past the lesion should be kept to a minimum. Low energy X-rays are a very well-established modality and extend over a range of 40–300 kVp. Superficial is between 50 and 150 kVp and orthovoltage ranges from 150 to 300 kVp. The difference in the energies is related to the falloff of dose in water, with the depth dose of the higher energy beams decreasing more gradually. Orthovoltage X-rays allow for relatively homogeneous dose distribution to 5 mm depth with the tradeoff of increased dose to deeper structures. Superficial X-rays show less homogeneity in the surface region and have a percent depth dose (PDD) curve that decreases very quickly (Fig. 9). All four realms of the kilovoltage energies deliver 100 % of their dose at the skin surface.

Beam Profiles

A beam profile is measured at multiple points on a plane perpendicular to the central beam axis. Measurement is usually performed in a water phantom using a cylindrical ionization chamber. A beam profile can be one dimensional (along one axis) or two dimensional (measuring in the *X* and *Y* axes). Beam profile may also be determined by film dosimetry or other dosimeters, particularly TLD or silicon diodes which have a small detection area. This is most beneficial for the penumbra region, which has rapid dose changes that may be above the resolution of a typical cylindrical ionization chamber. Penumbra areas are very tight and uniform at the edge in kilovoltage energies, a significant advantage over electron therapy which can be in the order of 6 mm or more [5].

Percentage Depth Dose (Depth Dose)

The absorbed dose of radiation deposited into matter, along the central axis, at a particular depth below the surface is defined as "percentage depth dose." The percentage depth dose, in kilovoltage energies, is found by dividing the percentage of dose measured at a depth by that measured dose at the surface. Kilovoltage surface dose is referenced as being 100 % (Fig. 10). The percentage depth dose increase in

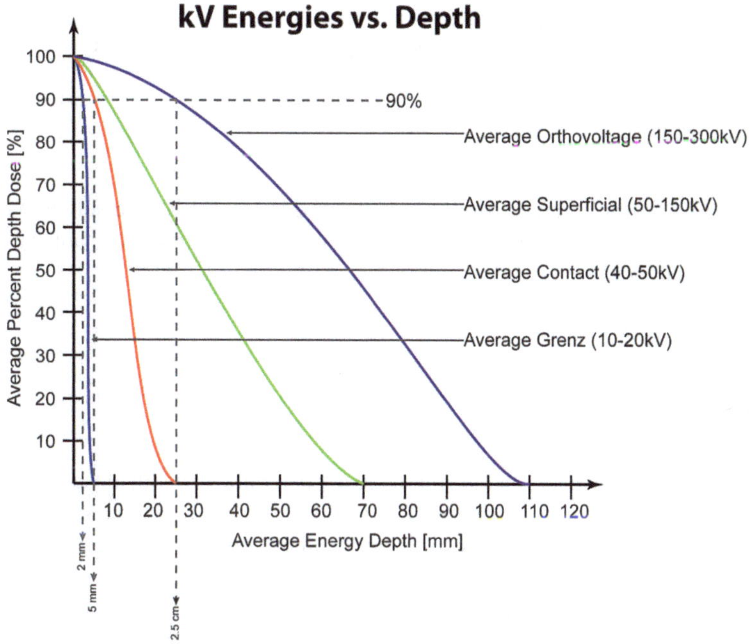

Fig. 9 kV energies deliver 100 % of the energies at the skin surface and then drop off quickly. The drop off in dose spares tissue beyond the lesions and helps maintain vascularity and an efficient healing process. There are four realms in the kV energies, Grenz, Contact, Superficial, and Orthovoltage

Percent Depth Dose

$$P = \frac{D_d}{D_{d_0}} x\ 100$$

Fig. 10 Percent depth dose formula can be used to normalize a dose to a selected depth other than to the surface. d is the depth of which one would want to raise the dose higher than the normal profile of the beam. d_0 represents the depth of maximum deposit of a selected energy, surface for kV energies

depth with beam energy, treatment field size, and source to surface distance. If the tumor is at a deeper depth, there will be lower percentage depth dose coverage. If tissue is other than the density of water, this will affect the percentage depth dose by either shallowing (density more than 1) or deepening the penetration (density of less than 1). The interactions of X-ray beams in this energy range (resulting in energy deposition in tissue) are very dependent on atomic number. This leads to dose inhomogeneities that become significant when there is bone and cartilage (calcium atomic number is 20) in the treated volume. For orthovoltage (up to about 300 kVp) and lower-energy X-rays, the reference depth is usually the surface ($do = 0$). For higher energies, particularly electron beams, the reference depth is taken at the position of the peak absorbed dose ($do = dm$, rather Dmax).

- Absorbed dose at any depth: d
- Absorbed dose at a fixed reference depth: d_0

The above formula can be used to calculated dose at depth, inversely to measure dose at the surface, and helpful in plotting out isodose curves in planning X-ray depth and field size.

Isodose Curves

When point that have the same depth dose (percentage depth dose) are joined together an isodose curve is created. The isodose curve is a graphic representation of point of the same dose joined together to show dosage coverage of tumor or organs of critical risk. Based upon the energy and field size of the beam, isodose curves can have varying distributions.

Isodose Charts (Depth Dose Distribution)

Isodose charts are two-dimensional representations of dose distribution. They are formed by lines drawn along equal increments of percent dose, relative to a particular point. Isodose charts represent a combination of the PDD and the beam profile at multiple points along the central axis. Beam symmetry refers to the ratio of dose at a pair of points located opposite each other from the central beam axis. Examples of depth dose distributions are shown in (Fig. 11).

D ½ vs. D90 Philosophy

D ½ (half-value depth (HVD)) is the depth in tissue at which the radiation dose equals 50 % of the surface dose. D ½ (HVD) is a clinical expression of the penetrating ability of a specified radiation beam. The D ½ concept provides an avenue to select the energy for superficial lesions based upon the depth of the 50 % isodose line. The correct energy's D ½ isodose line should lie at a depth past the deepest portion of the lesion in tissue. D ½ is considered in the planning of intermediate or deep therapy, in relation to dose percentage of organ of critical risk.

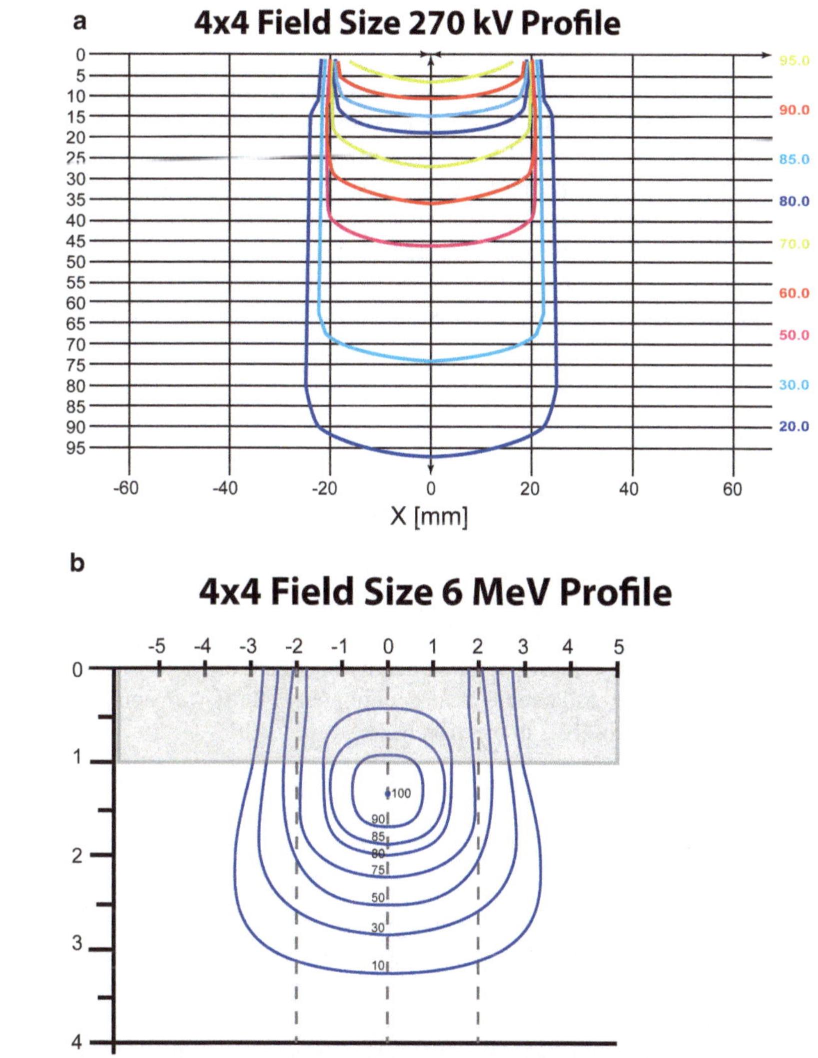

Fig. 11 Dose profiles are a graphic representation of isodose curves with field size, energy, and depth penetration. (**a**) kV energy with 100 % being delivered at the surface and very tight penumbra fine (edge of field). (**b**) Electron energy with 100 % not being delivered to the surface due to the high energy. These high energies require a region of buildup, Dmax, before a 100 % value can be obtained. Note that the penumbra regions at the edge of electron fields are much large, yielding a need for larger therapeutic margins when electrons are used for skin lesion treatment

The D90 is that dose that covers the depth and width of the volume, with no more than a 10 % variation from the top of the tumor to the bottom, and side to side across the lesion. The D90 philosophy is mainly used in high energy treatment planning and electron energy treatments.

Normalization

Normalization is best defined as prescribing to an isodose line or percentage depth dose (other than 100 %). Normalization is used for deep seeded lesion in correlation with planning base procedures, or with electron therapy were the fields are small and a large gradient may be present across the lesion volume. An example of normalization could be were the 80 % isodose line covers the back of a lesion and the physician only wants a 10 % gradient. The dose per fraction would be divided by the 90 %, thus raising the dose by 10 %, making the 90 % = 100 % and the 80 % isodose line 90 %. By contrast this will raise the dose to the surface 10 %, respectively.

Penumbra

The penumbra is the region of rapid dose falloff located at the edge of a beam. In kilovoltage and electron energies the penumbra is between the 20 and 80 % isodose lines. Photon beam of this energy usually has a 1–2 mm area of penumbra. Whereas electron beam has a significant penumbra region, which decreases with increase MeV. Small treatment field and superficial depth tumors are often best treated with kilovoltage energy. Whereas large fields, deeper tumors or those with complex topographic feature lead themselves to electron beam.

How Radiation is Measured

Biological effect depends on how much energy is absorbed from the radiation beam and deposited in the tissue. The absorbed dose is defined as the energy absorbed per unit mass of material. It's used to describe the interactions of all types of ionizing radiation with both directly ionizing (charged particles such as electrons and protons) and indirectly ionizing (gamma and X-ray). Since it is difficult to measure absorbed dose in tissue-like material directly, radiation dosimetry is typically performed by measuring ionization in air (radiation exposure) and then converting this measurement into absorbed dose.

Radiation Exposure

One way to measure the intensity of X-rays is to measure the amount of ionization they cause in air. The amount of ionization in air produced by the radiation is called the exposure. Exposure is expressed in terms of a scientific unit called a roentgen (R). This can only be used to describe an amount of gamma and X-rays, and only in air. One roentgen is equal to depositing in dry air enough energy to cause 2.58E^{-4} C/kg. It is a measure of the ionizations of the molecules in a mass of air. The main advantage of this unit is that it is easy to measure directly, but it is limited because it is only for deposition in air, and only for gamma and X rays. One roentgen of X-ray exposure produces approximately 1 cGy (Centigray) tissue dose [6].

Absorbed Dose

Ionizing radiation interacts with the human body; it transfers its energy to the body tissues. Absorbed dose is the radiation quantity used to express the concentration of radiation energy actually absorbed in the body tissue. This is the quantity that is most directly related to biological effects. The amount of energy deposited per unit of weight of human tissue is expressed in units of gray (Gy). Radiation doses are described in units of Gray (Gy) or centiGray (cGy): 1 Gy = 100 cGy. One gray dose is equivalent to one joule of radiation energy absorbed per kilogram of tissue. The unit Gy can be used for any type of radiation, but it does not describe the biological effects of the different radiations. Absorbed dose cannot be calculated unless a state of electronic equilibrium exists, which only occurs some distance into the medium (tissue).

Electronic Equilibrium (Dmax)

Low energy beams have the maximum dose absorbed at the surface. As energy is increased above 1 MeV, this maximum dose moves slowly to a point at a distance below the skin surface. These energies are associated with gamma and electron energies. Absorbed dose cannot be calculated unless a state of electronic equilibrium exists, which only occurs some distance into the medium (tissue), depending upon the energy. The superficial X-ray energies acquire electronic equilibrium at the surface of the medium. Electrons are liberated predominantly in the forward direction; initially there is a dose buildup. When the same numbers of liberated electrons are set in motion as come to rest in the same volume, electronic equilibrium has been obtained [7]. Not having Dmax at the surface of the skin with electron beams means a gradient of dose across the surface of a lesions leading to areas of under dosage. Electrons have a buildup region anywhere from 10 to 20 mm depending upon the energy. The use of bolus, known as tissue equivalent, is used to bring electronic equilibrium to the surface [8].

Energies of X-ray in Radiation Therapy

Grenz Rays

Grenz rays are part of the electromagnetic spectrum comprising low energy X-rays and are produced by X-ray machines generally operating in the 10–20 kV range. Grenz rays usually produce X-rays with HVL less than 0.035 mm Al. They have a HVD of 0.5 mm and essentially absorbed within the first 2 mm of skin. Grenz the German word for boundary, and refers to its position in the spectrum between the ultraviolet rays and the ordinary X-rays in the electromagnetic spectrum [9]. These energies were mainly used for a variety of inflammatory skin disorders other than skin lesions, although their use for actinic keratosis, Bowen's disease, and melanoma in situ have been reported.

Contact Therapy

X-ray machines that operate at potentials of 40–50 kV are referred to as contact units. They typically operate at tube currents of 2 mA. The beams are usually filtered with 0.5–1.0 mm aluminum in order to remove the very low energy X-rays in the beam, which only serve to breakdown the superficial epidermis. Treating is at a typical source-to-skin (SSD) distance of 15 cm. The dose in this beam drops off to 50 % of its surface value in less than 5 mm of water or soft tissue. Contact therapy is useful for lesions that are very superficial. The lead cutout is placed on the surface of the patient and should be a close relationship to the applicator. The energies of 50 kV and less have a lower percentage of backscatter (less than 6 %), so wax is not needed to lower scatter from the surface lead cutouts.

Superficial Therapy

Units with X-ray beam energies between 50 and 150 kV are usually referred to as superficial therapy units. These units normally are filtered with 0.5–4 mm aluminum and treated at distances of 15–25 cm SSD. Superficial units usually use an mA between 5 and 10. The 50 % depth in water or soft tissue in this energy range would be around 5 mm to 2 cm. Superficial units can be very useful for treatment of skin lesions up to the depth of 22 mm. Applicators sizes can run from 1.5 to 10 cm. Lead cutouts are usually placed on the skin to define the treatment area and reduce scatter to normal tissue.

Orthovoltage Therapy

Orthovoltage X-ray units are defined as those that operate in the 150–300 kV range. Typical SSDs for orthovoltage is 50 cm which by virtue of the inverse square distance makes them useful for convex or concave topography. Field sizes start from 1 cm up to 20 cm. The filters of this energy are usually made of copper and range from 1 to 4 mm. Depths of 50 % (D ½) are usually between 5 and 7 cm depending on filter thickness and field size. Regular fields are defined with detachable cones or adjustable collimators and irregular fields with lead cutouts or special hand blocking. Before 1950, these were the main units used in radiation therapy. Orthovoltage therapy was useful for treating disease in thin sections of the body such as the neck and arms. Thicker areas of the body where tumors are at greater depth, dose to the surface and normal tissue would become very high, resulting in significant acute reactions. Very few of these machines remain in current use in radiation therapy centers, but can be used in conjunction with electron beam for tumors that are complex by virtue of the depth, anatomic involvement, or topography.

Brachytherapy

The sealed source radiation therapy is named as brachytherapy. The primary sources in brachytherapy are gamma rays. Gamma rays are the short-wavelength or high-frequency on the electromagnetic (EM) spectrum, which ranges from gamma rays (short) to radio (long). Gamma rays are high-energy electromagnetic radiation emitted from the atomic nucleus. The treatment of skin cancer with brachytherapy by dermatologist was one of the first medical applications of radioactivity, dating back to the early 1890s. Decades of experience, combined with the latest state-of-the-art equipment and techniques make brachytherapy highly effective treatment, with minimal risk of complications. The dose rate of brachytherapy refers to the level or "intensity" with which the radiation is delivered to the surrounding medium and is expressed in Grays per hour (Gy/h). Brachytherapy is divided into three categories based upon this dose rate, low-dose rate (LDR), medium-dose rate (MDR), and high-dose rate (HDR). LDR brachytherapy involves implanting radiation sources that emit radiation at a rate of up to 2 Gy/h. LDR brachytherapy is commonly used for cancers of the oral cavity, oropharynx, sarcomas, and prostate cancer. MDR brachytherapy is characterized by a medium rate of dose delivery, ranging between 2 Gy/h and 12 Gy/h and is used for cancer of the cervix. HDR brachytherapy is when the rate of dose delivery exceeds 12 Gy/h and is used in tumors of the cervix, esophagus, lungs, breasts, and prostate. Most HDR treatments are performed on an outpatient basis, but this is dependent on the treatment site.

Brachytherapy for skin lesions can be delivered by surface molds and flaps and by external applicators or interstitially. In the treatment named interstitial brachy-therapy, the radioactive sources are placed into the body tissues. Interstitial brachy-therapy is a method for radiation delivery to tumors that maximizes exposure to the tumor volume while minimizing toxicity to adjacent normal tissue. This technique delivers a controlled, concentrated, LDR to the tumor based upon the fact the sources are located in the lesion. Custom-made surface molds, to be used in conjunction with HDR brachytherapy equipment, make possible a uniform dose distribution, with a sharp dose gradient in the limits of applicators. Thermoplastic molds are great for irregular surfaces and fit very accurately for daily treatment. A custom surface flap applicator can be used with non-irregular surfaces, and lesions up to 4 cm. The dose distribution was uniform in the surface of the skin and at 5 mm depth in the whole area of the applicator. The external applicator is used for treatment of small superficial lesions (with diameters <25 mm) together with 192Ir HDR source. Up until the 1908s dermatologist employed brachytherapy in their office for skin cancers typically with one treatment session.

Electron Beams

Electron radiotherapy fields were originally designed to be skin sparing, but are commonly used to treat superficial cancers. Electrons are produced by megavoltage linear accelerators which are used to treat various internal malignancies. An electron beam is characterized by a finite range of penetration with a rapid dose fall through tissues. This characteristic makes electron beams suitable for treating lesions at or close to the surface using a single field while sparing the underlying tissues. The use of electron beam irradiation requires additional technical details in considering the prescription depth, bolus, and sufficient margin (due to penumbra width at field edge). In many clinical skin radiotherapy cases it is necessary to employ electron beams of small dimensions and/or shaped fields. The energy of electron therapy is chosen so that the target volume is encompassed by the 90 % depth dose, which is termed the 90 % isodose philosophy. The percentage depth dose and output depends on the energy, the field dimensions, and the collimation system. The primary goal is to select the minimal beam energy and optimal bolus design to conform to the 90 % dose contour to the distal surface of the target volume so that there is minimal dose to nearby normal structures.

Electrons lose energy constantly as they pass through a medium, and their rate of energy loss and amount of scattering is dependent on their energy. Lower energy electrons scatter more and at larger angles, which causes more of a rapid buildup between the surface dose and Dmax. Higher energies scatter less and at smaller angles leading to less of a buildup region between the surface dose and the energies Dmax depth. Higher energy electron beams tend to undergo minimal scattering near the surface and continue forwards, losing their energy over a greater distance. This leads to significantly broader region of dose distribution, and Dmax rises closer to the surface. The final outcome of these interactions is that high energy electrons have a high surface dose relative to low energy electrons. By selecting appropriate beam energy, a uniform dose may be delivered from the surface to the desired depth, with relative sparing of deep normal structures. Unlike superficial X-rays, electron beam is used to give a greater depth dose with appropriate energy to treat large or thick lesions or those with a high risk of deep penetration.

In electron therapy the dose can be low at the surface due to electron equilibrium being achieved at depth. For treatment of superficial lesions, "bolus" is necessary to bring up the surface dose. Appropriate bolus for 6–12 MV electron is necessary (0.5–1 cm) to ensure a dose at the surface.

Penumbra is a width or measurement of dose gradient or blur. The penumbra for electron beams is defined as the distance between two isodose values (80 and 20 %) on a beam profile at the depth of maximum dose. The penumbra is typically broader for electron beams than for a photon beam, mostly due to lateral scatter of high energy electrons. The electron field penumbra increased at lower energies and decreased for higher energies. When the cut-out is used, the field size becomes smaller and that very small field may be inappropriate for treatment because of under dosage of lateral tissues. Small field sizes require even more margin because of changes in the beam profile. Special care of superficial lesions surrounding critical structures, such as an eye, may require tight margins. When this is the case, small megavoltage electron treatment fields and nonstandard treatment distances may become necessary. When the field size is found to be less than the practical range of the electron beam, dosimetric measurements should be performed or other modalities such as superficial or orthovoltage therapy may be considered.

References

1. Clerk J. Calculations in a level chemistry, Chapter 2 Basic calculations involving formulae and equations.
2. Johns HE, Cunningham JR. The physics of radiology, The structure of matter and radiation. 3rd edn. p. 13–21.
3. Khan FM. The physics of radiation therapy, Production of X-rays. p. 41–2.
4. Selman J. The fundamentals of X-ray and radium physics, The X-rays. 6th edn. p. 170–4.
5. Polston GK. A Dosimetric model for small-field electron radiation, Chapter 4: experimental results. p. 18.
6. Selman J. The fundamentals of X-ray and radium physics, The X-rays. 6th edn. p. 166–7.
7. Martin JE. Physics for radiation protection: a handbook, Energy transfer and absorption of photon. p. 353.
8. Perez HC, Brady LW. Principles and practice of radiation oncology, Chapter 7. p. 202–4.
9. Selman J. The fundamentals of X-ray and radium physics, The X-rays. 6th edn. p. 179.

Radiation Protection

Jeffrey M. Long

Radiation safety consists of two levels. The first level consists of physical solutions. The second level consists of people's attitudes. The first level is by far the easier of the two to accomplish. The second requires continuous work. It is important to establish a culture of radiation safety. The difficulty is convincing people to avoid a behavior that has consequences that might not be realized for 20 years or more.

Historically the development of radiation safety was a slow process even though Wilhelm Conrad Röntgen, who in 1895 discovered X-ray radiation, was known to use lead shielding when working with radiation producing equipment [1]. Most pioneers used the X-ray generating apparatus without shielding. In 1944 an article written in *Radiology* by Herman C. March, M.D. speaks of the realization that people exposed to small amounts of radiation over a prolonged period were developing leukemia at a higher rate than a similar nonexposed population [2]. It was at this time that the protection of radiation workers was beginning to be taken seriously. Then on August 6, 1945 an atomic bomb was dropped on Hiroshima, Japan and on August 9, 1945 a second bomb was dropped on Nagasaki, Japan. This exposed a huge population to both high and low levels of radiation. Many of the regulations now in effect have been based on studies of the survivors of these attacks.

One of the principles of radiation protection is the mnemonic "A.L.A.R.A." This stands for "As Low As Reasonably Achievable." In radiation protection the common practice is to believe that the effects of radiation start at zero and increase with increasing dose from that point. Even though studies of mammalian cell cultures indicate that there is a dose under which no harmful effects are seen A.L.A.R.A. serves the radiation protection community well. So, it is on this principle that the establishment of a radiation protection program is founded. One of the important tenants of this principle is the statement of reasonably achievable. This is open to

J.M. Long (✉)
Pearlman Comprehensive Cancer Center, South Georgia Medical Center,
2501 North Patterson Street, Valdosta, GA 31602, USA
e-mail: Jlong49342@yahoo.com

A.B. Cognetta and W.M. Mendenhall (eds.), *Radiation Therapy for Skin Cancer*,
DOI 10.1007/978-1-4614-6986-5_4, © Springer Science+Business Media New York 2013

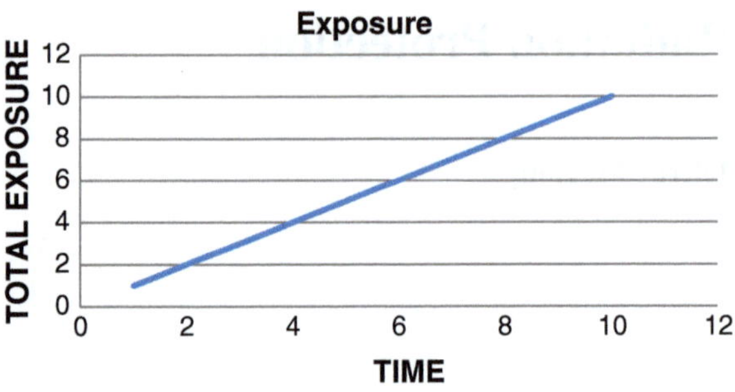

Fig. 1 Graph of exposure at a given point vs. time spent at that point

interpretation. What might be reasonable for one person is unreasonable for another. Each site must work out the best solution for the existing circumstances.

With the above guiding principle in mind, governing bodies must still be satisfied.

Manufacturers of electronic radiation-emitting products sold in the United States are responsible for compliance with the Federal Food, Drug and Cosmetic Act (FFDCA), Chapter V, Subchapter C—Electronic Product Radiation Control [3]. Manufacturers of X-ray machines submit an application to this agency and if found to be in compliance with the act are able to sell the machines in the United States. It is the states that control the use of the machines. Each state has regulations that pertain to that state.

Most, if not all, states require a shielding design and radiation survey done by a qualified expert before an X-ray machine can be used to treat patients. This is almost always under the Department of Health. These experts are usually a medical physicist or a health physicist. To find a person that is qualified in any given state the state office that is responsible for regulating the use of X-ray machines in that state should be contacted. The purpose is to quantitate the amount of radiation that can be measured outside the treatment room including the operator's area, as well as contiguous rooms and outside walls.

Often the decisions concerning location of the X-ray unit are made far in advance of needing the actual shielding evaluation. A wise choice of location can save thousands of dollars in building or renovation costs. A few principles can help with these types of decisions. The corner stone of radiation protection is time, distance, and shielding.

The consideration of time is a linear function. That is, if the time at a point in space of radiation exposure is doubled the dose at that point is doubled. This linearity of the effect is seen in Fig. 1. The slope of the line is the dose rate at the considered point in space. It is then an advantage to place the X-ray machine in a room with walls adjacent to areas of low occupancy or exposure time. These areas are hallways, storage rooms, restrooms, and the outdoors.

Distance is a physical property of the X-ray room to consider. Dosage is the function of the inverse square of the distance. That is an increase of double the distance results in a 75 % reduction of exposure from one point in space to another.

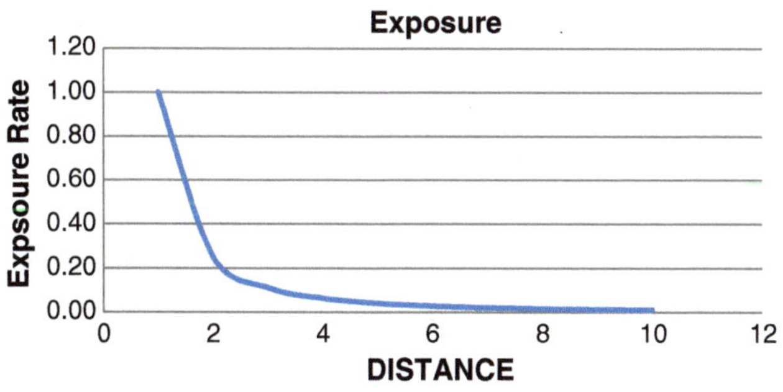

Fig. 2 Graph of exposure rate vs. distance from the radiation source

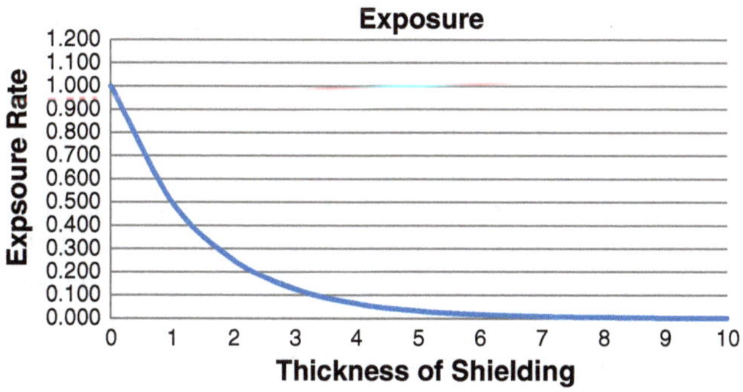

Fig. 3 Exposure at a given point vs. shielding thickness imposed between the source of radiation and the point

This effect is seen in Fig. 2. When space is at a premium, distance is often hard to achieve. Placing the X-ray machine in the corner of a large room certainly reduces the exposure outside the room, but may not be practical and call for other solutions.

The second physical property of the room for consideration is shielding. Shielding is any material imposed between a source of radiation and a point in space. All materials attenuate radiation. High density materials attenuate radiation more than low density materials of the same thickness. A solid concrete wall will attenuate more radiation than a wooden wall. When adding shielding, lead is the most commonly used material because of its high density. This allows thin sheets to be applied to the walls and doors. Shielding reduces the exposure in an exponential way. The effects of shielding are seen in Fig. 3. The determination of the correct shielding is the job of the qualified expert. Getting the qualified expert involved at the earliest possible time can, in the end, save money (i.e., it can be incorporated into the sheetrock phase, door construction, electrical, and computer line design. Leaded glass is available and routinely used).

Table 1 Annual allowable personal radiation dose for occupationally exposed persons

Annual radiation exposure limits	
Whole body, blood forming organs, gonads	5,000 mrem/year
Lens of eye	15,000 mrem/year
Extremities and skin	50,000 mrem/year
Fetal	500 mrem/gestation period
General public	100 mrem/year

The second part of radiation safety is the people involved. For any employer there are only two types of employees when radiation is concerned. The first is a non-radiation worker and therefore a member of the public. The second type is an occupationally exposed worker or radiation worker. In Table 1 the dose limits for different parts of the body are listed. These dose limits are from the USNRC regulations, Title 10, Part 20, Code of Federal Regulations. Many states have incorporated these dose limits into their own regulations; however, some might have other dose levels. The local qualified expert or the individual state regulatory agency can provide the dose limits applicable to the individual circumstance.

The doses in Table 1 are yearly doses. Some regulatory agencies require the dose limits to be on a quarterly basis. For these agencies all doses would be divided by four except the fetal dose which remains as a limit for the gestation period. In some cases the dose reporting must be in sieverts or millisieverts. The conversion factor for millirem (mrem) to millisievert (mSv) is 0.01. Therefore, the whole body dose would be 50 mSv/year. In order to show compliance with the regulations personal dosimeters are used. For the purposes of an office providing dermatologic radiation treatments, personal dosimeters would be required if there is a possibility for an individual to receive 25 % of the allowable limit. All companies that provide personal dosimetry services provide a control with each shipment. The control is a dosimeter kept in a non-radiation exposure area. The reason for the control dosimeter is to measure the background radiation at the work place and during shipment. When the personal dosimeters are returned to the provider for evaluation it is important to return the control. If the control is not returned the dosimeters are evaluated and the dose that is determined is recorded on the individual participant's record without background being removed. The normal average background radiation is about 360 mrem/year. Once it is established that no monitored person has received 25 % of allowable exposure limit, most regulatory agencies will allow the termination of monitoring.

In the context of radiation protection any non-radiation worker is a member of the public. This fact means all offices that use radiation for diagnosis or treatment of patients will have two types of areas: (1) controlled and (2) noncontrolled. The difference between the two is the allowable exposure in each. The dose of 100 mrem/year is allowed in noncontrolled areas and the other doses in Table 1 are for controlled areas. The areas referred to as controlled and noncontrolled are often misunderstood. Because dermatologic radiation therapy uses low energy X-rays and the rooms can be shielded easily, all areas except the inside of the radiation treatment room can be declared as a noncontrolled area. This then requires that the walls of the treatment room are shielded such that any area outside the room receives an exposure of less than 100 mrem/year. As above, the dose levels of noncontrolled areas can be established either by the qualified expert's calculation or by monitoring.

Radiation protection as applied to the patient is a straightforward topic (see Chapter 20). That is, the disease should be treated without miss while limiting the dose to normal tissue. This is done by insuring that the X-ray unit used to treat the patient is properly shielded and calibrated and only the areas of treatment receive primary radiation. If major repairs are made to the machine, a new survey of the unit might be needed to make certain that machine shielding has not been disturbed or removed.

Patient shielding is an important facet of patient protection. The shielding of the patient falls into two categories. One category is external field shaping. This entails the use of lead foil with an area cut out to treat the disease (photo 1). Lead foil can be purchased in rolls as thin as 0.006 in. (0.15 mm); however, it is more commonly seen in thicknesses of 0.03 in. (0.762 mm) and 0.125 in. (3.18 mm). However, many other thicknesses are found. The foils are easy to work and can be cut with standard scissors. Shields are made such that the opening covers the area to be treated with approximately 1.5 cm lead past the cone or field edge. This allows the radiation field to cover the opening and allow for some minor patient movement. The thicknesses of shielding required are dependent on the kVp of the X-ray beam used. The attenuation coefficients are listed in Table 2. These attenuation coefficients were derived from half value layer thicknesses found in NCRP 49. The attenuations can be seen in Fig. 4. The thickness of lead for a patient shield should reduce the radiation by 95 % or more. Therefore for 50, 70, and 100 kVp the thicknesses would be 0.26 mm, 0.74 mm, and 1.17 mm of lead foil, respectively.

In some circumstances such as the eyeball special shielding consideration is warranted. This is done using eye shields. They can be obtained from a number of medical supply sources. The thickness of the shields is 1.7 mm. This is sufficient for the energies normally used in dermatology. In use the shields are normally covered with wax and placed beneath the upper and lower eyelids. The wax protects the delicate tissues of the eye and inside eyelid from physical damage. Other areas that can be protected by custom shielding are the inside of the nose and mouth.

For the nose, a cylindrical shield is fashioned and placed in the nostril for each treatment. For the mouth, shields can be fashioned in small plates to fit inside the check or lip. These too can be covered in a thin layer of wax or rubber cot (rubber glove).

Table 2 Attenuation coefficients as derived from NCRP 49

kVp	50	70	100
Exponent	−11.55	−4.08	−2.57

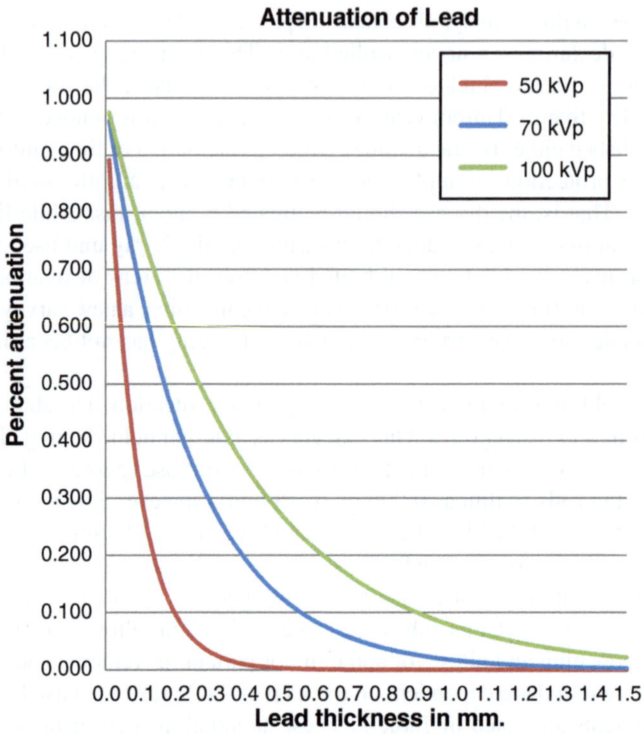

Fig. 4 Percent attenuation for indicated kVp vs. thickness of lead

Calibration

All discussion of patient treatment assumes a correctly calibrated machine. The machine must be calibrated by a medical physicist certified as a qualified expert in the state in which the machine is located. There are 50 states and each has their own definitions and qualifications for this person. It cannot be stressed enough that a qualified expert must be associated with each radiotherapy program. In addition the unit must be calibrated using a recognized protocol. The American Association of Physicists in Medicine (AAPM) is an organization of physicist dedicated to the application of physics to medicine. The AAPM publishes protocols for calibration and use of radiation producing machines in medicine. Their current protocol for low energy calibrations was published as report 76 which is the work of the task group 61. It is common for states to require annual calibration of treatment machines as a minimum. Along with calibration quality control is important. Some new machines have built-in radiation measurement devices. These devices are used to measure the radiation output each morning the machine will be used. In order to use the machine it must pass this check. Older machines do not have this feature. For these older machines a program can be set up with the consultation of the medical physicist to accomplish the same goal; of assuring an accurate treatment. Some physicians, including the editor, used a monthly check on older machines to assure that the calibration stayed accurate. The calculation of dose should have a redundancy. This can be accomplished by having two people check the calculations. In contrast some modern machines have added an automatic time calculation. That is, the desired dose for the patient is entered into the machine and it will calculate the correct time. Before treatment begins this time should be compared to a time previously calculated for that patient by hand using one's printed calibration tables for the specific KV, TSD, and cone size supplied by one's physicist. The two times should be less than 1 % different. With older machines the time to deliver the dose should be calculated by two different people independently. These times should be compared, and be within 1 % of each other. Following the above recommendations can minimize the possibility of a radiation mistreatment. Both under-treatment and over-treatment are equally harmful. Some believe under-treatment is not as bad as over-treatment. When it is true over-treatment can result in disastrous results such as fistulas and radio necrosis or death, while under-treatment results in less than optimal cure rates. Radiation given without maximum benefit to the patient is indeed unfortunate. In addition to the requirement of accurate treatment, the fact is that many of the harmful effects of the incorrect dose might not be evident for years after the treatment. Every effort should be made to give a treatment that delivers the prescribed dose to plus or minus 5 %.

Record Keeping

The question of record keeping is often discussed by administrator looking to reduce or eliminate the storage of records. With the advent of digital storage, this should be less important. Each state has specific requirements for these records. Some common sense rules can be discussed. For patient records, they should be kept until the statute of limitations for legal action is ended. Yet as a practical matter since tissues previously treated with radiation might not tolerate retreatment, they should be kept forever. It has been my experience that patients will return, often 20 years or more after initial radiation treatment, with diseases requiring new radiation treatment. It is then important to know the precise location and dose of any previous treatment. Personal dosimeter records should be kept as long as possible, even past the time required by a state. This philosophy can be applied to the room shielding report and survey. Even if a state requires a shorter time period, the reports should be kept as long as the room is being used for radiation treatments. Calibration reports should be kept for at least 5 years from the date of calibration; however, each state has regulations pertaining to this time period.

References

1. Hasse A, Landwehr G, Umbach E, editors. Röntgen centennial: X-rays in natural and life sciences. Singapore: World Scientific; 1997. p. 7–8.
2. March HC. Leukemia in radiologists. Radiology. 1944;43(3):275–8.
3. U.S. Food and Drug Administration. Radiation-emitting products. http://www.fda.gov/radiation-emittingproducts

Staging of Squamous Cell Carcinoma and Basal Cell Carcinoma

Armand B. Cognetta Jr. and Christopher M. Wolfe

Introduction

The principal purposes of staging cancer are to aid in treatment planning, indicate prognosis, to assist in the evaluation of treatment results, and through the use of a "common language," facilitate the exchange of information between treatment centers and aid the investigation of human cancer. For solid tumors by far the most common system of staging is the TNM classification of malignant tumors. T describes the size or direct extent of the primary tumor, N represents the degree of spread to regional lymph nodes, and M represents the presence of metastasis. TNM is dual system that includes a clinical (pretreatment) classification denoted by a prefix "c" cTNM and a pathologic (postsurgical histopathologic) classification given the prefix "p" pTNM. Even though biopsy of the primary tumor is performed, pathologic staging refers to excision of the primary tumor and/or lymph nodes; therefore, dermatologists and radiation oncologists utilizing radiotherapy in the treatment of non-melanoma skin cancer (NMSC) are only able to stage tumors clinically. Additional modifiers may be applied depending on the tumor type or to increase the degree of specificity. After assigning TNM the scores are combined to give an overall stage, denoted by roman numerals 0 (carcinoma in situ), I (localized), II (early locally advanced), III (late locally advanced), and IV (metastasized), which is considered essential for selecting and evaluating therapy.

A.B. Cognetta Jr. (✉)
Dermatology Associates of Tallahassee, Chief, Division of Dermatology,
Florida State University College of Medicine, 1707 Riggins Road, Tallahassee, FL 32308, USA
e-mail: acognetta@gmail.com

C.M. Wolfe
Lake Erie College of Osteopathic Medicine, 1858 West Grandview Boulevard,
Erie, PA 16509-1025, USA

A.B. Cognetta and W.M. Mendenhall (eds.), *Radiation Therapy for Skin Cancer*,
DOI 10.1007/978-1-4614-6986-5_5, © Springer Science+Business Media New York 2013

Squamous Cell Carcinoma and Basal Cell Carcinoma of the Skin

Collectively, squamous cell carcinoma (SCC) and basal cell carcinoma (BCC) comprise the majority of carcinomas encountered in the dermatologic setting and together are staged according to the TNM classification (Tables 1, 2, 3, 4, 5, 6, and 7). High-risk features have been identified for primary tumor staging of cutaneous (non-eyelid) carcinoma (Table 2). New to the seventh edition of the American Joint Committee on Cancer's (AJCC) *AJCC Cancer Staging Manual* for carcinomas are separate staging systems for the eyelid vs. other skin surfaces [1, 2]. The staging system is primarily designed for SCCs because of their ability to metastasize but includes basal cell carcinoma. For purposes of this section cutaneous carcinomas refer to non-eyelid carcinoma.

In general, radial size for both SCC and BCC is thought to mirror biologic behavior. Overall staging is based on radial size (stage I <2 cm and stage II >2 cm). As the carcinomas extend vertically, with invasion into deeper tissue such as bone and beyond to lymph nodes, they receive a higher overall stage (III–IV). Based solely on T (tumor) component of the TNM classification system, invasion into the maxilla, mandible, orbit, or temporal bone automatically receives an overall stage III (T3 N0 M0) and direct or perineural invasion into the skull base or axial skeleton receives an overall stage IV (T4 N0 M0). Similarly, based solely on N (nodal involvement) of the TNM classification system, involvement of a single ipsilateral node ≤3 cm in size receives an overall stage III and involvement of nodes ≥3 cm in size or multiple nodes receives an overall stage IV. Metastasis is categorized as either M0 (no metastasis) or M1 (distant metastasis, which if present, is assigned an overall stage IV) for SCC and BCC.

Table 1 Primary tumor (T) for cutaneous carcinoma (non-eyelid)[a]

TX	Primary tumor cannot be assessed
T0	No evidence of primary tumor
Tis	Carcinoma in situ
T1	Tumor ≤2 cm in greatest dimension with <2 high-risk features[b]
T2	Tumor >2 cm in greatest dimension or Tumor any size with ≥2 high-risk features[b]
T3	Tumor with invasion of maxilla, mandible, orbit, or temporal bone
T4	Tumor with invasion of skeleton (axial or appendicular) or perineural invasion of skull base

Reprinted with permission from AJCC: Cutaneous squamous cell carcinoma and other cutaneous carcinomas. In: Edge SB, Byrd DR, Compton CC, et al., eds.: AJCC Cancer Staging Manual. 7th ed. New York, NY: Springer, 2010, pp 301–14

[a]Excludes cutaneous squamous cell carcinoma of the eyelid

[b]High-risk features for the primary tumor (T) staging

Table 2 High-risk features for primary tumor (T) staging for cutaneous non-eyelid carcinoma

Depth/invasion	>2 mm thickness (Breslow thickness)
	Clark level ≥IV
	Perineural invasion
Anatomic location	Primary site ear
	Primary site non-hair-bearing lip
Differentiation	Poorly differentiated or undifferentiated

Reprinted with permission from AJCC: Cutaneous squamous cell carcinoma and other cutaneous carcinomas. In: Edge SB, Byrd DR, Compton CC, et al., eds.: AJCC Cancer Staging Manual. 7th ed. New York, NY: Springer, 2010, pp 301–14

Table 3 Regional lymph nodes (N) for cutaneous carcinoma

NX	Regional lymph nodes cannot be assessed
N0	No regional lymph node metastases
N1	Metastasis in a single ipsilateral lymph node, ≤3 cm in greatest dimension
N2	Metastasis in a single ipsilateral lymph node, >3 cm but ≤6 cm in greatest dimension; or in multiple ipsilateral lymph nodes, ≤6 cm in greatest dimension; or in bilateral or contralateral lymph nodes, ≤6 cm in greatest dimension
N2a	Metastasis in a single ipsilateral lymph node, >3 cm but ≤6 cm in greatest dimension
N2b	Metastases in multiple ipsilateral lymph nodes, ≤6 cm in greatest dimension
N2c	Metastases in bilateral or contralateral lymph nodes, ≤6 cm in greatest dimension
N3	Metastasis in a lymph node, >6 cm in greatest dimension

Reprinted with permission from AJCC: Cutaneous squamous cell carcinoma and other cutaneous carcinomas. In: Edge SB, Byrd DR, Compton CC, et al., eds.: AJCC Cancer Staging Manual. 7th ed. New York, NY: Springer, 2010, pp 301–14

Table 4 Anatomic stage/prognostic groups for cutaneous carcinoma

Stage	T	N	M
0	Tis	N0	M0
I	T1	N0	M0
II	T2	N0	M0
III	T3	N0	M0
	T1	N1	M0
	T2	N1	M0
	T3	N1	M0
IV	T1	N2	M0
	T2	N2	M0
	T3	N2	M0
	Any T	N3	M0
	T4	Any N	M0
	Any T	Any N	M1

Reprinted with permission from AJCC: Cutaneous squamous cell carcinoma and other cutaneous carcinomas. In: Edge SB, Byrd DR, Compton CC, et al., eds.: AJCC Cancer Staging Manual. 7th ed. New York, NY: Springer, 2010, pp 301–14

Table 5 Primary tumor (T) for eyelid carcinoma

TX	Primary tumor cannot be assessed
T0	No evidence of primary tumor
Tis	Carcinoma in situ
TX	Primary tumor cannot be assessed
T1	Tumor ≤5 mm in greatest dimension Not invading the tarsal plate or eyelid margin
T2a	Tumor >5 mm but not >10 mm in greatest dimension Or, any tumor that invades the tarsal plate or eyelid margin
T2b	Tumor >10 mm but not >20 mm in greatest dimension Or, involves full thickness eyelid
T3a	Tumor >20 mm in greatest dimension Or, any tumor that invades adjacent ocular or orbital structures Any T with perineural tumor invasion
T3b	Complete tumor resection requires enucleation, exenteration, or bone resection
T4	Tumor is not resectable because of extensive invasion of ocular, orbital, craniofacial structures, or brain

Reprinted with permission from AJCC: Carcinoma of the Eyelid. In: Edge SB, Byrd DR, Compton CC, et al., eds.: AJCC Cancer Staging Manual. 7th ed. New York, NY: Springer, 2010, pp 523–526

Table 6 Regional lymph nodes (N) for eyelid carcinoma

NX	Regional lymph nodes cannot be assessed
cN0	No regional lymph node metastasis based upon clinical evaluation or imaging
pN0	No regional lymph node metastasis based upon lymph node biopsy
N1	Regional lymph node metastasis

Reprinted with permission from AJCC: Carcinoma of the Eyelid. In: Edge SB, Byrd DR, Compton CC, et al., eds.: AJCC Cancer Staging Manual. 7th ed. New York, NY: Springer, 2010, pp 523–526

Table 7 Anatomic stage/prognostic groups for eyelid carcinoma

Stage 0	Tis	N0	M0
Stage IA	T1	N0	M0
Stage IB	T2a	N0	M0
Stage IC	T2b	N0	M0
Stage II	T3a	N0	M0
Stage IIIA	T3b	N0	M0
Stage IIIB	Any T	N1	M0
Stage IIIC	T4	Any N	M0
Stage IV	Any T	Any N	M1

Reprinted with permission from AJCC: Carcinoma of the Eyelid. In: Edge SB, Byrd DR, Compton CC, et al., eds.: AJCC Cancer Staging Manual. 7th ed. New York, NY: Springer, 2010, pp 523–526

Staging for Squamous Cell Carcinoma Treated by Dermatologists Utilizing Radiotherapy

As mentioned previously, AJCC staging primarily applies to SCC as BCC has a different biological behavior and is limited mainly to local destruction with very little chance of distant metastasis (see Chaps. 7, 8 and 9 for histologic features considered to be radio-resistant). For dermatologists utilizing radiotherapy to treat cutaneous SCC, primary tumor (T) classification will determine the overall stage and will include Tis, T1, and T2 classification, with an overall stage of 0 (Tis), I (T1 N0 M0), or II (T2 N0 M0). Tumors beyond T2 or with certain aggressive features (perineural invasion, poorly differentiated, or undifferentiated tumors) are better managed with surgery and adjuvant radiotherapy using more deeply penetrating radiation by radiation oncologists [3–7]. Recently published data from researchers at the University of Florida in a comparison of patients with SCC and perineural invasion receiving Mohs surgery plus radiotherapy vs. non-Mohs resection plus radiotherapy noted improved 5-year local control rates and improved cause-specific survival rates when Mohs surgery was the surgical method utilized [8].

The main factor in differentiating T1 and T2 for SCC is the presence of two or more high-risk features. T1 includes carcinomas (not in situ) ≤2 cm in greatest dimension with one aggressive feature, whereas T2 includes carcinomas with two or more aggressive features or diameter greater than 2 cm. Of note, the AJCC includes Clark level≥IV (used in the past for melanoma staging) as a high-risk feature which by definition includes invasion into the reticular dermis [9]. It should be taken into consideration that the AJCC believes the prognostic contribution of Breslow thickness and Clark level in staging will depend on future studies, however sufficient evidence exists that depth of tumor invasion correlates with prognosis [1]. Multi-professional guidelines published by the British Association of Dermatologists for the management of patients with primary cutaneous SCC have noted that a tumor depth greater than 4 mm and Clark level V were more likely to recur and metastasize (45.7 % metastatic rate) compared with thinner tumors (2 mm or less rarely metastasize) [10]. Additional studies have also found a correlation between SCC behavior and tumor depth with similar findings, noting increased risk of recurrence or metastasis with tumor thickness greater than 4 mm [11, 12].

Staging of eyelid SCC likely to be treated by dermatologists is based on lesion diameter or extension into the tarsal plate or eyelid margin. The primary tumor (T) staging utilized in dermatologic radiotherapy will include Tis, T1 (less than 5 mm), T2a (5–10 mm or invades tarsal plate or eyelid margin), or T2b (11–20 mm or full-thickness eyelid). It is important to note that tumors suspected of invading the tarsal plate or deep medial canthus lesions, due to potential lacrimal infiltration, are not treated with radiotherapy in our practice. Mohs micrographic surgery is utilized or patients are referred to our radiation oncology colleagues for radiologic studies and more deeply penetrating radiation qualities. Overall staging for eyelid SCC treated with radiotherapy by dermatologists includes 0 (Tis), IA (T1 N0 M0), IB (T2a N0 M0), IC (T2b N0 M0), or II (T3a N0 M0).

Clinical Examples for Staging SCC and BCC in Dermatologic Radiotherapy

Examples of TNM staging for the most commonly treated BCC/SCC encountered by dermatologists using radiotherapy are provided below. The goal is to provide a quick reference for dermatologists documenting TNM classification and overall stage in radiation treatment reports. Metastasis is categorized as either M0 (no metastasis) or M1 (distant metastasis) for SCC and BCC.

1. Head/neck lesion other than eye-lid
   (a) SCCIS any size: Tis N0 M0; Stage 0
   (b) SCC/BCC ≤2 cm no more than 1 high-risk feature: T1 N0 M0; Stage I
   (c) SCC/BCC ≤2 cm with two or more high-risk features: T2 N0 M0; Stage II
   (d) SCC/BCC >2 cm: T2 N0 M0; Stage II
2. High-risk features (applies to non-eyelid tumors)
   (a) Depth/invasion: >2 mm thickness (Breslow thickness), Clark level≥IV, perineural invasion
   (b) Anatomic location: primary site ear or non-hair baring lip
   (c) Differentiation: poorly differentiated or undifferentiated
      - Presence of one high-risk feature = Automatically Stage I (T1 N0 M0)
      - Presence of two or more high-risk features = Automatically Stage II (T2 N0 M0)
3. Eyelid lesion
   (a) SCCIS any size: Tis N0 M0; Stage 0
   (b) SCC/BCC ≤5 mm: T1 N0 M0; Stage IA
   (c) SCC/BCC 6–10 mm: T2a N0 M0; Stage IB
   (d) SCC/BCC any size invading the tarsal plate or eyelid margin: T2a N0 M0; Stage IB
   (e) SCC/BCC 10–20 mm: T2b N0 M0; Stage IC
   (f) SCC/BCC any size involving full-thickness eyelid: T2b N0 M0; Stage IC
   (g) SCC/BCC >20 mm: T3a N0 M0; Stage II
   (h) SCC/BCC any size with perineural invasion or invading adjacent ocular or orbital structures: T3a N0 M0; Stage II
4. Staging based on key features of TNM classification that may be encountered
   (a) T: Invasion into the maxilla, mandible, orbit, or temporal bone = T3 N0 M0; Stage III
   (b) T: Direct or perineural invasion into the skull base or axial skeleton = T4 N0 M0; Stage IV
   (c) N: Involvement of a single ipsilateral node ≤3 cm in size = Stage III
   (d) N: Involvement of nodes ≥3 cm in size or multiple nodes = Stage IV
   (e) M: Distant metastasis = Stage IV

Half-Value Depth (D ½ Philosophy) and Depth Assessment

Prior histologic review of each lesion by the dermatologist using radiotherapy allows for evaluation of the cancer providing more precise information that can be used to prescribe treatment and predict treatment response and outcomes. If a shave biopsy does not allow for adequate depth assessment, a repeat punch biopsy may be warranted since adequate staging requires evaluation of the aggressive features used to stage SCC/BCC (depth greater than 2 mm and Clark level ≥IV). This also allows the clinician to assess the lesion's appropriateness for radiotherapy according to the D ½ philosophy or half-value depth.

Another modality that may be used to confirm and assess tumor depth is high-frequency ultrasound (HFUS). HFUS has been used to assess BCC depth and tumor response to photodynamic therapy in the treatment of nevoid basal cell carcinoma syndrome patients [13, 14]. Prior studies involving the use of HFUS in delineating Mohs surgical margins (horizontal diameter) for SCC and BCC noted difficulty in determining the horizontal extension of superficial tumors or those deeper tumors with lateral extension within the epidermis (sclerosing or morpheaform BCC) [15]. Typically this is not an issue as horizontal diameter is easily assessed clinically for NMSC amenable to dermatologic radiotherapy (BCC nodular, BCC superficial, SCCIS, and SCC invasive). Thinner tumors, such as SCCIS and superficial BCC, need not be assessed for depth as they are confined to the epidermis and do not extend beyond the 5.8 mm treatment depth of the lowest (50 kV) setting of most X-ray machines. In our own pilot study comparing HFUS determined depth to histological depth measured from biopsy specimens, we found HFUS measured depth comparable to microscopically measured histologic depth for nodular BCC and invasive/hyperkeratotic SCC. Ultimately HFUS, optical coherence tomography, and confocal microscopy (in reflectance or fluorescence mode) may prove to be useful for the purpose of confirming or evaluating depth in dermatologic radiotherapy.

The half-value depth (D ½) has been established as a practical guideline to select the radiation qualities (kilovoltage, filter, and half-value layer) most appropriate to treat an individual lesion at a given depth. The D ½ is the tissue depth in mm at which the absorbed dose is 50 % of the surface dose. Therapeutic efficacy has been established when radiation qualities place the D ½ equal to or greater than the lesion depth [16–18]. Table 8 shows calibration data of the beryllium-window superficial X-ray unit currently used in our practice. Radiation qualities are calibrated by our physicist and preset within the unit. Treatment depth (D ½) is changed based on selecting one of the three set kV values (50, 70, or 100) with automatic rotary insertion of the aluminum filter specific to each kV within the unit. The source-to-surface distance (SSD) is fixed based on the cone (applicator) length, which is uniform for all cones except the 10 cm cone (25 cm SSD). The lower 50 kV setting (see Table 8), with a corresponding D ½ of 5.8 mm, is adequate for the treatment of superficial BCC and SCCIS. Accurate depth assessment is important for nodular BCC and SCC that are between 5.8 and 20.0 mm in depth in order to select the appropriate kilovoltage (70 or 100 kV) and to minimize irradiation of non-tumorous tissue.

Table 8 Calibration data of the beryllium-window superficial X-ray unit currently used in our practice

Tube voltage (kV)	SSD (source to surface distance) (cm)	Field size (cm)	D ½ (mm)	HVL (half-value layer) (mm) aluminum	Output (cGy/min)	Dose rate (Gy/min)
50	15	1.0	**5.8**	0.44	762.3	0.13
	15	1.5	**5.8**	0.44	779.1	0.13
	15	2.0	**5.8**	0.44	791.4	0.13
	15	2.5	**5.8**	0.44	806.9	0.12
	15	3.0	**5.8**	0.44	811.7	0.12
	15	4.0	**5.8**	0.44	822.6	0.12
	15	5.0	**5.8**	0.44	824.2	0.12
	25	10.0	**6.4**	0.44	284.4	0.35
70	15	1.0	**13.3**	1.05	597.5	0.17
	15	1.5	**13.3**	1.05	614.1	0.16
	15	2.0	**13.3**	1.05	628.8	0.16
	15	2.5	**13.3**	1.05	643.3	0.16
	15	3.0	**13.3**	1.05	654.7	0.15
	15	4.0	**13.3**	1.05	665.7	0.15
	15	5.0	**13.3**	1.05	678.0	0.15
	25	10.0	**14.2**	1.05	240.3	0.42
100	15	1.0	**17.9**	2.0	568.6	1.23
	15	1.5	**17.9**	2.0	588.9	1.19
	15	2.0	**17.9**	2.0	606.0	1.16
	15	2.5	**17.9**	2.0	627.7	1.12
	15	3.0	**17.9**	2.0	637.8	1.10
	15	4.0	**17.9**	2.0	652.7	1.07
	15	5.0	**17.9**	2.0	669.6	1.05
	25	10.0	**20.0**	2.0	245.6	2.85

None of the tumors selected for superficial radiotherapy were 2 cm or greater in depth in our treatment series [19]. In these exceptional cases referral to radiation oncologists who have at their disposal more deeply penetrating radiation may be appropriate if surgery is declined or not advised. Atkinson [20] summarized the data on the depth of cutaneous carcinomas treated with X-ray therapy by Strandqvist ($n=280$) [21], Ebbehoj ($n=195$) [22], and Polano ($n=170$) [23] from biopsy specimens treated with superficial radiotherapy. Seventy five percent of all BCC and selected SCC reached a depth of 5 mm or less and 50 % reached 2 mm or less. Measuring the depth of 67 randomly submitted surgical excisions of BCC, Newell [24] found that 95.5 % of BCC reached a depth of 2.9 mm and only 1.5 % exceeded 5 mm. Zacarian [25] reporting on the depth of 123 BCC found that 96 % extended to 3 mm and 0.8 % extended beyond 5 mm. In light of this the lowest kilovoltage (50 kV) will be adequate to treat the majority of lesions and deeper lesions up to 20 mm in depth can be treated using the 100 kV setting.

References

1. Cutaneous squamous cell carcinoma and other cutaneous carcinomas. In: Edge SB, Byrd DR, Compton CC, Fritz AG, editors. AJCC cancer staging manual. 7th ed. New York, NY: Springer; 2010. p. 301–14.
2. Carcinoma of the eyelid. In: Edge SB, Byrd DR, Compton CC, Fritz AG, editors. AJCC cancer staging manual. 7th ed. New York, NY: Springer; 2010. p. 523–6.
3. Kyrgidis A, Tzellos TG, Kechagias N, Patrikidou A, Xirou P, Kitikidou K, et al. Cutaneous squamous cell carcinoma (SCC) of the head and neck: risk factors of overall and recurrence-free survival. Eur J Cancer. 2010;46(9):1563–72.
4. Jackson JE, Dickie GJ, Wiltshire KL, Keller J, Tripcony L, Poulsen MG, et al. Radiotherapy for perineural invasion in cutaneous head and neck carcinomas: toward a risk-adapted treatment approach. Head Neck. 2009;31(5):604–10.
5. Mendenhall WM, Amdur RJ, Hinerman RW, Cognetta AB, Mendenhall NP. Radiotherapy for cutaneous squamous and basal cell carcinomas of the head and neck. Laryngoscope. 2009; 119(10):1994–9.
6. Leibovitch I, Huilgol SC, Selva D, Hill D, Richards S, Paver R. Cutaneous squamous cell carcinoma treated with Mohs micrographic surgery in Australia II. Perineural invasion. J Am Acad Dermatol. 2005;53(2):261–6.
7. Han A, Ratner D. What is the role of adjuvant radiotherapy in the treatment of cutaneous squamous cell carcinoma with perineural invasion? Cancer. 2007;109(6):1053–9.
8. Kropp L, Balamucki CJ, Morris CG, et al. Mohs resection and postoperative radiotherapy for head and neck cancers with incidental perineural invasion. Am J Otolaryngol. Feb 12 2013 [Epub ahead of print].
9. National Cancer Institute at the National Institutes of Health. Clark level IV skin cancer; 2012. http://www.cancer.gov/dictionary?cdrid=630772. Accessed 28 July 2012.
10. Motley R, Kersey P, Lawrence C. Multiprofessional guidelines for the management of the patient with primary cutaneous squamous cell carcinoma. Br J Plast Surg. 2003;56(2):85–91.
11. Rowe DE, Carroll RJ, Day Jr CL. Prognostic factors for local recurrence, metastasis, and survival rates in squamous cell carcinoma of the skin, ear, and lip implications for treatment modality selection. J Am Acad Dermatol. 1992;26(6):976–90.
12. Friedman HI, Cooper PH, Wanebo HJ. Prognostic and therapeutic use of microstaging of cutaneous squamous cell carcinoma of the trunk and extremities. Cancer. 1985;56(5):1099–105.
13. Loncaster J, Swindell R, Slevin F, Sheridan L, Allan D, Allan E. Efficacy of photodynamic therapy as a treatment for Gorlin syndrome-related basal cell carcinomas. Clin Oncol (R Coll Radiol). 2009;21(6):502–8.
14. Loncaster JA, Moore JV, Allan D, Allan E. An ultrasound analysis of the response of Gorlin syndrome-related and sporadic basal cell carcinomas to aminolaevulinic acid photodynamic therapy. Photodiagnosis Photodyn Ther. 2005;2(2):149–55.
15. Jambusaria-Pahlajani A, Schmults CD, Miller CJ, Shin D, Williams J, Kurd SK, et al. Test characteristics of high-resolution ultrasound in the preoperative assessment of margins of basal cell and squamous cell carcinoma in patients undergoing Mohs micrographic surgery. Dermatol Surg. 2009;35(1):9–15; discussion 6.
16. Goldschmidt H, Breneman JC, Breneman DL. Ionizing radiation therapy in dermatology. J Am Acad Dermatol. 1994;30(2 Pt 1):157–82; quiz 183–6.
17. Jennings WA. A survey of depth dose data for X rays from 6 to 75kVp; half value layers from 0.01 to 1.0 MM AL. Br J Radiol. 1953;26(309):481–7.
18. Schirren CG. Rontgentherapie gutartiger und bosartiger Geshwulste der Haut. In: Jadassohn J, editor. Handbuch der Haut-und Geschlechtskrankheiten. Berlin: Springer; 1959. p. 289–463.
19. Cognetta AB, Howard B, Heaton H, Stoddard E, Hong HG, Green WH. Superficial X-ray in the treatment of basal and squamous cell carcinomas: a viable option in select patients. J Am Acad Dermatol. 2012;67(6):1235–41.

20. Atkinson HR. Skin carcinoma depth and dose homogeneity in dermatological x-ray therapy. Aust J Dermatol. 1962;6:208–16.
21. Strandqvist M. Studien uber die kumulative Wirkung der Rontgenstrahlen bei Fraktionierung. Acta Radiol. 1944; Suppl 55:1–300.
22. Ebbehoj E. Bucky-rays and other ultrasoft x-rays. Acta Derm Venereol. 1952;32(2):117–30.
23. Polano MK. Investigations on the optimal dosage in the treatment of skin carcinoma. J Belge Radiol. 1958;41(1):37–58.
24. Newell GB. Depth of basal cell epithiolomas. Personal communication to S.A. Zacarian cited in cryosurgery of skin cancer: fundamentals of technique and application. Cutis. 1975;16: 449–60.
25. Zacarian SA. Cryosurgery of skin cancer: fundamentals of technique and application. Cutis. 1975;16:449–60.

Acute and Chronic Cutaneous Reactions to Radiotherapy

Michele N. Edison and Carolyn M. Johns

Introduction

Radiation therapy is a core treatment modality for many types of cancer. Approximately two-thirds of oncology patients will receive radiation therapy during the course of their treatment [5]. Irradiation damages cellular DNA thereby impairing DNA replication and triggering apoptosis [3, 6]. The goal of radiotherapy is to deliver a lethal dose of radiation to the tumor cells while minimizing damage to normal tissue. Rapidly proliferating cells, such as epidermal keratinocytes, are highly radiosensitive. Consequentially, skin within the radiation field is susceptible to radiation-induced changes, or radiodermatitis. Approximately 90–95 % of radiation oncology patients will experience radiodermatitis during or after their treatment [1, 7].

Radiodermatitis may be acute or chronic and includes localized erythema and edema, the shedding of skin (desquamation), hair loss (epilation), fibrosis, and necrosis. These skin changes may be painful and are associated with decreased quality of life [2, 4, 6]. Furthermore, severe radiodermatitis necessitates treatment modifications or delays that may compromise the efficacy of radiotherapy [3, 8]. Given the scope and potential consequences of radiodermatitis, it is crucial that clinicians are familiar with its risk factors, clinical presentation, and evidenced-based interventions for the management of symptoms.

M.N. Edison (✉)
Florida State University, 1115 West Call Street, Tallahassee, FL 32306, USA
e-mail: Mne09@med.fsu.edu

C.M. Johns
Smilow Cancer Hospital Care Center, 111 Goose Lane, Suite 1300, Guilford, CT 06437, USA

A.B. Cognetta and W.M. Mendenhall (eds.), *Radiation Therapy for Skin Cancer*,
DOI 10.1007/978-1-4614-6986-5_6,

Risk Factors

Risk factors for radiodermatitis may be classified as either treatment-related or individual-related. Treatment-related risk factors include: type of radiation beam, total dose and fractionation, the location and size of the treatment field, presence of overlapping fields, and concurrent use of chemotherapy or radiosensitizers [3, 9, 10]. Individual-related risk factors for radiodermatitis include: presence of skin folds, poor nutritional status, tobacco use, individual radiosensitivity, and comorbid conditions such as diabetes and some autoimmune diseases [1, 3, 11].

In general, an individual's risk for radiodermatitis is proportional to the degree of skin exposure to radiation. The type of radiation beam correlates with the amount of radiation delivered to the skin. Radiation beams with a shorter wavelength and with lower energy photons and electrons deposit greater doses of radiation in the skin as compared to megavoltage linear accelerators. Accordingly, short wavelength photon and electron beams are associated with greater risk for radiodermatitis [11].

Greater cumulative doses, larger treatment fields, and overlapping treatment fields increase total skin irradiation and therefore increase risk for skin toxicity. Large treatment areas are more likely to damage a critical mass of epidermal stem cells, thus impairing the skin's ability to regenerate. Tangential treatment fields are associated with dose inhomogeneity in "hot spot" areas where tangents overlap. These "hot spots" are at increased risk for skin toxicity [12, 13].

Intensity-modulated radiation therapy (IMRT) minimizes risk for radiodermatitis by more precisely targeting tumor and sparing normal tissue. IMRT delivers a more homogenous dose throughout the target tissue, thus minimizing "hot spot" areas [4, 14, 15]. Skin toxicity may also be minimized by 3-dimensional treatment planning and 3-dimensional conformal radiation therapy. Divided radiation dosing, or fractionation, decreases an individual's risk for radiodermatitis by allowing normal tissue to repair between treatments [10].

Many radiation oncology patients will also receive chemotherapy as part of their treatment plan. Chemotherapy, like radiation therapy, interferes with mitosis in rapidly dividing normal and malignant cells. Chemotherapy may be associated with neutropenia, increased risk for infection, and impaired wound healing. Concurrent chemoradiation therapy may therefore increase and prolong radiodermatitis [16]. Additionally, there are specific medications, including some chemotherapy agents, that potentiate the effect of radiation. These medications are known as radiosensitizers. Oncologists may utilize combined modality treatment with radiotherapy and a radiosensitizer medication, such as Xeloda, to increase tumor cell kill [17]. Unfortunately, radiosensitizers also increase the incidence and severity of radiodermatitis [18, 19].

Several individual-related risk factors also impact the development of radiodermatitis. The presence of skin folds within the radiation field, as found in areas such as the neck and axilla, potentially increase the radiation dose to the skin due to a "bolus" effect. This "bolus" effect is believed to increase risk for radiodermatitis [16, 20]. Poor nutritional status, tobacco use and other illnesses, such as diabetes, may exacerbate radiodermatitis by impairing wound healing [10, 11]. Autoimmune illnesses, such as scleroderma and systemic lupus erythematosus, are believed to be indicators of individual radiosensitivity and therefore may increase one's risk for radiodermatitis [3]. Additionally, there are several rare genetic syndromes that predispose individuals to severe radiodermatitis, including ataxia telangiectasia and nevoid basal cell carcinoma syndrome [3, 10].

Pathophysiology

The high mitotic rate of the skin renders it susceptible to radiation. Irradiation damages keratinocyte DNA, resulting in cell apoptosis and impaired re-epithelialization of the epidermis. DNA damage may occur from direct exposure to radiation, and indirectly, via water ionization and free radical production [3]. Repeated insults from irradiation overwhelm the skin's ability to regenerate, leading to radiodermatitis.

Acute skin changes, including erythema and swelling, occur as a result of cytokine-mediated inflammation [3, 21]. Irradiation triggers the release of cytokines that lead to capillary dilation, leukocyte infiltration, and localized swelling and erythema [1, 3]. Dryness and epilation may occur within days to weeks of radiation treatment due to damage to the sebaceous glands and hair follicles in the dermis [1]. Dry desquamation, characterized by dryness, scaling, and pruritus, typically occurs within three weeks of initiating radiotherapy or after a cumulative dose of 20–30 Gy due to destruction of regenerative keratinocytes [22]. Dry desquamation typically resolves within one to two weeks [1]. Moist desquamation, evidenced by red, exposed dermis and serous oozing, occurs after four to five weeks or with a cumulative dose of 45–60 Gy as the keratinocytes are further depleted [22]. Moist desquamation is associated with altered skin integrity that compromises the barrier function of the epidermis and increases risk for superinfections by *Staphylococcus aureus* or *Candida albicans*. *S. aureus* may also act as a superantigen and trigger a cytokine cascade that results in inflammation and impaired wound healing. Acute radiodermatitis usually resolves within four weeks of completing radiotherapy [1].

Late radiation-induced skin changes include atrophy, fibrosis, telangiectasias, and pigmentation changes that occur as a result of permanent damage to the skin. Radiation decreases the population of fibroblasts in the dermis that is, not are responsible for the synthesis of connective tissue and plays an important role in wound healing. Consequentially, collagen is reabsorbed and atrophy develops. The remaining fibroblasts are stimulated by the up-regulation of the cytokine TGF-*B* to produce dense, fibrous tissue [23]. Radiation-induced fibrosis is characterized by progressive induration, edema, and thickening of the dermis. Radiation also damages the vasculature of the dermis, leading to prominent, dilated, and tortuous blood vessels, also known as telangiectasias. Pigmentation changes may vary depending on the extent of damage to the melanocytes of the epidermis. Irradiation may eradicate the skin's population of melanocytes, resulting in hypopigmentation, or it may trigger post-inflammatory production of melanin leading to hyperpigmentation [21].

Histology of Irradiated Skin

The microscopic appearance of late skin changes to irradiation mirrors the macroscopic changes described above. The normal wavy border of the rete ridges at the junction of the epidermis and dermis is replaced by a flat and atrophic epidermis [24]. The presence of sebaceous glands and hair follicles is reduced and there is atrophy of the eccrine glands [25]. Telangiectasias, identified by tortuous vasculature, are prominent against the hypocellular and fibrotic dermis. Fibrotic changes that occur shortly after radiotherapy, termed "young-type fibrosis" demonstrate an abundance of fibroblasts. Fibrotic changes that occur years after radiation, or "old-type fibrosis," are characterized by decreased number of fibroblasts and degenerative changes of the connective tissue [25].

Assessment of Radiodermatitis

Acute radiodermatitis is defined as any adverse skin effect secondary to radiation exposure that occurs within 90 days of initiating treatment. A persistent, pink-hued erythema is often the initial sign of radiodermatitis. Patients may report pruritus, epilation, scaling, and/or change in skin pigmentation in the effected area [3]. These complaints often coincide with dry desquamation. Moist desquamation is differentiated from dry desquamation by the presence of serous exudates. In addition, moist desquamation is often painful and increases one's risk for *S. aureus* and *C. albicans* superinfections. Prolonged pain or foul musty odor should prompt a culture and KOH preparation to assess for bacterial versus yeast infection.

Evaluating the severity of radiodermatitis is controversial because it is subjective. Objective scoring criteria are essential to forming guidelines that monitor the severity of symptoms, determine appropriate interventions, and assess when it is prudent to withhold radiotherapy. The Radiation Therapy Oncology Group (RTOG) and the National Cancer Institute (NCI) have established objective scoring criteria which allow for classification of radiodermatitis by clinical presentation (Tables 1, 2, and 3) [26–28].

For acute radiodermatitis, the RTOG grade zero is equivalent to no skin change from baseline [26]. The lowest grade on the NCI Cancer Therapy Evaluation Program (CTEP) Common Terminology Criteria for Adverse Events (CTCAE) is a grade one [28]. The RTOG and NCI CTCAE both equate a grade one with skin that has mild erythema or follicular erythema and/or dry desquamation [26, 28]. Grade two is associated with significant erythema, patchy moist desquamation within the skin folds, and/or edema [26, 28]. Grade three denotes confluent moist desquamation not isolated to intertriginous zones and bleeding with minor trauma. Grade four on the NCI CTCAE and RTOG scales is characterized by ulceration, spontaneous bleeding, and/or necrosis [3]. Grade five is given when radiodermatitis is associated with death [26, 28].

Table 1 RTOG acute radiation morbidity scoring criteria

	0	1	2	3	4
Skin	No change from baseline	Follicular, faint, or dull erythema/ epilation/dry desquamation/ decreased sweating	Tender or bright erythema, patchy moist desquamation/ moderate edema	Confluent, moist desquamation other than in skin folds/ pitting edema	Ulceration, hemorrhage, necrosis

Adapted from the RTOG Acute Radiation Morbidity Scoring Criteria. Philadelphia: American College of Radiology; [updated 2012, cited 2012 Nov 4]. Available from http://www.rtog.org/ResearchAssociates/AdverseEventReporting/AcuteRadiationMorbidityScoringCriteria.aspx

Table 2 NCI: common terminology criteria for adverse events v3.0

Adverse event	1	2	3	4
Radiation dermatitis	Faint erythema or dry desquamation	Moderate to brisk erythema/patchy moist desquamation, mostly confined to skin folds and creases/ moderate edema	Moist desquamation other than skin folds and creases/bleeding induced by minor trauma or abrasion	Skin necrosis or ulceration of full thickness dermis/ spontaneous bleeding from involved site

Adapted from NCI Common Terminology Criteria for Adverse Events v3.0. Bethesda, MD: Cancer Therapy Evaluation Program, DCTD, NCI, NIH, DHHS; 2003 Dec 12 [cited 2012 Nov 4]. NIH Publication #03-5410. Available from: http://ctep.cancer.gov/protocolDevelopment/electronic_applications/docs/ctcaev3.pdf

Table 3 RTOG late radiation morbidity scoring criteria

	0	1	2	3	4
Skin	No change from baseline	Slight atrophy/ pigmentation change/some hair loss	Patchy atrophy/moderate telangiectasia/total hair loss	Marked atrophy/gross telangiectasia	Ulceration

Adapted from the RTOG Late Radiation Morbidity Scoring Criteria. Philadelphia: American College of Radiology; [updated 2012, cited 2012 Nov 4]. Available from: http://www.rtog.org/ResearchAssociates/AdverseEventReporting/RTOGEORTCLateRadiationMorbidityScoringSchema.aspx

Chronic radiodermatitis is defined as any adverse skin effects of radiation exposure that occur more than 90 days after treatment. Chronic radiodermatitis is classified according to the RTOG Late Radiation Morbidity Scoring Schema (Table 3). According to the RTOG, a score of zero is consistent with no change from baseline. A score of one is consistent with loss of some hair, slight atrophic changes, and change in pigmentation (together known as poikilodermatous changes) [3, 28]. A score of two is associated with patchy atrophy, moderate telangiectasia, and complete alopecia. A score of three is consistent with significant atrophy and gross telangiectasias [28]. A score of four is associated with ulceration of the formerly irradiated skin [3, 28]. According to the RTOG, a score of five is assigned for radiodermatitis-associated death [28]. The symptoms of chronic radiodermatitis can change and progress for up to ten years [29].

Radiation-recall dermatitis is defined as radiodermatitis that occurs days to years after radiation exposure secondary to concomitant drug administration (usually chemotherapeutic medications) which affects the epithelia and mucosa of many organs including the heart, lungs, gastrointestinal tract, and bladder [30]. Symptoms typically progress from erythema to a dry desquamation. In more severe cases, radiation-recall dermatitis may result in vesicular lesions, ulceration, and necrosis.

Management of Radiodermatitis

The overarching goals for the management of radiodermatitis include preventing or minimizing symptoms, preventing or identifying and treating infection, reducing healing time, and maximizing quality of life. The prevention and management of radiodermatitis is challenging as there is no universally accepted set of guidelines.

There is a general consensus regarding hygiene of the irradiated skin. The skin should be routinely washed with a gentle soap that has a low pH, like Dove or Aveeno, and warm water [3, 31, 32]. Studies by Roy et al. and Campbell and Illingworth, showed that the severity of radiodermatitis did not significantly vary with or without washing the affected area [33, 34]. Although not statistically significant, Roy et al. concluded that washing should not be discouraged as there was a lower incidence of moist desquamation and less pain, burning, and itching reported in the group that washed [35]. In addition, patients should also be encouraged to wash their hair as this does not affect the severity of radiodermatitis, even in patients undergoing cranial radiotherapy [36]. In the past, patients were cautioned to avoid deodorant with a metallic base due to concern for a radiation "bolus" effect. Many patients who refrained from deodorant use during radiation treatment have expressed concerns about body odor [36]. According to studies by Burch et al. and Theberge et al., deodorant does not affect the severity of radiodermatitis [37, 38]. Thus, normal hygiene including washing with mild soaps and using topical deodorants and lotions should be encouraged.

Management of Acute Radiodermatitis

There are many research trials that test and compare agents to prevent and treat acute radiodermatitis [31]. Unfortunately, none have been proven by double-blind, randomized clinical trials with high statistical power to be the best management strategy.

Topical Agents

Natural Products

Natural products are used by many different cultures to treat a variety of disease states. Unfortunately, research has shown that many natural products are not effective in the management of radiodermatitis. A study that compared chamomile cream with almond ointment found no significant difference in the severity of radiodermatitis between these two treatment modalities [39]. Another natural agent, calendula ointment which is an extract of the marigold plant, has been found to significantly reduce pain and frequency of grade two or higher acute radiodermatitis compared to Biafine (see next section) [20]. The effect of drinking wine has also been studied. A retrospective study found that women who drink one glass of wine per day, but no more or less, have a reduced incidence of grade two or higher radiodermatitis [40].

Aloe vera extract has long been used to treat cuts and burns. Aloe vera has been touted to have anti-inflammatory and antibacterial effects that, in theory, would benefit irradiated epidermis [29]. The available data, however, suggests that aloe vera is not effective for the prevention or treatment of radiodermatitis [23, 29, 41, 42]. One study suggested that aloe vera may delay the onset of skin symptoms in patients with fewer risk factors for radiodermatitis and in those with skin that is more resistant to radiodermatitis [43]. The preponderance of evidence suggests that aloe vera does not reduce dermatologic adverse effects caused by radiation exposure.

Biafine

Biafine, a trolamine containing compound commonly used in France for radiodermatitis prophylaxis, also lacks support for its use in the management of acute radiodermatitis. According to Fisher et al., in a comparison of Biafine to four other standards of care (aloe vera, Aquaphor, no treatment, other) for prophylaxis of radiodermatitis, there was no statistically significant difference in average of RTOG grade criteria between these groups [2]. The RTOG Trial 99-13 showed that the use of a trolamine emulsion versus standard of care did not reduce grade two or higher radiodermatitis [44]. Yet another study comparing Biafine, Lipiderm, and no treatment showed no significant difference among the groups with regard to ratings by the patients, nurses, and radiotherapists [45].

Topical Corticosteroids

Topical corticosteroids have been trialed for the prevention and management acute radiodermatitis, but results have varied. Mometasone furoate, a medium potency corticosteroid, has shown promising results in reducing radiodermatitis severity [46]. Furthermore, it is dosed once daily and causes less cutaneous atrophy than other topical steroids [46]. Another medium potency corticosteroid, betamethasone, as compared to petrolatum, has demonstrated a reduced severity of acute radiodermatitis [47]. Beclomethasone spray has also been shown to reduce the incidence of wet desquamation [48]. Conversely, the use of very high potency corticosteroids, like clobetasone, is associated with significantly higher rates of severe skin reactions as compared to a low potency steroid-like hydrocortisone [49]. Low dose corticosteroids do not appear to effect the presentation and symptoms of radiodermatitis [50, 51]. These results suggest that there may be a role for medium potency corticosteroids in the management of acute dermatitis. More research is required before steroids may be accepted as a standard of care [3].

Sucralfate

Sucralfate cream is another product that has evidence to both support and negate its use in clinical practice for the treatment of radiodermatitis. Sucralfate has been shown to be better than placebo in reducing radiodermatitis severity, yet results are comparable to that of aqueous creams and sorbolene creams [52–55]. Oral Sucralfate tablets have also been tested and have not been found to be superior to placebo in reducing radiodermatitis [56].

Hyaluronic Acids

Hyaluronic acids stimulate the process of healing. In a comparison of a cream containing sodium hyaluronate and silver sulfadiazine to placebo, the hyaluronic acid cream was found to reduce the incidence of high-grade radiation dermatitis and was favored by both patients and physicians [57]. To date, this is the only human study using hyaluronic acids for the management of acute radiation dermatitis, thus, further research is required [31].

Other Topical Products

Various other products including a dexpanthenol containing cream, a gel product containing reduced glutathione, a vitamin C solution, and a cream containing CM-glucan, methylsilanol hydroxyproline aspartate and matrikines, have been trialed in the management of radiodermatitis, but none of these significantly affected the incidence or severity of radiation dermatitis [58–61]. Hydrolytic enzymes have been shown to significantly reduce the severity and duration of radiodermatitis when compared to no treatment [62]. MAS065D, a water-in-oil cream with hydrating and anti-inflammatory characteristics, has also been shown to reduce skin toxicity, burning, and desquamation associated with radiodermatitis when compared to placebo [63].

Dressings

A moist environment is believed to be beneficial to wound healing [31]. However, in the case of moist desquamation, too much moisture may result in maceration. Dry dressings are preferred to hydrogel dressings for moist desquamation as hydrogel dressings prolong healing time and do not provide symptom relief [64]. Gentian violet, an antifungal agent, is associated with significantly less pain and smaller wounds compared to a moist hydrocolloid dressing for the management of moist desquamation [65]. The old adage "if it's dry, wet it, and if it's wet, dry it" appears to hold true for radiodermatitis.

Silver-leaf nylon dressings, a silver-coated nanocrystalline material, are used to treat burns and/or skin grafts. A study that tested the efficacy of this dressing versus no dressing, showed significantly reduced severity of radiodermatitis [66]. In a study of 12 patients comparing silver sulfadiazine and silver-leaf dressings, the silver-leaf dressings did not improve healing in patients with RTOG grade two or higher radiodermatitis, although patient reported pain was reduced [67]. Silver sulfadiazine cream has been shown to reduce radiodermatitis severity when compared to no topical treatment [68]. These agents need to be avoided in patients with known sulfa sensitivity.

Management of Chronic Radiodermatitis

Chronic radiodermatitis is a serious sequela of radiation exposure. The signs include tissue fibrosis, atrophy, ulceration, and pain. Chronic radiodermatitis is the dose-limiting side effect of radiotherapy [69–71]. Thus, prevention of chronic radiodermatitis is crucial to avoiding treatment delays that may compromise the effectiveness of radiotherapy. Unfortunately, there are no proven methods to prevent chronic radiodermatitis. There are, however, some promising potential treatment options for chronic skin changes related to radiation.

Pentoxifylline

Pentoxifylline is a hemorheologic agent that is commonly used to treat intermittent claudication and other vaso-occlusive disease processes. Pentoxifylline increases red blood cell membrane flexibility, stimulating fibrinolysis, inhibiting platelet aggregation, and altering both fibroblast physiology and immune modulation [72]. It has been shown to increase healing of soft tissue necrosis and formerly nonhealing, radiation-induced necrotic ulcers [73]. Pentoxifylline is associated with reduced radiation-induced fibrosis and fibrosis-associated pain [69, 71]. Other studies have demonstrated significant regression in fibrotic scarring with the use of pentoxifylline plus α-tocopherol [70, 74].

Hyperbaric Oxygen

Hyperbaric oxygen therapy promotes revascularization within irradiated tissues to heal radiation injury to soft tissues. A study from M. D. Anderson Cancer Center showed improved soft tissue texture, increased sensation, and increased mucosal secretions in patients who underwent hyperbaric oxygen treatments [75]. Hyperbaric oxygen therapy is also associated with significant reduction in erythema, pain, and edema, but no reduction in fibrosis or telangiectasia [76]. Unfortunately, compliance is a potential issue with hyperbaric oxygen therapy as these treatments are often over an hour long and must be completed multiple times per week.

Superoxide Dismutase

Superoxide dismutase (SOD) is a group of enzymes that are known for their antioxidant effects in neutralizing free radicals. SOD has also been shown to reduce radiation-induced fibrosis. SOD is associated with fibrotic tissue softening, a significant reduction in the length, width, and depth of fibrosis, and histologically, demonstrates replacement of fibrotic tissue with normal tissues [77, 78].

Conclusion

Radiodermatitis is a common side effect of radiotherapy that is associated with pain, decreased quality of life, and treatment delays that may compromise the delivery and effectiveness of radiation treatment [1–3]. Radiodermatitis ranges from mild to severe and may be acute or chronic. Symptom severity is influenced by the degree of exposure to irradiation as well as several treatment-related and individual-related risk factors. Familiarity with these risk factors will allow dermatologists and radiation oncologists to anticipate the potential for skin toxicity and to plan treatment accordingly.

A multitude of interventions have been studied for the prevention and management of radiodermatitis with varied results. The use of many natural products, including aloe vera and calendula for the management of acute radiodermatitis is not supported by research. Washing the skin with a mild soap and the use of deodorant is recommended as these interventions do not increase toxicity but do improve patient comfort. Medium potency topical corticosteroids have been shown to reduce symptoms and severity of acute radiodermatitis. Interestingly, low potency corticosteroids are less effective and high potency steroids may be associated with increased incidence of severe radiodermatitis. Hydrogel dressings may be appropriate for the management of dry desquamation but result in maceration and prolonged healing in moist desquamation. Instead, dry dressings or gentian violet dressings should be used for the management of moist desquamation. Pentoxifylline and hyperbaric oxygen therapy promote healing of chronic wounds related to radiodermatitis. Preliminary data for the use of several newer agents, including hyaluronic acids and SOD, is favorable. Additional randomized controlled trials with large sample size and standardized assessment tools are needed to develop practice guidelines for the prevention and management of radiodermatitis.

References

1. McQuestion M. Evidenced-based skin care management in radiation therapy. Semin Oncol Nurs. 2006;22(3):163–73.
2. Fisher J, Scott C, Stevens R, Marconi B, Champion L, Freedman GM, et al. Randomized phase III study comparing best supportive care to Biafine as a prophylactic agent for radiation-induced skin toxicity for women undergoing breast irradiation: radiation therapy oncology group (RTOG) 97-13. Int J Radiat Oncol Biol Phys. 2000;48(5):1307–10.
3. Hymes SR, Strom EA, Fife C. Radiation dermatitis: clinical presentation, pathophysiology, and treatment. J Am Acad Dermatol. 2006;54(1):28–46.
4. Pignol J, Olivotto I, Rakovitch E, Gardner S, Sixel K, Beckham W, et al. A multicenter randomized trial of breast intensity-modulated radiation therapy to reduce acute radiodermatitis. J Clin Oncol. 2008;26(1):2085–92.
5. American Society for Radiation Oncology. Statistics about radiation therapy. 2010. Retrieved from http://www.rtanswers.org/statistics/aboutradiationtherapy.aspx.
6. De Conno F, Ventafridda V, Saita L. Skin problems in advanced and terminal cancer patients. J Pain Symptom Manage. 1991;6:247–56.
7. Lopez E, Nunez MI, Guerrero MR, del Moral R, de Dios Luna J, del Mar Rodriguez M, et al. Breast cancer acute radiotherapy morbidity evaluated by different scoring systems. Breast Cancer Res Treat. 2002;73:127–34.
8. Hansen O, Overgaard J, Hansen H, Overgaardd M, Hoyer M, Jorgensen K, et al. Importance of overall treatment time for the outcome of radiotherapy of advanced head and neck carcinoma: dependency on tumor differentiation. Radiother Oncol. 1996;43:47–51.
9. Bernier J, Bonner J, Vermorken JB, Bensadoun RJ, Dummer R, Giralt J, et al. Consensus guidelines for the management of radiation dermatitis and coexisting acne-like rash in patients receiving radiotherapy plus EGFR inhibitors for the treatment of squamous cell carcinoma of the head and neck. Ann Oncol. 2008;19(1):142–9.
10. Porock D. Factors influencing the severity of radiation skin and oral mucosal reactions: development of a conceptual framework. Eur J Cancer Care. 2002;11:33–43.
11. Noble-Adams R. Radiation-induced reactions 1: an examination of the phenomenon. Br J Nurs. 1999;8:1134–40.

12. Chen M, Chen WC, Lai CH, Hung CH, Liu KC, Cheng YH. Predictive factors of radiation-induced skin toxicity in breast cancer patients. BMC Cancer. 2010;10:508.
13. Das I, Cheng C, Fein D, Fowble B. Patterns of dose variability in radiation prescription of breast cancer. Radiother Oncol. 1997;43:83–9.
14. Freedman G, Li T, Nicolaou N, Chen YMC, Anderson P. Breast intensity modulated radiation therapy reduces time spent with acute dermatitis for women of all breast sizes during radiation. Int J Radiat Oncol Biol Phys. 2009;74(3):689–94.
15. McDonald M, Godette K, Butler E, Davis L, Johnstone P. Long-term outcomes of IMRT for breast cancer: a single-institution cohort analysis. Int J Radiat Oncol Biol Phys. 2009;72(4): 1031–40.
16. Back M, Guerrieri M, Wratten C, Steigler A. Impact of radiation therapy on acute toxicity in breast conservation therapy for early breast cancer. Clin Oncol. 2004;16:12–6.
17. Krishnan S, Janjan N, Skibber J, Rodriguez-Bigas M, Wolff R, Das P, et al. Phase II study of capecitabine (Xeloda®) and concomitant boost radiotherapy in patients with locally advanced rectal cancer. Int J Radiat Oncol Biol Phys. 2006;66(3):762–71.
18. Giro C, Berger B, Bolke E, Giernik F, Duprez F, Locati L, et al. High rates of severe radiation dermatitis during radiation therapy with concurrent cetuximab in head and neck cancer: results of survey of EORTC institutes. Radiother Oncol. 2009;90:166–71.
19. Studer G, Brown M, Salgueiro E, Schmuche H, Romahcuk N, Winkler G, et al. Grade 3/4 dermatitis in head and neck cancer patients treated with concurrent cetuximab and IMRT. Int J Radiat Oncol Biol Phys. 2011;81(1):110–7.
20. Pommier P, Gomez F, Sunyach MP, D'Hombres A, Carrie C, Montbarbon X. Phase III randomized trial of *Calendula officinalis* compared with trolamine for the prevention of acute dermatitis during irradiation for breast cancer. J Clin Oncol. 2004;22(8):1447–53.
21. Harper J, Franklin L, Jenrette J, Aguero E. Skin toxicity during breast irradiation: pathophysiology and management. South Med J. 2004;97(10):989–93.
22. Muller K, Khan FM, Port M, Abend M, Molls M, Ring J, et al. Intercellular adhesion molecule-1: a consistent inflammatory maker of the cutaneous radiation reaction both in vitro and in vivo. Br J Dermatol. 2006;155:670–9.
23. Richardson J, Smith JE, McIntyre M, Thomas R, Pilkington K. Aloe vera for preventing radiation-induced skin reactions: a systematic literature review. Clin Oncol. 2005;17:478–84.
24. Archambeau J, Pezner R, Wasserman T. Pathophysiology of irradiated skin and breast. Int J Radiat Oncol Biol Phys. 1995;31:1171–85.
25. Panizzon RG, Cooper JS. Radiation treatment and radiation reactions in dermatology. Germany: Springer; 2004.
26. Group RTO. Acute radiation morbidity scoring criteria. Philadelphia: American College of Radiology [updated 2012, cited 2012 Nov 4]. http://www.rtog.org/ResearchAssociates/AdverseEventReporting/AcuteRadiationMorbidityScoringCriteria.aspx2012.
27. Group RTO. RTOG/EORTC late radiation morbidity scoring schema. Philadelphia: American College of Radiology; [updated 2012, cited 2012 Nov 4]. http://www.rtog.org/ResearchAssociates/AdverseEventReporting/RTOGEORTCLateRadiationMorbidityScoringSchema.aspx2012.
28. National Cancer Institute. Common terminology criteria for adverse events v3.0. Bethesda, MD: Cancer Therapy Evaluation Program, DCTD, NCI, NIH, DHHS; 12 Dec 2003 [cited 2012 Nov 4]. NIH Publication #03-5410.
29. Heggie S, Bryant GP, Tripcony L, Keller J, Rose P, Glendenning M, et al. A phase III study on the efficacy of topical aloe vera gel on irradiated breast tissue. Cancer Nurs. 2002;25(6): 442–51.
30. Yeo W, Johnson PJ. Radiation-recall skin disorders associated with the use of antineoplastic drugs pathogenesis, prevalence, and management. Am J Clin Dermatol. 2000;2:113–6.
31. McQuestion M. Evidence-based skin care management in radiation therapy: clinical update. Semin Oncol Nurs. 2012;27(2):e1–17.
32. Frosch PJ, Klingman AM. The soap chamber test. A new method for assessing the irritancy of soaps. J Am Acad Dermatol. 1979;1(1):35–41.

33. Roy I, Fortin A, Larochelle M. The impact of skin washing with water and soap during breast irradiation: a randomized study. Radiother Oncol. 2001;58:333–9.
34. Campbell IR, Illingworth MH. Can patients wash during radiotherapy to the breast or chest wall? A randomized controlled trial. Clin Oncol. 1992;4(2):78–82.
35. Westbury C, Hines F, Hawkes E, Ashley S, Brada M. Advice on hair and scalp care during cranial radiotherapy: a prospective randomized trial. Radiother Oncol. 2000;54:109–16.
36. Graham PH, Graham JL. Use of deodorants during adjuvant breast radiotherapy: a survey of compliance with standard advice, impact on patients, and a literature review on safety. J Med Imaging Radiat Oncol. 2009;53:569–73.
37. Burch SE, Parker SA, Vann AM, Arazie JC. Measurement of 6-MV X-ray surface dose when topical agents are applied prior to external beam irradiation. Int J Radiat Oncol Biol Phys. 1997;38(2).
38. Theberge V, Harel F, Dagnault A. Use of axillary deodorant and effect on acute skin toxicity during radiotherapy for breast cancer: a prospective randomized noninferiority trial. Int J Radiat Oncol Biol Phys. 2009;75(4):1048–52.
39. Maiche AG, Grohn P, Maki-Hokkonen H. Effect of chamomile cream and almond ointment on acute radiation skin reaction. Acta Oncol. 1991;30(3):395–6.
40. Morganti AG, Digesù C, Panunzi S, De Gaetano A, Macchia G, Deodato F, et al. Radioprotective effect of moderate wine consumption in patients with breast carcinoma. Int J Radiat Oncol Biol Phys. 2009;74(5):1501–5.
41. Olsen DL, Raub W, Bradley C, Johnson M, Macias JL, Love V, et al. The effect of aloe vera gel/mild soap versus mild soap alone in preventing skin reactions in patients undergoing radiation therapy. Oncol Nurs Forum. 2001;28(3):543–7.
42. Merchant TE, Bosley C, Smith J, Baratti P, Pritchard D, Davis T, et al. A phase III trial comparing an anionic phospholipid-based cream and aloe vera-based gel in the prevention of radiation dermatitis in pediatric patients. Radiat Oncol. 2007;2:45.
43. Vogler BK, Ernst E. Aloe vera: a systematic review of its clinical effectiveness. Br J Gen Pract. 1999;49(447):823–8.
44. Elliott EA, Wright JR, Swann RS, Nguyen-Tan F, Takita C, Bucci MK, et al. Phase III trial of an emulsion containing trolamine for the prevention of radiation dermatitis in patients with advanced squamous cell carcinoma of the head and neck: results of Radiation Therapy Oncology Group Trial 99-13. J Clin Oncol. 2006;24(13):2092–7.
45. Fenig E, Brenner B, Katz A, Sulkes J, Lapidot M, Schacter J, et al. Topical biafine and lipiderm for the prevention of radiation dermatitis: a randomized prospective trial. Oncol Rep. 2001;8(2):305–9.
46. Bostrom A, Lindman H, Swartling C, Berne B, Bergh J. Potent corticosteroid cream (mometasone furoate) significantly reduces acute radiation dermatitis: results from a double-blind, randomized study. Radiother Oncol. 2001;59:257–65.
47. Omidvari S, Saboori H, Mohammadianpanah M, Mosaleai A, Ahmadloo N, Mosley-Shirazi MA, et al. Topical betamethasone for prevention of radiation dermatitis. Indian J Dermatol Venereol Leprol. 2007;73(3):209.
48. Shukla PN, Gairola M, Mohanti BK, Rath GK. Prophylactic beclomethasone spray to the skin during postoperative radiotherapy of carcinoma breast: a prospective randomized study. Indian J Cancer. 2006;43(4):180–4.
49. Glees JP, Mameghan-Zadeh H, Sparkes CG. Effectiveness of topical steroids in the control of radiation dermatitis: a randomised trial using 1% hydrocortisone cream and 0.05% clobetasone butyrate (Eumovate). Clin Radiol. 1979;30(4):397–403.
50. Potera ME, Lookingbill DP, Stryker JA. Prophylaxis of radiation dermatitis with a topical cortisone cream. Radiology. 1982;143:775–7.
51. Schmuth M, Wimmer MA, Hofer S, Sztankay A, Weinlich G, Linder DM, et al. Topical corticosteroid therapy for acute radiation dermatitis: a prospective, randomized double-blind study. Br J Dermatol. 2002;146:983–91.
52. Maiche A, Isokangas O-P, Grohn P. Skin protection by sucralfate cream during electron beam therapy. Acta Oncol. 1994;33(2):201–3.

53. Wells M, Macmillan M, Raab G, MacBride S, Bell N, MacKinnon K, et al. Does aqueous or sucralfate cream affect the severity of erythematous radiation skin reactions? A randomised controlled trial. Radiother Oncol. 2004;73:153–62.
54. Delaney G, Fisher R, Hook C, Barton M. Sucralfate cream in the management of moist desquamation during radiotherapy. Australas Radiol. 1997;41:270–5.
55. Falkowski S, Trouillas P, Duroux J-L, Bonnetblanc J-M, Clavere P. Radiodermatitis prevention with sucralfate in breast cancer: fundamental and clinical studies. Support Care Cancer. 2011;19(1):57–65.
56. Lievens Y, Haustermans K, Van den Weyngaert D, Van den Bogaert WS, Pierre Hutsebaut L, Fowler J, et al. Does sucralfate reduce the acute side-effects in head and neck cancer treated with radiotherapy? A double-blind randomized trial. Radiother Oncol. 1998;47:149–53.
57. Liguori V, Guillemin C, Pesce GF, Mirimanoff RO, Bernier J. Double-blind, randomized clinical study comparing hyaluronic acid cream to placebo in patients treated with radiotherapy. Radiother Oncol. 1997;42:155–61.
58. Roper B, Kaisig D, Auer F, Mergen E, Molls M. Theta-cream versus bepanthol lotion in breast cancer patients under radiotherapy. Strahlenther Onkol. 2004;5:315–22.
59. Lokkevik E, Skovlund E, Reitan JB, Hannisdal E, Tanum G. Skin treatment with bepanthen cream versus no cream during radiotherapy. Acta Oncol. 1996;35(8):1021–6.
60. Enomoto TM, Johnson T, Peterson N, Homer L, Walts D, Johnson N. Combination glutathione and anthocyanins as an alternative for skin care during external-beam radiation. Am J Surg. 2005;189(5):627–31.
61. Halperin EC, Gaspar L, George S, Darr D, Pinnell S. A double-blind, randomized, prospective trial to evaluate topical vitamin C solution for the prevention of radiation dermatitis. Int J Radiat Oncol Biol Phys. 1993;26:413–6.
62. Gujral MS, Patnaik PM, Kaul R, Parikh HK, Conradt C, Tamhankar CP, et al. Efficacy of hydrolytic enzymes in prevention radiation therapy-induced side effects in patients with head and neck cancers. Cancer Chemother Pharmacol. 2001;47:S23–8.
63. Leonardi MC, Gariboldi S, Ivaldi GB, Ferrari A, Serafini F, Didier F, et al. A double-blind, randomised, vehicle-controlled clinical study to evaluate the efficacy of MAS065D in limiting the effects of radiation on the skin: interim analysis. Eur J Dermatol. 2008;18(3):317–21.
64. MacMillan MS, Wells M, MacBride S, Raab GM, Munro A, MacDougall H. Randomized comparison of dry dressings versus hydrogel in management of radiation-induced moist desquamation. Int J Radiat Oncol Biol Phys. 2007;68(3):864–72.
65. Mak SS, Molassiotis A, Wan W-M, Lee I, Chan E. The effects of hydrocolloid dressing and gentian violet on radiation-induced moist desquamation wound healing. Cancer Nurs. 2000;23(3):220–9.
66. Vuong T, Franco E, Lehnert S, Lambert C, Portelance L, Nasr E, et al. Silver leaf nylon dressing to prevent radiation dermatitis in patients undergoing chemotherapy and external beam radiotherapy to the perineum. Int J Radiat Oncol Biol Phys. 2004;59(3):809–14.
67. Vavassis P, Gelinas M, Chabot J, Nguyen-Tan PF. Phase 2 study of silver leaf dressing for treatment of radiation-induced dermatitis in patients receiving radiotherapy to the head and neck. J Otolaryngol Head Neck Surg. 2008;37(1):124–9.
68. Hemati S, Asnaashari O, Sarvizadeh M, Motlagh BN, Akbari M, Tajvidi M, et al. Topical silver sulfadiazine for the prevention of acute dermatitis during irradiation for breast cancer. Support Care Cancer. 2011;20(8):1613–8.
69. Futran ND, Trotti A, Gwede C. Pentoxifylline in the treatment of radiation related soft tissue injury: preliminary observations. Laryngoscope. 1997;107(3):391–5.
70. Delanian S, Balla-Makias S, Lefaix J-L. Striking regression of chronic radiotherapy damage in a clinical trial of combined pentoxifylline and tocopherol. J Clin Oncol. 1999;17(10): 3283–90.
71. Aygenc E, Celikkanat S, Kaymakci M, Aksaray F, Ozdem C. Prophylactic effect of pentoxifylline on radiotherapy complications: a clinical study. Otolaryngol Head Neck Surg. 2004;130(3): 351–6.

72. Samlaska CP, Winfield EA. Pentoxifylline. J Am Acad Dermatol. 1994;30(4):603–21.
73. Dion MW, Hussey DH, Doornbos JF, Vigliotti AP, Wen B-C, Anderson B. Preliminary results of a pilot study of pentoxifylline in the treatment of late radiation soft tissue necrosis. Int J Radiat Oncol Biol Phys. 1990;19(2):401–7.
74. Lefaix J-L, Delanian S, Vozenin M-C, Leplat J-J, Tricaud Y, Martin M. Striking regression of subcutaneous fibrosis induced by high doses of gamma rays using a combination of pentoxifylline and -tocopherol: an experimental study. Int J Radiat Oncol Biol Phys. 1999;43(4):839–47.
75. King GE, Scheetz J, Jacob RF, Martin JW. Electrotherapy and hyperbaric oxygen: promising treatments for postradiation complications. J Prosthet Dent. 1989;62(3):331–4.
76. Carl UM, Feldmeier JJ, Schmitt G, Hartmann KA. Hyperbaric oxygen therapy for late sequelae in women receiving radiation after breast-conserving surgery. Int J Radiat Oncol Biol Phys. 2001;49(4):1029–31.
77. Lefaix J-L, Delanian S, Leplat J-J, Tricaud Y, Martin M, Nimrod A, et al. Successful treatment of radiation-induced fibrosis using Cu/Zn-SOD and Mn-SOD: an experimental study. Int J Radiat Oncol Biol Phys. 1996;35(2):305–12.
78. Delanian S, Baillet F, Huart J, Lefaix J-L, Maulard C, Housset M. Successful treatment of radiation-induced fibrosis using liposomal Cu/Zn superoxide dismutase: a clinical trial. Radiother Oncol. 1994;32(1):12–20.

Efficacy of Superficial Radiotherapy

W. Harris Green and Armand B. Cognetta Jr.

Efficacy for Primary BCC and SCC

Dermatologists have been utilizing cathode tube-induced radiation in the treatment of skin cancers for over a century. In the early decades, the recurrence rates were high while the long-term sequelae were unfavorable. With more consistent and reliable tubes and a better understanding of dosimetry, cure rates have steadily improved over the decades while late side effects have lessened allowing an overall improved degree of cure and cosmesis. The following reported cure rates are from the larger studies in the last several decades.

The 5-year cure rate published by the New York Skin and Cancer Unit for 500 histologically proven primary basal cell carcinomas was 93 % [1]. In contrast, for 468 BCCs treated with surgical excision, the recurrence rate was 6.8 % with the highest recurrence rates found in the periocular, scalp, nose, and perinasal areas [2]. Dubin and Kopf updated these results in 1983 reporting recurrence rates for 2,064 patients with 3,531 primary BCCs. Radiotherapy was employed in 21 % of the tumors yielding recurrence rates of 9.3 % while excision yielded 9 % recurrence rates [3]. Silverman and Kopf further reviewed the experience in the Skin and Cancer Unit, from 1955 through 1982, with the treatment of 862 primary BCCs irradiated by a "standardized" (i.e., NYU protocol 680 × 5) X-ray therapy schedule [4]. The overall 5-year recurrence rate for these lesions, as determined by the modified life table method, was 7.4 %. Additional analysis showed that BCCs on the

W.H. Green (✉)
Division of Dermatology, Florida State University College of Medicine, 1707 Riggins Road, Tallahassee, FL 32308, USA
e-mail: DATresearch@gmail.com

A.B. Cognetta Jr.
Dermatology Associates of Tallahassee, Chief, Division of Dermatology, Florida State University College of Medicine, 1707 Riggins Road, Tallahassee, FL 32308, USA

A.B. Cognetta and W.M. Mendenhall (eds.), *Radiation Therapy for Skin Cancer*,
DOI 10.1007/978-1-4614-6986-5_7,

head less than 10 mm in diameter had a 5-year recurrence rate of 4.4 % whereas those 10 mm or greater in diameter had a rate of 9.5 %. In 1989, Rowe et al. systematically reviewed the previous 40 years of literature and employed 5-year life table analyses (which also adjust recurrence rates for the number of patients lost to follow-up each year) comparing the therapeutic results of various treatment modalities [5]. Five-year recurrence rates were as follows: surgical excision, 10.1 % (264 of 2,606 patients); radiation therapy, 8.7 % (410 of 4,695 patients); curettage and electrodessication, 7.7 % (274 of 3,573 patients); cryotherapy, (insufficient data) 7.5 % (20 of 269 patients); and Mohs micrographic surgery, 1 % (73 of 7,670 patients).

In a large Australian study published in 1989, Ashby et al. reported 5-year Kaplan-Meier recurrence rates of 10 % for 434 basal and squamous cell carcinomas treated with SXRT [6]. Similarly, in 1992, Panizzon reported estimated recurrence rates of 5.1 % in 297 non-sclerosing BCCs and 22 % in 36 BCCs with a sclerosing component during a follow-up of 7.9 years [7]. In 2003, Zagrodnik et al. reported 5-year Kaplan-Meier recurrence rates of 8.2 % for 103 nodular BCCs, 26.1 % for 25 superficial BCCs, and 27.7 % for 47 sclerosing BCCs treated with SXRT in 154 patients [8]. In 2007, Chan et al., in a large British study involving 1,005 lesions (986 BCC and 19 SCC) in 806 patients, reported a raw recurrence rate of 4.4 % and 5-year Kaplan-Meier recurrence estimates of 10 % using a single fraction of SXRT up to 2,250 cGy [9]. Finally, Cognetta et al. in a systematic review of 1,715 nonaggressive BCCs and SCCs and treated at Dermatology Associates of Tallahassee over a 10-year period, 45 were considered to be recurrent (using very liberal inclusion criteria) at follow-up with a raw recurrence rate for all tumors treated was 2.6 % [10]. Because of the variation in follow-up lengths among patients, Kaplan-Meier estimates were used to estimate the control rates for all tumors at 2- and 5-year intervals and were found to be 98.1 % and 95.0 %, respectively. Kaplan-Meier estimates of cumulative control rates of BCCs at 2 and 5 years were 98 % (96.9–99.2 %) and 95.8 % (93.6–98.1 %), respectively, of all SCC (including SCC in situ) at 2 and 5 years were 98.2 % (97.2–99.2 %) and 94.2 % (91.3–97.1 %), respectively, of invasive SCC at 2 and 5 years were 98.8 % (96.3–100 %) and 93.3 % (85.5–100 %), respectively, and of SCC in situ were 98.1 % (97.0–99.3 %) and 94.5 % (91.7–97.5 %), respectively. Cognetta employed 700 cGy×5 for a total of 3,500 cGy for the vast majority of the tumors in the study. Additionally, all of the tumors were reviewed prior to treatment and considered nonaggressive and amenable to superficial radiotherapy.

The recurrence estimates in Cognetta's 10-year study are conservative for a number of reasons. Any tumor in the study which arose within or contiguous to the treatment site was counted as a recurrence. Many of these patients in the study had extreme sun damage and, at baseline, were exhibiting multiple skin cancers arising synchronously or meta-synchronously in individual areas of the head and neck. Any occurrence in or contiguous to the radiation treatment field could represent a de novo cancer but was always counted as a recurrence. Similarly, in any case where an MOHS layer cleared a tumor near a previous radiation site and the postoperative defect encroached into the outer umbra of the radiotherapy site, this was counted as a recurrence. Furthermore, the Kaplan-Meier estimates tend to overestimate recurrence rates in the context of high follow-up drop out by patients who either continued subsequent care under their referring physician, who experienced no reportable problems with the treatment site, or who had passed on from other health problems in their advanced age. Because of the tight referral base and patterns of Dermatology Associates of Tallahassee, it would be common practice for the referring physician or patient to report back with any problems in that area. In this way, the proportion of patients in follow-up at 5 years without recurrences to those who have a suspected recurrence is very low often creating what may have been an overestimation of the proportion of patients with recurrence in the Kaplan-Meier estimations. Nevertheless, the success rates in Cognetta's study remain favorable and are comparable to the success rates of SXRT reported in previous smaller studies in the last few decades [6, 8, 9, 11–18]. In summary, the overall cure rates for primary BCC in most of the larger studies over the past several decades is in the 90–96 % range.

Efficacy in Aggressive or Recurrent BCC and SCC

As the cure rate of aggressive and recurrent BCC decreases significantly with superficial radiotherapy reaching recurrence rates near 33 %, it is in the authors' opinion that these tumors are best treated with Mohs surgery or by a radiation oncologist if the patient is a poor surgical candidate.

Cosmesis

While cure rates have been relatively easy to quantify for various treatment methods, cosmesis has proved more difficult to assess and quantify. In 1954, Churchill-Davidson and Johnson, in an assessment of 664 irradiated patients, found excellent cosmetic results in 15.8 % of patients and good cosmetic results in 76.5 % of patients [19]. They stated that excellent results cannot be expected in very penetrating lesions larger than 5 cm^2. Bart and associates from their experience from the New York Skin and Cancer Unit emphasized that cosmetic results tend to worsen with time and advised against radiotherapy in patients under 40 years of age [1]. Excellent to good cosmetic results were observed in 74 % of the 500 lesions within the first year of treatment, in 68 % in the third to fifth years of treatment, and in 49 % in the ninth to twelfth years. It is noteworthy that the treatments in this study were limited to five fractions (680 cGy × 5 fractions for a total of 3,400 cGy) as the patients often had a significant distance to travel for the treatment sessions and in this way, cosmesis could have been improved via a regimen with more fractions [20]. In fact, according to Silverman et al., because of the less favorable results observed at the Skin and Cancer Unit over the past few years, they adopted a modified regimen of ten treatments of 400 cGy for a total dose of 4,000 cGy [4]. In Cognetta's 10-year experience, no patients under age 65 were treated with radiotherapy and all cosmetic results were good to very good [10].

Most authors agree that optimal cosmetic results occur when the overall dosage is spread out over a higher number of fractions. The poorest results occur on the neck, trunk, and extremities. In the experience of the senior editor, the cosmetic results of radiotherapy for a BCC on the alar rim of a phymatous nose are unparalleled, surpassing plastic surgical repair results after Mohs surgery and, in our practice, is

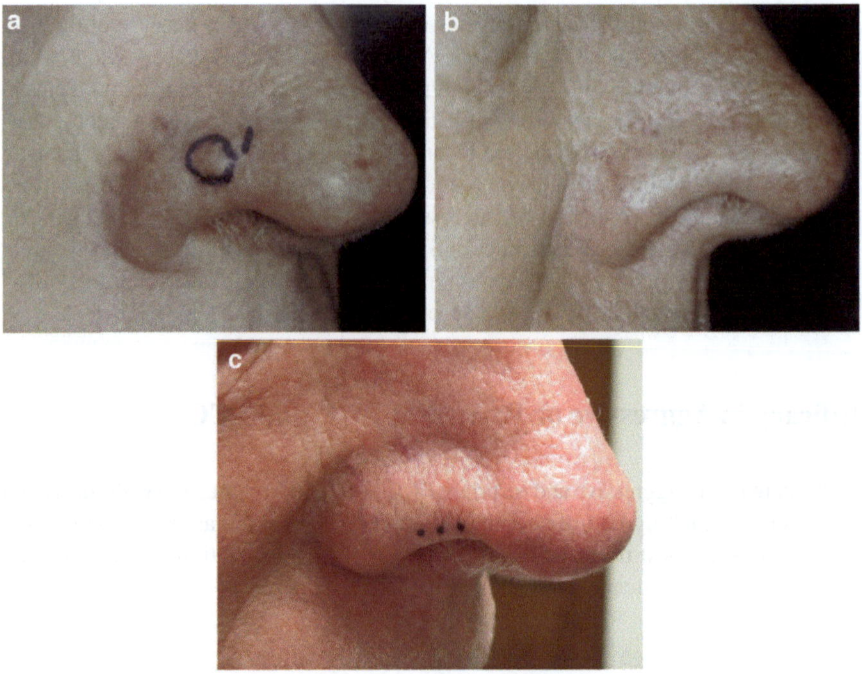

Fig. 1 Patient with nodular basal cell carcinoma of right ala before (**a**), 3 years after (**b**), and 6 years after (**c**) superficial radiation therapy

strongly considered in patients 65 years old and older (Figs. 1, 2, 3, and 4). Similarly, the cosmetic results of large squamous cell carcinoma in situ of the scalp are superior to those of surgical resection and skin grafting and far gentler on elderly and frail patients who are poor surgical candidates. Furthermore, ectropion of the eyelid and retraction of the lip are not uncommon occurrences after surgery and are not seen with superficial radiotherapy.

The initial scarring with resulting hypopigmentation, permanent alopecia, and telangiectasias which typically arise within treatment sites over the decades should be discussed and compared to the scarring, pain, and potential disfigurement of surgical excision and repair. One should discuss with the patient improved cosmesis with increased fractionation (and increased cost) and how scars from surgery generally improve with time compared to the skin changes from radiotherapy. As discussed in greater detail in Chap. 9, logistical variables such as age of the patient, medical comorbidities, transportation, and cosmetic concerns all go into the decision process when choosing treatment regimens and fractionation schemes.

In contrast to surgery, the initial scarring from radiation therapy is minimal the first 1 or 2 years after radiation. It starts out gradually with hypopigmentation, followed by atrophy, and eventually telangiectasia occurs many years later. These lesions are discoid in appearance and can become very prominent over time. As discussed, the thick rhinophymatous skin of the nose holds up better to radiation

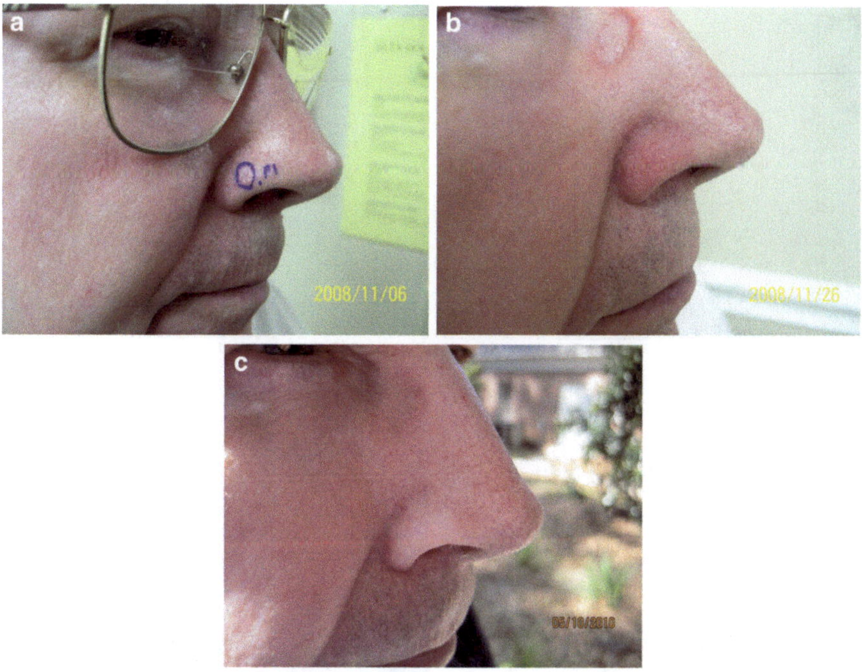

Fig. 2 A patient with a nodular BCC of the right ala before (**a**), during (final treatment) (**b**), and 350 days after radiation therapy (**c**)

than the thin skin of the cheek or forehead. In this location, short and long-term scars are often far superior than surgery and complex closure. Scarring from radiation is dependent on fractionation. If scarring is a prime factor or concern for the patient, one can utilize 10, 15, or even 20 fractions to minimize this.

Comparison to Electron Beam Radiotherapy

Photon SXRT differs from electron beam radiotherapy in that light is the energy source rather than a charged particle. The machines are smaller and less expensive as a linear accelerator is not required, and the applied physics and dosimetry are inherently simpler. With SXRT, a complex physics calculation and bolus are not needed in order to deliver 100 % of the dose to the skin surface as is required with electron beam therapy. Additionally, the beam and delivered dose with SXRT have far less lateral edge beam drop-off in the umbra of the treatment site [21, 22]. Technical factors such as these may have contributed to the inferior cure rates of electron beam therapy reported in the literature [21]. Lastly, SXRT is more cost-effective in terms of equipment and patient costs. Electron beam therapy, however, can be used to treat broader areas of the skin than can typically be utilized with

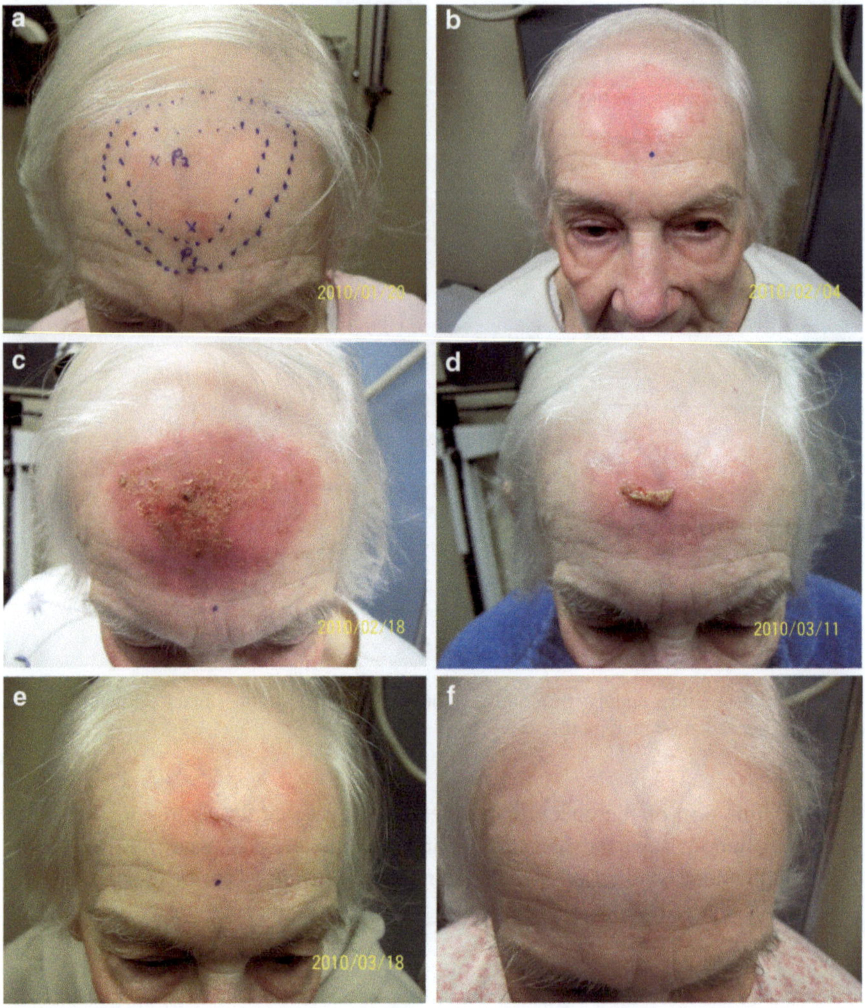

Fig. 3 Patient with SCC in situ of the forehead on day of first treatment. The *inner marked circle* represents the clinical lesion while the *outer circle* represents a 10 mm clinical margin (**a**), the day of final treatment (**b**), 14 days after with normal desquamation (**c**), 37 days after (**d**), 44 days after (**e**), and 106 days after radiation treatment (**f**)

SXRT and by virtue of its long TSD, may be superior in delivering a homogenous dose in complex topographical treatment sites (i.e., Perforating lesions of the nares). Electron beam therapy also has an established role in adjunctive therapy in tumors with perineural invasion, in the treatment of cutaneous T-cell lymphoma, merkel cell carcinoma, dermatofibrosarcoma protuberans, and in select melanomas of the head and neck [18, 23, 24].

It is our standard practice to review the histological slides of all patients that are referred to us for Mohs surgery and at the same time review their medical history,

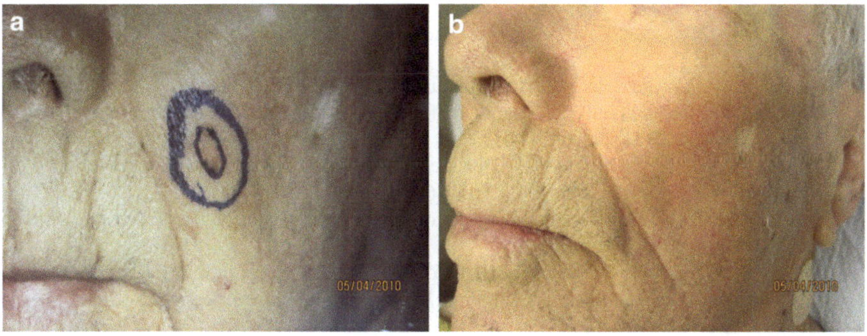

Fig. 4 A patient with biopsy proven SCC in situ of the left cheek prior to (**a**) and 4 years after radiation therapy (**b**)

age, and location of tumors. Each tumor is looked at histologically to ascertain tumor depth and to identify aggressive features or lack thereof. On the appointed day of surgery, patients are given during informed consent the option for Mohs surgery and repair. In patients over age 65 where the tumor is nonaggressive and we can delineate it well, we will offer them superficial X-ray for tumors on the head and face. In cases of aggressive tumors in patients whom we do not think are good surgical candidates, we typically refer them to our local radiation oncologist or our regional colleagues. If the tumor is highly aggressive, we typically refer the patient to a tertiary care referral center tumor board. We work closely with our radiation oncologist colleagues for patients who have aggressive squamous cells and require postoperative radiation for perineural invasion or other factors.

We have seen and reported multiple SCC in situs and other tumors (e.g., atypical fibroxanthomas) arising in the radiation field for scalp lesions treated with electron beam for perineural invasion and attribute it to the widened 80–20 % penumbra that occurs on convex surfaces resulting in a paradoxical subtherapeutic carcinogenic dose to the periphery of the treatment field [25]. Nevertheless, it remains in invaluable tool in adjunctive therapy for aggressive tumors with perineural invasion.

Conclusion

In conclusion, the literature and collective experience of the authors of this text suggest that superficial X-ray therapy continues to serve as a reasonable nonsurgical option with good cosmetic results for the treatment of primary, nonaggressive BCC and SCC in patients where surgical intervention is either declined, unadvisable due to comorbidities, or potentially associated with significant cosmetic or functional limitations. Although not superior to Mohs surgery in terms of tumor recurrence rates, superficial radiation therapy, when utilized properly and responsibly, continues to serve as an important tool in the dermatologic armamentarium for the management of skin cancer amidst an increasing elderly and frail patient population.

References

1. Bart RS, Kopf AW, Petratos MA. X-ray therapy of skin cancer: evaluation of a "standardized" method for treating basal cell epitheliomas. In: Proceedings of the sixth national cancer conference. Philadelphia, PA: JB Lippincott; 1968.
2. Bart RS, Kopf AW, Gladstein AH. Treatment of morphea-type basal cell carcinomas with radiation therapy. Arch Dermatol. 1977;113(6):783–6.
3. Dubin N, Kopf AW. Multivariate risk score for recurrence of cutaneous basal cell carcinomas. Arch Dermatol. 1983;119(5):373–7.
4. Silverman MK, Kopf AW, Gladstein AH, Bart RS, Grin CM, Levenstein MJ. Recurrence rates of treated basal cell carcinomas. Part 4: X-ray therapy. J Dermatol Surg Oncol. 1992; 18(7):549–54.
5. Rowe DE, Carroll RJ, Day Jr CL. Long-term recurrence rates in previously untreated (primary) basal cell carcinoma: implications for patient follow-up. J Dermatol Surg Oncol. 1989;15(3): 315–28.
6. Ashby MA, Smith J, Ainslie J, McEwan L. Treatment of nonmelanoma skin cancer at a large Australian center. Cancer. 1989;63(9):1863–71.
7. Goldschmidt H, Breneman JC, Breneman DL. Ionizing radiation therapy in dermatology. J Am Acad Dermatol. 1994;30(2 Pt 1):157–82; quiz 83–6.
8. Zagrodnik B, Kempf W, Seifert B, Muller B, Burg G, Urosevic M, et al. Superficial radiotherapy for patients with basal cell carcinoma: recurrence rates, histologic subtypes, and expression of p53 and Bcl-2. Cancer. 2003;98(12):2708–14.
9. Chan S, Dhadda AS, Swindell R. Single fraction radiotherapy for small superficial carcinoma of the skin. Clin Oncol (R Coll Radiol). 2007;19(4):256–9.
10. Cognetta A, Howard B, Heaton H, Stoddard E, Hong G, Green WH. Superficial X-ray in the treatment of basal cell and squamous cell carcinoma: a viable option. American Academy of Dermatology, annual meeting, San Diego, CA; 2012.
11. Olschewski T, Bajor K, Lang B, Lang E, Seegenschmiedt MH. [Radiotherapy of basal cell carcinoma of the face and head: importance of low dose per fraction on long-term outcome]. J Dtsch Dermatol Ges. 2006;4(2):124–30.
12. Wilder RB, Kittelson JM, Shimm DS. Basal cell carcinoma treated with radiation therapy. Cancer. 1991;68(10):2134–7.
13. Lovett RD, Perez CA, Shapiro SJ, Garcia DM. External irradiation of epithelial skin cancer. Int J Radiat Oncol Biol Phys. 1990;19(2):235–42.
14. Rodriguez JM, Deutsch GP. The treatment of periocular basal cell carcinomas by radiotherapy. Br J Ophthalmol. 1992;76(4):195–7.
15. Abbatucci JS, Boulier N, Laforge T, Lozier JC. Radiation therapy of skin carcinomas: results of a hypofractionated irradiation schedule in 675 cases followed more than 2 years. Radiother Oncol. 1989;14(2):113–9.
16. Mazeron JJ, Chassagne D, Crook J, Bachelot F, Brochet F, Brune D, et al. Radiation therapy of carcinomas of the skin of nose and nasal vestibule: a report of 1676 cases by the Groupe Europeen de Curietherapie. Radiother Oncol. 1988;13(3):165–73.
17. Locke J, Karimpour S, Young G, Lockett MA, Perez CA. Radiotherapy for epithelial skin cancer. Int J Radiat Oncol Biol Phys. 2001;51(3):748–55.
18. Mendenhall WM, Amdur RJ, Hinerman RW, Cognetta AB, Mendenhall NP. Radiotherapy for cutaneous squamous and basal cell carcinomas of the head and neck. Laryngoscope. 2009;119(10):1994–9.
19. Churchill-Davidson I, Johnson E. Rodent ulcers: an analysis of 711 lesions treated by radiotherapy. Br Med J. 1954;1(4877):1465–8.
20. Kopf AW. Personal communication; 2012.
21. Griep C, Davelaar J, Scholten AN, Chin A, Leer JW. Electron beam therapy is not inferior to superficial x-ray therapy in the treatment of skin carcinoma. Int J Radiat Oncol Biol Phys. 1995;32(5):1347–50.

22. Goldschmidt HP, Panizzon RG. Modern dermatologic radiation therapy. New York: Springer; 1991.
23. Ling SM, Roach III M, Fu KK, Coleman C, Chan A, Singer M. Local control after the use of adjuvant electron beam intraoperative radiotherapy in patients with high-risk head and neck cancer: the UCSF experience. Cancer J Sci Am. 1996;2(6):321–9.
24. de Sanctis V, Persechino S, Fanelli A, Valeriani M, Bracci S, D'Arienzo M, et al. Role of radiation therapy in mycosis fungoides refractory to systemic therapy. Eur J Dermatol. 2011;21(2):213–7.
25. Wolfe CM, Green WH, Hatfield HK, Shakar TJ, Baniahmad O, Cognetta AB. Multiple secondary cutaneous tumours following electron beam radiotherapy for cutaneous malignancies of the scalp. Australas J Dermatol. 2012;53(3):233–8.

Treatment Selection for Superficial Radiotherapy

Armand B. Cognetta Jr. and Christopher M. Wolfe

Introduction

Non-melanoma skin cancer (NMSC) is the most common malignancy in the United States [1, 2]. Basal cell carcinoma (BCC) makes up 75–90 % of all NMSC, with squamous cell carcinoma (SCC) accounting for the remainder [3, 4]. These cutaneous carcinomas are most often related to ultraviolet light exposure occurring most commonly on the head and neck of middle-age to elderly patients. With thorough screening, these NMSCs can be identified at an early stage and with appropriate treatment can result in excellent local control and cosmesis in most patients. Common treatments include surgery, electrodessication & curettage, cryosurgery, carbon dioxide laser ablation, off-label use of imiquimod, 5-fluorouracil, photodynamic therapy, and radiotherapy. Radiotherapy has been used by dermatologists for over 100 years; however, its use within dermatology has declined due to multiple factors. Selection of treatment is contingent on multiple factors such as tumor characteristics, patient preference, physical condition of the patient, cosmetic considerations, availability of treatment options, and the preference, education, and skill of the treating physician. The recommendation for radiotherapy is generally limited to patients who are either poor surgical candidates, those whose outcome with radiotherapy is expected to be better due to the site or size of the lesion compared to surgical intervention, those who refuse or wish to avoid surgery, and those who are being cared for by a physician who is knowledgeable in its use or is amenable to referring the patient to someone who is. Despite the low recurrence rates, favorable

A.B. Cognetta Jr. (✉)
Dermatology Associates of Tallahassee, Chief, Division of Dermatology,
Florida State University College of Medicine, 1707 Riggins Road, Tallahassee,
FL 32308, USA
e-mail: acognetta@gmail.com

C.M. Wolfe
Lake Erie College of Osteopathic Medicine, 1858 West Grandview Boulevard,
Erie, PA 16509-1025, USA

A.B. Cognetta and W.M. Mendenhall (eds.), *Radiation Therapy for Skin Cancer*,
DOI 10.1007/978-1-4614-6986-5_8, © Springer Science+Business Media New York 2013

cosmesis, ease of use, lack of patient discomfort, and relatively low costs of outpatient superficial X-ray therapy (SXRT), the percentage of dermatology clinics in the United States administering SXRT has decreased significantly over the years for a variety of reasons, including the development and availability of Mohs surgery, a relinquishment on the part of dermatologists of radiotherapy to radiation oncologists, and until recently a lack of modern radiation equipment designed to be used in dermatology offices [5, 6].

Overview of Superficial Radiotherapy

It is useful to have a broad view of the types of radiotherapy available now and in the past for the treatment of NMSC (Table 1). Superficial radiotherapy (SRT) utilizing low-voltage X-ray (photon) is used primarily by dermatologists to treat BCC

Table 1 Classification of radiotherapy methods based on energy/voltage/generator

Type	Sources & synonyms	Type of generator	kV	D ½ (mm tissue)	Surface dose (%)[a]
Megavoltage electron therapy	Electron beam radiation	Linear accelerator (LINAC)	>1,000 (6,000–9,000)	90 % Isodose method used for electrons[b]	78–86
Megavoltage photon therapy (not routinely used to treat NMSC)	Megavoltage X-ray	Linear accelerator (LINAC)	>1,000	150–200	6–30
Supervoltage therapy	Gamma (γ)-ray	Isotope teletherapy machines (^{60}Cobalt)	>1,000	80–110	40–90
Orthovoltage therapy	Deep X-ray	X-ray machine	200–400	50–80	100
Intermediate therapy	Half-deep therapy	X-ray machine	110–130	30	100
Superficial/soft X-ray therapy[c]	Pyrex (glass) window (older units), Beryllium window (modern units)	X-ray machine	20–100	1–20	100
Grenz therapy	Ultrasoft therapy, Supersoft therapy	X-ray machine	5–20	0.2–0.8	100

Adapted from Goldschmidt [7]

[a]Surface dose is the percent of radiation dose delivered to the skin surface

[b]90 % Isodose method is used by radiation oncologists for electron beam radiotherapy

[c]Superficial/soft X-ray therapy is the type most often utilized in dermatology office-based radiotherapy for SCC, SCCIS, and BCC

and SCC in an outpatient setting. Electrons are accelerated towards a target such as tungsten in order to yield a resultant beam of photon radiation typically in the range of 50–100 kV. At this energy, and due to photon characteristics (100 % dose delivered to the skin surface), this is ideal for the primary treatment of superficial malignancies such as BCC and SCC. Other radiotherapy methods typically employed in hospital settings by radiation oncologists as primary or adjuvant therapy for skin cancer include orthovoltage photons 200–400 kV, megavoltage photons or electrons typically in the range of 1,000–9,000 kV, and occasionally brachytherapy, a form of radiotherapy that places gamma ray-emitting radioactive isotopes close to the treatment area through the use of plastic molds or implants [8]. Most BCC and SCC demonstrate sensitivity to ionizing radiation. In a recent study Cognetta et al., reported recent 5-year recurrence rates of primary BCCs and SCCs treated with SRT. Utilizing very liberal criteria for recurrence for the 1,715 tumors treated with SRT, cumulative 5-year recurrence rates for all tumors were 5 %, BCC 4.2 %, and SCC 5.8 % (95 % CI) [9], demonstrating efficacious treatment when SRT is utilized properly. In a review of all studies (since 1947) Rowe et al. [10] compares 5-year recurrence rates by treatment modality for primary BCC with the following results; 1 % Mohs micrographic surgery, 10.1 % surgical excision, 7.7 % curettage and electrodessication, 7.7 % radiation therapy, and 7.5 % cryotherapy, illustrating the effectiveness of radiation therapy in comparison to other modalities. The recurrence rate for SRT can be further reduced when selection criteria is based on histological tumor review. Cognetta et al., who utilize histological review of all biopsy specimens prior to radiotherapy, report a 4.2 % recurrence rate for primary BCC, whereas Rowe et al. report a 7.7 % recurrence rate in their review of literature. Conventional excision for SCC has long been the standard of care with a reported cure rate of 92 % increasing up to 98 % when Mohs surgery is utilized [11]. For SCC, direct comparison of cure rates among treatment modalities is difficult due to the complex and variable aggressiveness of SCC and differences in study designs, nevertheless the overall 5.8 % 5-year recurrence rate reported by Cognetta et al. suggest that SRT is effective in select patients [9]. Most recurrences in this study were SCC in situ (SCCIS), which are often multicentric and occur in areas of severe sun damage.

General Indications for Superficial Radiotherapy of BCC/SCC

1. Location of the skin cancer in the central face, including the eyelids, nasal tip, nasal ala, ears, the lips, and in patients with rhinophyma where surgical extirpation leaves complex skin/cartilage defects and surgical repair leaves a noticeable scar. Advantages of SRT in these areas are the tissue sparing effect, with retention of pretreatment function as well as preservation of these cosmetically sensitive facial aesthetic units. SRT is considered less advantageous on the trunk and even less so on the extremities due to late-sequelae changes (telangiectasias and pigmentary changes), lower oxygen saturation leading to wound healing issues, and the general ease and expediency of surgical removal.

Table 2 Eastern Cooperative Oncology Group (ECOG) performance status

Grade	ECOG
0	Fully active, able to carry on all pre-disease performance without restriction
1	Restricted in physically strenuous activity but ambulatory and able to carry out work of a light or sedentary nature, e.g., light house work, office work
2	Ambulatory and capable of all self-care but unable to carry out any work activities. Up and about more than 50 % of waking hours
3	Capable of only limited self-care, confined to bed or chair more than 50 % of waking hours
4	Completely disabled. Cannot carry on any self-care. Totally confined to bed or chair
5	Dead

From Oken MM, Creech RH, Tormey DC, Horton J, Davis TE, McFadden ET, et al. Toxicity and response criteria of the Eastern Cooperative Oncology Group. Am J Clin Oncol. 1982;5(6): 649–55

2. Older age. To minimize the synergistic effects of ultraviolet radiation, superficial radiation should not be considered in patients younger than 60 years of age [12]. In our practice the age of patients considered for SRT is 65 years of age and above and our median patient age is 78.
3. Tumor size. Medium size tumors up to 5 cm in diameter may be adequately treated with SRT. Tumors larger than 5 cm treated with SRT demonstrate higher recurrence rates [13, 14], and may be best treated with Mohs surgery or at tertiary centers where imaging and complex treatment planning (hyperfractionation schedules) and multiple modalities are available to the patient.
4. Tumor type/depth of invasion. Superficial and nodular BCCs, SCCIS, and SCC that are nonaggressive are amenable to SRT. We and others before us avoid SRT for aggressive BCCs (sclerosing, morpheaform, infiltrative) [15, 16]. SCCs with aggressive features such as poorly/undifferentiated, spindle cell, sarcomatous, deeply invasive, or those exhibiting perineural invasion should, whenever possible, be approached with Mohs surgery with consideration of postoperative radiotherapy to the appropriate depth and field in selected cases [17–21]. Tumors secondary to osteomyelitis arising in previous sites of RT, burn scars, and chronic ulcers are also avoided due to risk of recurrence. SRT is typically not indicated for tumors that invade bone, cartilage.
5. Frailty and medical status. Patients who are unable to tolerate surgery due to poor health, multiple comorbidities, and who are on anticoagulant therapy. Such patients may incur a higher risk of adverse events with surgery. Eastern Cooperative Oncology Group (ECOG) performance status [22] may be used to document patient functional status and aid decision of radiotherapy vs. surgery (see Table 2). Typically ECOG grades of 2–4 indicate varying degrees of frailty, poor health, or comorbidities associated with a higher risk of adverse events in surgery.
6. Patient choice. When patients, as part of an informed consent, decide to avoid surgery when radiotherapy is a cost-effective and viable option.

Relative and Absolute Contraindications for Superficial Radiotherapy of BCC/SCC

1. Aggressive tumor histology. BCC at increased risk for recurrence include sclerosing, morpheaform, and infiltrative BCC. Aggressive SCC include those with perineural invasion, arising in previous sites of RT, burn scars, chronic ulcers, spindle cell carcinoma, poorly/undifferentiated, or those secondary to osteomyelitis.
2. Deep tumor invasion. Tumors that invade bone, cartilage, or arise within the mucosal surfaces of the inner nares or intraorally. However, these may be treated successfully using other radiation methods capable of penetrating deeper (orthovoltage, megavoltage photon, megavoltage electron beam radiation) or capable of delivering the radiation dose specifically to the tumor bypassing healthy tissue (intensity modulated radiation therapy) [19, 23].
3. Previously irradiated site. Second courses of radiotherapy to the same site or contiguous to a prior site increase incidence of late-term sequelae (ulcer, radionecrosis of cartilage and bone), result in unsatisfactory cosmesis, recurrence, and second primary tumors [24, 25].
4. Genetic anomalies. Nevoid basal cell carcinoma syndrome (NBCCS), xeroderma pigmentosum (XP), Garner's syndrome, Li-Fraumeni syndrome, scleroderma, and others with increased radiosensitivity or where radiation can induce new malignancies [26, 27].
5. Organ transplant recipients. The mainstay in healthy transplant recipients of treatment is surgery. Radiation should be considered as an adjuvant in SCC with perineural invasion with devices capable of delivering more deeply penetrating radiation qualities such as orthovoltage or megavoltage radiation. SRT or electron beam radiotherapy should also be considered in situations when diffuse SCCIS of the scalp would require extensive surgery and skin grafts or flaps [28, 29].
6. Diffuse large fields of SCC and SCCIS and periadnexal SCCIS. Goldberg and Kimyai-Asadi [30] ascribed the appellation "diffuse epidermal and periadnexal squamous cell carcinoma in situ" (DEPS) to this condition. The authors describe large areas of skin affected by atypical keratinocytes that grow beneath the epidermis and encase adnexal epithelia, noting that normal differentiation of the overlying epidermis and adnexal epithelium was present. Extirpation of large areas would result in severe disfigurement (large scalp lesions) or significant functional impairment (dorsal hands). In this setting hyper-fractionated radiotherapy methods able to treat such large fields may be advisable.

Considerations for Surgery of BCC/SCC

1. Small lesions. Smaller lesions when excision is simple, quick, affords high cure rate, and satisfactory cosmesis. This is especially true of the trunk or extremities.
2. Younger patients. Age less than 65 when a surgical scar is less noticeable and preferable to the discoid hypopigmented scar of RT, or on areas where SRT will

induce noticeable alopecia (i.e., eyebrows). The risk of radiogenic carcinomas is rare for dosages used to treat skin cancer and has been reported to be 0.3 % by Halpern [31]. At smaller dosages that were used in the past to treat benign conditions such as tinea capitis and acne the risk of radiogenic carcinoma appears to be most prevalent 30 years after RT with BCC the predominant tumor [12]. Shore et al. [32] posit that the mutagenic alterations induced by ultraviolet radiation following earlier lower doses of ionizing radiation used to treat tinea capitis act synergistically to promote tumors.

3. Presence of relative contraindications for SRT listed above that would be better managed with Mohs micrographic surgery or alternative methods of radiotherapy (orthovoltage, megavoltage electron beam, or megavoltage photon radiotherapy).

Conclusion

SRT is an appropriate reasonable nonsurgical option for the treatment of primary nonaggressive BCC and SCC in patients where surgical intervention is contraindicated, declined, unadvisable due to poor health, when surgery would result in significant functional limitations, or when cosmesis would be considered poor with surgery. When SRT is discussed as part of informed consent and utilized properly and responsibly, it serves as an important tool in the dermatologic armamentarium for the management of BCC and SCC in the frail and expanding elderly population. With the exception of Mohs micrographic surgery, cure rates for primary carcinoma when treated with SRT meet or exceed other modalities [10, 11]. The greatest impact on cure rates will be observed when histological review of the tumor slide is performed to ascertain the depth and presence or absence of aggressive features and the appropriate choice of radiotherapy or surgery plus radiotherapy is performed.

References

1. Parkin DM, Muir CS. Cancer incidence in five continents comparability and quality of data. IARC Sci Publ. 1992;120:45–173.
2. MacDonald EJ, Bubendorf E. Some epidemiologic aspects of skin cancer. In: Cumley RW MJ, Aldridge D, et al., editors. Tumors of the skin. St. Louis, MO: Mosby-Year Book; 1964. p. 23–65.
3. Finizio L, Vidali C, Calacione R, Beorchia A, Trevisan G. What is the current role of radiation therapy in the treatment of skin carcinomas? Tumori. 2002;88(1):48–52.
4. Lovett RD, Perez CA, Shapiro SJ, Garcia DM. External irradiation of epithelial skin cancer. Int J Radiat Oncol Biol Phys. 1990;19(2):235–42.
5. Schalock PC, Carter J, Zug KA. Use of ionizing radiation in dermatologic training centers. J Am Acad Dermatol. 2006;55(5):912–3.
6. Kingery FA. Radiation therapy in dermatologic training centers. J Am Acad Dermatol. 1986;14(6):1108–10.

7. Goldschmidt H. Treatment planning: selection of physical factors and radiation techniques. In: Goldschmidt H, Panizzon RG, editors. Modern dermatologic radiation therapy. New York: Springer; 1991.
8. Alam M, Nanda S, Mittal BB, Kim NA, Yoo S. The use of brachytherapy in the treatment of nonmelanoma skin cancer: a review. J Am Acad Dermatol. 2011;65(2):377–88.
9. Cognetta AB, Howard B, Heaton H, Stoddard E, Hong HG, Green WH. Superficial X-ray in the treatment of basal and squamous cell carcinomas: a viable option in select patients. J Am Acad Dermatol. 2012;67(6):1235–41.
10. Rowe DE, Carroll RJ, Day Jr CL. Long-term recurrence rates in previously untreated (primary) basal cell carcinoma: implications for patient follow-up. J Dermatol Surg Oncol. 1989;15(3):315–28.
11. Rowe DE, Carroll RJ, Day Jr CL. Prognostic factors for local recurrence, metastasis, and survival rates in squamous cell carcinoma of the skin, ear, and lip implications for treatment modality selection. J Am Acad Dermatol. 1992;26(6):976–90.
12. Shore RE, Moseson M, Harley N, Pasternack BS. Tumors and other diseases following childhood x-ray treatment for ringworm of the scalp (Tinea capitis). Health Phys. 2003;85(4): 404–8.
13. Wilder RB, Kittelson JM, Shimm DS. Basal cell carcinoma treated with radiation therapy. Cancer. 1991;68(10):2134–7.
14. Caccialanza M, Piccinno R, Grammatica A. Radiotherapy of recurrent basal and squamous cell skin carcinomas: a study of 249 re-treated carcinomas in 229 patients. Eur J Dermatol. 2001;11(1):25–8.
15. Bart RS, Kopf AW, Petratos MA. X-ray therapy of skin cancer: evaluation of a "standardized" method for treating basal-cell epitheliomas. Proc Natl Cancer Conf. 1970;6:559–69.
16. Bart RS, Kopf AW, Gladstein AH. Treatment of morphea-type basal cell carcinomas with radiation therapy. Arch Dermatol. 1977;113(6):783–6.
17. Kyrgidis A, Tzellos TG, Kechagias N, Patrikidou A, Xirou P, Kitikidou K, et al. Cutaneous squamous cell carcinoma (SCC) of the head and neck: risk factors of overall and recurrence-free survival. Eur J Cancer. 2010;46(9):1563–72.
18. Jackson JE, Dickie GJ, Wiltshire KL, Keller J, Tripcony L, Poulsen MG, et al. Radiotherapy for perineural invasion in cutaneous head and neck carcinomas: toward a risk-adapted treatment approach. Head Neck. 2009;31(5):604–10.
19. Mendenhall WM, Amdur RJ, Hinerman RW, Cognetta AB, Mendenhall NP. Radiotherapy for cutaneous squamous and basal cell carcinomas of the head and neck. Laryngoscope. 2009; 119(10):1994–9.
20. Leibovitch I, Huilgol SC, Selva D, Hill D, Richards S, Paver R. Cutaneous squamous cell carcinoma treated with Mohs micrographic surgery in Australia II. Perineural invasion. J Am Acad Dermatol. 2005;53(2):261–6.
21. Han A, Ratner D. What is the role of adjuvant radiotherapy in the treatment of cutaneous squamous cell carcinoma with perineural invasion? Cancer. 2007;109(6):1053–9.
22. Oken MM, Creech RH, Tormey DC, Horton J, Davis TE, McFadden ET, et al. Toxicity and response criteria of the Eastern Cooperative Oncology Group. Am J Clin Oncol. 1982;5(6): 649–55.
23. Mendenhall WM, Parsons JT, Mendenhall NP, Million RR. T2-T4 carcinoma of the skin of the head and neck treated with radical irradiation. Int J Radiat Oncol Biol Phys. 1987;13(7): 975–81.
24. Friedman DL, Whitton J, Leisenring W, Mertens AC, Hammond S, Stovall M, et al. Subsequent neoplasms in 5-year survivors of childhood cancer: the Childhood Cancer Survivor Study. J Natl Cancer Inst. 2010;102(14):1083–95.
25. Newhauser WD, Durante M. Assessing the risk of second malignancies after modern radiotherapy. Nat Rev Cancer. 2011;11(6):438–48.
26. Gatti RA. The inherited basis of human radiosensitivity. Acta Oncol. 2001;40(6):702–11.
27. Kleinerman RA. Radiation-sensitive genetically susceptible pediatric sub-populations. Pediatr Radiol. 2009;39 Suppl 1Suppl 1:S27–31.

28. Veness MJ, Harris D. Role of radiotherapy in the management of organ transplant recipients diagnosed with non-melanoma skin cancers. Australas Radiol. 2007;51(1):12–20.
29. Mendenhall WM, Amdur RJ, Williams LS, Mancuso AA, Stringer SP, Price MN. Carcinoma of the skin of the head and neck with perineural invasion. Head Neck. 2002;24(1):78–83.
30. Goldberg LH, Kimyai-Asadi A. Diffuse epidermal and periadnexal squamous cell carcinoma in situ: a report of 13 patients. J Am Acad Dermatol. 2005;53(4):623–7.
31. Halpern JN. Radiation therapy in skin cancer. A historical perspective and current applications. Dermatol Surg. 1997;23(11):1089–93.
32. Shore RE, Albert RE, Reed M, Harley N, Pasternack BS. Skin cancer incidence among children irradiated for ringworm of the scalp. Radiat Res. 1984;100(1):192–204.

Superficial Radiation Therapy Treatment Planning

W. Harris Green, Kenneth F. Morse, Jeremy L. Edwards, and Armand B. Cognetta Jr.

Part I: Theoretical Considerations

Therapeutic Index

The main objective in radiation oncology for skin lesions is to eradicate the lesion while maintaining the patient's present and future quality of life. Delivering precisely measured dose of radiation to a defined tumor volume with minimal damage to surrounding tissue is the main goal. The success of eradicating a tumor depends on the radiosensitivity of the tumor as well as tolerance of surrounding normal tissue. Normal tissue toxicity factors that should be considered in selecting a dose scheme should depend on the size or volume of the area, vascularity, and the underlying and supporting tissues. The tissues of the body have individual variation of absorption and tolerance to ionizing radiation. Therapeutic indexes (also known as therapeutic ratios) are a good tool for dose selection.

In radiation therapy a tumor cell is always irradiated with normal healthy cells in the margin. The reactions to the tumor volume as compared to surrounding can be

W.H. Green (✉)
Division of Dermatology, Florida State University College of Medicine, 1707 Riggins Road, Tallahassee, FL 32308, USA
e-mail: DATresearch@gmail.com

K.F. Morse
Clinical Applications, Sensus Healthcare, 851 Broken Sound Parkway NW #215, Boca Raton, FL 33487, USA

J.L. Edwards
Dermatology Associates of Tallahassee, 1707 Riggins Road, Tallahassee, FL 32308, USA

A.B. Cognetta Jr.
Dermatology Associates of Tallahassee, Chief, Division of Dermatology, Florida State University College of Medicine, 1707 Riggins Road, Tallahassee, FL 32308, USA
e-mail: acognetta@gmail.com

A.B. Cognetta and W.M. Mendenhall (eds.), *Radiation Therapy for Skin Cancer*, DOI 10.1007/978-1-4614-6986-5_9, © Springer Science+Business Media New York 2013

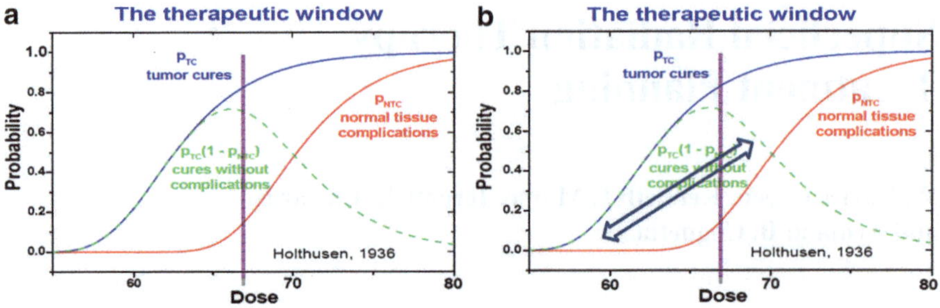

Fig. 1 Therapeutic window. (**a**) The optimal dosage range lies along the vertical purple line where the probability of cure is high while normal tissue reactions are minimal (Modified from Matthew Beasley, David Driver and H Jane Dobbs, Complications of radiotherapy: improving the therapeutic index, *Cancer Imaging* (2005) **5,** 78–84.). (**b**) The therapeutic index lies within the area denoted by the *blue arrow*

illustrated by sigmoid curves with dissimilar slopes [1] (Fig. 1a). The P_{TC} (tumor cure) slope represented in blue illustrates the probability of cure (*y* axis) as dependent on dose (*x*-axis). Similarly, the P_{NTC} (normal tissue complications) slope represented in red illustrates how increases in dose eventually lead to increased tissue complications.

The optimal dosage range lies along the vertical purple line where the probability of cure is high while normal tissue reactions are minimal. The therapeutic index lies within the area denoted by the *blue arrow* (Fig. 1b).

Treatment Factors

In order to eradicate a tumor in radiation therapy while staying within the desired therapeutic index, several factors play an important role including dose of radiation, time of dose delivery, and fractionation of dose. As described in a previous chapter, dose is a physical quantity of radiation. Dose refers to the amount of energy absorbed from a beam of radiation at a given point in a medium. The two SI units of dose are in gray (Gy) or centigray (cGy). 1 Gy = 1 J/kg (joule/kilogram) and 1 cGy = 0.01 J/kg, so 1 Gy = 100 cGy.

Choice of dose and fractionation depend upon the radiosensitivity of the tumor, size of the treatment volume, proximity of dose limiting structures (i.e., bone and brain), vascularity of the area, and cosmesis desired.

Time, Dose, and Fractionation

Time, dose, and fractionation refer to the schedule of the radiation treatments to be administered. The probability of tumor control obviously increases with a higher total dose, but so does the issues of early and late complications. To mitigate this problem, multiple fractions of dose with specific intervals are delivered. The different intervals and doses per fraction should be specifically based upon the area and size treated. When dose is administered in fractions and not all at once, it is referred to as dose

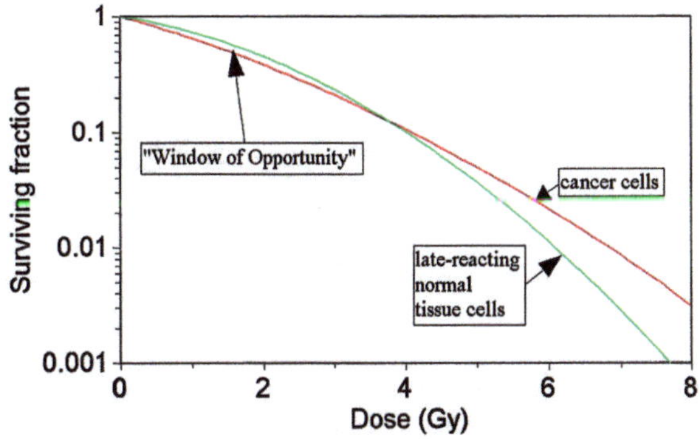

Fig. 2 Surviving fraction "window of opportunity" (Modified from Theodore T. Puck, Dimitry Morkovin, Philip I. Marcus, Steven J. Cieciura, Action of X-rays on Mammalian Cells II: Survival Curves of Cells from Normal Human Tissues. J Exp Med. 1957 September 30; 106(4): 485–500)

fractionation. Fractionation of dose in radiotherapy is largely concerned with improving tissue tolerance. Much larger cumulative doses can be administered with less long-term adverse effects if the total dose is divided into fractions or increments and spread over a period of days or weeks.

The increased tissue tolerance provided by fractionation is principally due to the multi-hit characteristics of cellular damage and death. Cell survival curves in relation to rapid repair and recovery of targets in the cells. Cellular repair is usually completed in less than 20 h with respect to those targets associated with the capability of a cell to divide, replicate, and clone. The time required for minimal repair is 6 h for most tissues [2]. Fractionation increases tumor damage through oxygenation and redistribution of tumor cells. Redistribution (assortment) is when radiotherapy is given to a population of cells. Cells in S-phase are typically radioresistant, whereas those in late G2 and M phase are relatively sensitive. A small dose of radiation delivered over a short time period (external beam or high dose brachytherapy) will kill a lot of the sensitive cells and less of the resistant cells. Over time, the surviving cells will continue to cycle. If a second dose of radiation is delivered some time later, some of these cells will have left the resistant phase and be in a more sensitive phase, allowing them to be killed more easily. With the proper fractionation scheme, a balance between the response of the tumor and early and late reactions to the normal tissue can be achieved. Cancer cells do not repair damage at low doses as do normal tissue cells. Fractionation of radiation doses spares slowly responding normal tissues as they have a greater capacity for tissue repair than rapidly responding tumor tissue. Tissue repair and the sparing of slowly responding normal tissues is the reason that most radiation therapy is delivered in multiple small fractions.

The Effect of Dose

At low doses, single-strand breaks and repair of sublethal hits dominate. High doses bring double-strand breaks with a higher percentage of repairs not completed before the next fraction. The higher doses will produce steeper survival curves. At low doses, the survival of normal tissue cells exceeds that of cancer cells while at high doses, the survival of cancer cells exceeds that of normal cells (see Fig. 2).

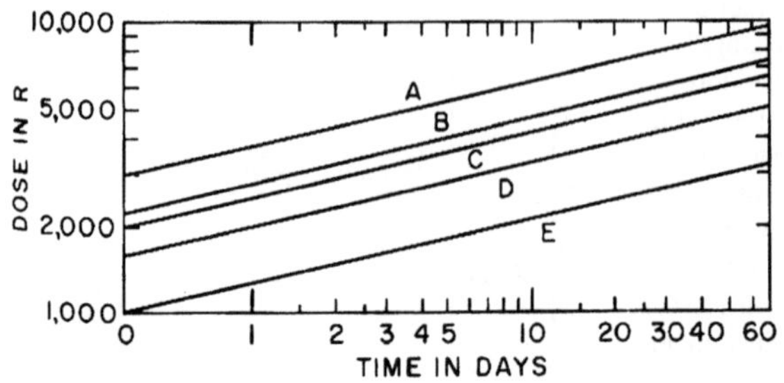

Fig. 3 Strandquist plot. *A* skin necrosis; *B* cure of skin carcinoma; *C* moist desquamation; *D* dry desquamation; *E* erythema (used with permission from Eric J. Hall and Amato J. Giaccia, Radiobiology for the Radiologist, Lippincott Williams & Wilkins, Philadelphia, PA, 6th ed., 2006)

Therefore there is a "window of opportunity" at lower doses where the dose more consistently delivers unrecoverable lethal damage to cancer cells and recoverable nonlethal injury to healthy cells. It is precisely within this window that radiation therapy functions best.

The Strandquist Plot

In 1944, Strandquist was the first to present the importance of fractionation based on acquired data and observation of the effects of tumor and normal surrounding skin over dosage and time. The observations were based on a 250 kV X-ray machine which was used to deliver 2.0 Gy/day 3–5 times a week to 280 carcinomas of the skin and lip. The plot was based upon overall time in relation to a single total dose and represents the iso-effective total dose, *D*, against the log of overall treatment time, *T*.

$$D \propto T^{0.33}$$

The fractions were 3–5 a week, so overall time in the plot would imply the number of fractions needed. The plot demonstrated that the iso-effect curve for skin was about 0.33 [3]. In the plot below (Fig. 3), the *y* axis is total dose in rad (R) and the *x* axis is time in days. The "B" curve represents dose at which cure was achieved, while overdose would occur if the dose lay above the "B" curve and skin necrosis (A curve) would occur. Similarly, should the dose lie below the "B" curve, cure may not be achieved although other milder skin reactions would be seen at subsequently lower doses such as moist desquamation (C), dry desquamation (D), and erythema (E). Strandquist's results indicated that 2,000 rad in 1 day was equivalent to 3,000 rad in 4 days, 4,000 rad in 11 days, 5,000 rad in 25 days, and 6,000 rad in 45 days. The take-home point from Strandquist's efforts was that total dose is most meaningful when the overall treatment time is known.

The Nominal Standard Dose

This led Ellis and colleagues in 1967 to develop the nominal standard dose (NSD) system which takes into account both time and number of fractions.

Total dose = $D = (\text{NSD}) \times T^{0.11} \times N^{0.24}$ where T is the overall time in days and N is the number of fractions. Herein, Ellis proposed fractionation is twice as important as time according to clinical observations. The formula projected that the tolerance dose for normal tissue (D cGy) could be related to the overall treatment time (T days) *and* the number of fractions (N). The formula became known as the Ellis NSD equation and was based on the iso-effect curve for skin, the slope of which is again 0.33 [3].

The disadvantage of the Ellis equation was it produced a number which described a complete course of fractionated radiotherapy which results in full connective tissue tolerance. If the values of D, T, and N, were substituted with numbers of less than full tolerance, then the NSD number would be meaningless.

The Time Dose Fractionation Factor

In 1973, Orton and Ellis developed the concept of time dose factor (TDF) which takes into account time, fractions, and interval between fractions. The NSD concept in radiotherapy has thus become simplified by the introduction of time, dose, and fractionation factors, which are proportional to partial tolerance, but not dependent upon any specific NSD value. Partial tolerance is related to NSD by a factor which is a function of overall time, the dose per fraction, and the fraction pattern. This factor is called the time, dose, and fractionation (TDF) factor. The TDF is related to the NSD as follows:

$$\text{TDF} = 10^{-3} \times \text{NSD}^{1.538} = Nd^{1.538}(T/N)^{-0.17} \times 10^{-3}$$

$$(N = \text{number of fractions}, d = \text{dose per fraction}, T = \text{overall treatment time in days})$$

The TDF numbers were evaluated for treatment schedules of 1, 2, 3, 4, and 5 fractions per week and corresponding tables containing TDF factors for various treatment regimens were presented. Orton and Ellis consolidated these numbers into corresponding tables based on the number of fractions per week. By using the TDF tables in treatment planning, it is possible to predict treatment outcome for cure, skin necrosis, and other effects. The cure for epithelial skin cancers requires a TDF number between 90 and 110 and thus the therapeutic index lies between these two numbers [4]. The TDF tables presented by Orton and Ellis afford a pre-calculated standardized optimal range for effective delivery of desired dose. Following the TDF tables, allows an increased number of fractions with improved cosmesis while not compromising efficacy. The importance and utility of these tables in planning curative treatment regimens that are precise and predictable cannot be overstated.

The following tables have a horizontal green row that gives total fractions and a vertical red row assigning dose per fraction in cGy. The cells between the two rows give a TDF number. The tables state how many fractions per week along the top. When a desired fractionation scheme is selected, it is important that the joining of the horizontal fractionation and the vertical dose per fraction converge to a number within the therapeutic index (highlighted in gold with green number). Please see Tables 1, 2, 3, 4, and 5 below.

Table 1 Time dose fractionation (TDF) for one treatment per week

FRACTION (cGy)	TDF # Between 90 and 110 for NMSC Skin Lesions NUMBER OF FRACTIONS																
	4	5	6	7	8	9	10	11	12	13	14	15	16	17	18	19	20
250	15	18	22	26	29	33	36	40	44	47	51	55	58	62	66	69	73
260	15	19	23	27	31	35	39	43	46	50	54	58	62	66	70	74	77
270	16	21	25	29	33	37	41	45	49	53	57	62	66	70	74	78	82
280	17	22	26	30	35	39	43	48	52	56	61	65	69	74	78	82	87
290	18	23	27	32	37	41	46	50	55	60	64	69	73	78	82	87	92
300	19	24	29	34	39	43	48	53	58	63	68	72	77	82	87	92	96
320	21	27	32	37	43	48	53	59	64	69	75	80	85	91	96	101	107
340	23	29	35	41	47	53	58	64	70	76	82	88	94	99	105	111	117
360	26	32	38	45	51	57	64	70	77	83	89	96	102	109	115	121	128
380	28	35	42	49	56	62	69	76	83	90	97	104	111	118	125	132	139
400	30	38	45	53	60	68	75	83	90	98	105	113	120	128	135	143	150
420	32	40	49	57	65	73	81	89	97	105	113	121	129	138	146	154	
440	35	43	52	61	70	78	87	96	104	113	122	130	139	148	156		
460	37	47	56	65	74	84	93	102	112	121	130	140	149	158			
480	40	50	60	70	80	89	99	109	119	129	139	149	159				
500	42	53	63	74	85	95	106	116	127	138	148	159					
520	45	56	67	79	90	101	112	124	135	146	157						
540	48	60	71	83	95	107	119	131	143	155							
560	50	63	76	88	101	113	126	139	151								
580	53	66	80	93	106	120	133	146	160								
600	56	70	84	98	112	126	140	154									
700	71	89	107	124	142	160	178										
800	87	109	131	153	174												
900	105	131	157														
1000	123	154															

Table 2 TDF for two treatments per week

DOSE/ FRACTION (cGy)	TDF # Between 90 and 110 for NMSC Skin Lesions NUMBER OF FRACTIONS																
	4	5	6	7	8	9	10	11	12	13	14	15	16	17	18	19	20
250	16	20	24	28	32	36	40	44	48	52	56	61	65	69	73	77	81
260	17	21	26	30	34	39	43	47	51	56	60	64	69	73	77	81	86
270	18	23	27	32	36	41	45	50	54	59	64	68	73	77	82	86	91
280	19	24	29	34	38	43	48	53	58	62	67	72	77	82	86	91	96
290	20	25	30	35	41	46	51	56	61	66	71	76	81	86	91	96	101
300	21	27	32	37	43	48	53	59	64	69	75	80	85	91	96	101	107
320	24	29	35	41	47	53	59	65	71	77	83	88	94	100	106	112	118
340	26	32	39	45	52	58	65	71	78	84	91	97	104	110	117	123	129
360	28	35	42	49	57	64	71	78	85	92	99	106	113	120	127	134	141
380	31	38	46	54	61	69	77	84	92	100	108	115	123	131	138	146	154
400	33	42	50	58	66	75	83	91	100	108	116	125	133	141	150	158	
420	36	45	54	63	72	81	90	99	107	116	125	134	143	152			
440	38	48	58	67	77	87	96	106	115	125	135	144	154				
460	41	52	62	72	82	93	103	113	124	134	144	155					
480	44	55	66	77	88	99	110	121	132	143	154						
500	47	59	70	82	94	105	117	129	141	152							
520	50	62	75	87	100	112	124	137	149	162							
540	53	66	79	92	105	119	132	145	158								
560	56	70	84	98	112	125	139	153									
580	59	74	88	103	118	132	147	162									
600	62	78	93	109	124	140	155										
700	79	98	118	138	157	177											
800	97	121	145	169													
900	116	145	174														
1000	136	170															

Table 3 TDF for three treatments per week

DOSE/ FRACTION (cGy)	TDF # Between 90 and 110 for NMSC Skin Lesions NUMBER OF FRACTIONS										
	4	5	6	8	10	12	14	15	16	18	20
250	17	21	26	34	43	51	60	64	69	77	86
260	18	23	27	36	46	55	64	68	73	82	91
270	19	24	29	39	48	58	68	72	77	87	96
280	20	25	31	41	51	61	71	76	82	92	102
290	22	27	32	43	54	65	75	81	86	97	108
300	23	28	34	45	57	68	79	85	91	102	113
320	25	31	38	50	63	75	88	94	100	113	125
340	27	34	41	55	69	82	96	103	110	124	137
360	30	38	45	60	75	90	105	113	120	135	150
380	33	41	49	65	82	98	114	122	131	147	163
400	35	44	53	71	88	106	124	132	141	159	
420	38	48	57	76	95	114	133	143	152		
440	41	51	61	82	102	123	143	153			
460	44	55	66	88	109	131	153				
480	47	58	70	93	117	140	164				
500	50	62	75	100	124	149	174				
520	53	66	79	106	132	159					
540	56	70	84	112	140	168					
560	59	74	89	118	148	178					
580	63	78	94	125	156						
600	66	82	99	132	165						
700	83	104	125	167							
800	103	128	154								
900	123	154									
1000	145	181									

Table 4 TDF for four treatments per week

DOSE/ FRACTION (cGy)	TDF # Between 90 and 110 for NMSC Skin Lesions NUMBER OF FRACTIONS										
	4	5	6	8	10	12	14	15	16	18	20
250	18	23	27	36	45	54	63	68	72	81	90
260	19	24	29	38	48	57	67	72	77	86	96
270	20	25	30	41	51	61	71	76	81	91	102
280	21	27	32	43	54	64	75	81	86	97	107
290	23	28	34	45	57	68	79	85	91	102	113
300	24	30	36	48	60	72	84	90	96	107	119
320	26	33	40	53	66	79	92	99	105	119	132
340	29	36	43	58	72	87	101	109	116	130	145
360	32	40	47	63	79	95	111	119	126	142	158
380	34	43	52	69	86	103	120	129	137	155	
400	37	46	56	74	93	112	130	139	149	167	
420	40	50	60	80	100	120	140	150	160		
440	43	54	65	86	108	129	151				
460	46	58	69	92	115	138	161				
480	49	61	74	98	123	148	172				
500	52	65	79	105	131	157					
520	56	70	83	111	139	167					
540	59	74	88	118	147	177					
560	62	78	94	125	156						
580	66	82	99	132	165						
600	69	87	104	139	173						
700	88	110	132	176							
800	108	135	162								
900	129	162									
1000	152										

Table 5 TDF for five treatments per week

DOSE/ FRACTION (cGy)	TDF # Between 90 and 110 for NMSC Skin Lesions NUMBER OF FRACTIONS										
	4	5	6	8	10	12	14	15	16	18	20
250	19	23	28	37	46	56	65	70	74	84	93
260	20	25	30	40	49	59	69	74	79	89	99
270	21	26	31	42	52	63	73	78	84	94	105
280	22	28	33	44	55	66	77	83	89	100	111
290	23	29	35	47	58	70	82	88	93	105	117
300	25	31	37	49	62	74	86	92	98	111	123
320	27	34	41	54	68	82	95	102	109	122	136
340	30	37	45	60	75	89	104	114	119	134	149
360	33	41	49	65	81	98	114	122	130	147	163
380	35	44	53	71	88	106	124	133	142	159	
400	38	48	57	77	96	115	134	144	153		
420	41	52	62	83	103	124	144	155			
440	44	55	67	89	111	133	155				
460	48	59	71	95	119	142	166				
480	51	63	76	101	127	152					
500	54	67	81	108	135	162					
520	57	72	86	115	143	172					
540	61	76	91	121	152						
560	64	80	96	128	161						
580	68	85	102	136	169						
600	71	89	107	143	179						
700	91	113	136	181							
800	111	139	167								
900	133	167									
1000	157										

Table 6 Table for calculating decay factor to account for intra-treatment delays

"Decay Factors" For Split-course Radiotherapy

T	Rest Period R (days)											
(days)	5	10	15	20	25	30	35	40	50	60	80	100
5	0.93	0.89	0.86	0.84	0.82	0.81	0.80	0.79	0.77	0.75	0.73	0.72
10	0.96	0.93	0.90	0.89	0.87	0.86	0.85	0.84	0.82	0.81	0.79	0.77
15	0.97	0.95	0.93	0.91	0.90	0.89	0.88	0.87	0.85	0.84	0.82	0.80
20	0.98	0.96	0.94	0.93	0.91	0.90	0.89	0.89	0.87	0.86	0.84	0.82
25	0.98	0.96	0.95	0.94	0.93	0.92	0.91	0.90	0.89	0.87	0.85	0.84
30	0.98	0.97	0.96	0.95	0.94	0.93	0.92	0.91	0.90	0.89	0.87	0.85
35	0.99	0.97	0.96	0.95	0.94	0.93	0.93	0.92	0.91	0.90	0.88	0.86
40	0.99	0.98	0.97	0.96	0.95	0.94	0.93	0.93	0.91	0.90	0.89	0.87
45	0.99	0.98	0.97	0.96	0.95	0.95	0.94	0.93	0.92	0.91	0.89	0.88
50	0.99	0.98	0.97	0.96	0.96	0.95	0.94	0.94	0.93	0.92	0.90	0.89

T = Total Days of TX before break

R = Total days of Rest

TDF x " Decay Factor"= Adjusted TDF for TX after break

TDF Decay Table

Courses of treatments in the elderly are sometimes interrupted by illness, inclement weather, or other unforeseen events. A decay table with "decay factors" is provided. The table is based upon radiobiological responses to cancer cells, a disruption in the course could possibly decay whatever portion of the TDF factor that had to that point, been delivered. In order to use a decay table, one needs to know the total days under treatment and the total days of rest. Table 6 is based upon total days under treatment until the interruption and the total day of rest before the treatment resumes.

Clinical Treatment Planning

Tumor Depth

Once the decision has been made to proceed with superficial X-ray therapy, several logistical issues need to be addressed prior to the beginning of therapy. The first consideration is the penetration depth of the beam needed to adequately treat the skin cancer. Slide review is essential as a means of appreciating the histologic characteristics and depth of the tumor. A simple micrometer can be used in conjunction with most standard microscopes. Our standard microscopes have a built-in program that can measure depth and assist in estimating tumor volume. Once the depth of the tumor has been determined, the penetrating quality of the beam can be selected to adequately treat the deepest portions of the tumor.

Beam Quality

The heterogeneous beam produced by superficial dermatologic X-ray units consists of X-rays of varying wavelengths. The distribution and proportion of short wavelengths (hard X-rays) vs. longer wavelengths (soft X-rays) determine the penetrating effect, or quality, of the radiation. The penetration of superficial quality X-rays is determined by three variables: the voltage (kV), the filtration, and the target skin distance (TSD). The combined effect of these variables has been traditionally expressed as the "half-value layer" (HVL). The HVL is the thickness of a given material (typically aluminum) that reduces the intensity of the photon beam to 50 % of the original exposure. The greater the HVL, the more penetrating the resulting beam. The HVL values in dermatologic therapy range from 0.01 mm Al (Grenz-ray range) to 2.0 mm Al. The range in which most dermatologic X-ray machines operate within is 10–100 kV which relates to an HVL range of 0.02–2.0 mm Al. As the kilovoltage increases, the potential difference between the cathode and the anode increases, resulting in a higher speed and energy of the electrons aimed at the tungsten target. This increase in kilovoltage results in a higher intensity photon beam with greater penetrating power.

Beam quality is also affected by the degree of filtration. An aluminum filter is typically employed to filter out the lower intensity portions of the heterogeneous beam, resulting in an emerging beam of less intensity but of greater average penetration. The choice of filtration is limited by most X-ray machine manufacturers to only four to five different choices of aluminum thicknesses (e.g., 0.1, 0.25, 0.5, and 1 mm). This limitation is desirable as it can avoid confusion and error as only a limited number of combinations of filter and kilovoltage are needed in daily dermatologic practice and all machines need to be calibrated at each and every combinational permutation of kilovoltage, TSD, and filtration.

Half-Value Depth (D ½)

The half-value depth (D ½) is a concept that has served as an invaluable guideline in dermatologic radiation therapy. In lieu of confusing arithmetic computations based on depth dose charts with varying combinations of radiation factors, the modern dermatologic radiotherapist takes advantage of calibrations based on the D ½. The D ½ is the tissue depth expressed in mm at which the absorbed dose is 50 % of the surface dose. In treating non-melanoma skin cancers, the goal is to deliver at least 50 % of the surface dose to the lesion's base (deepest portion of tumor). The D ½ concept helps ensure adequate dosage to the tumor and decreases the possibility of radiation damage to deeper underlying structures (see Fig. 4).

In our experience and with the calibration settings of our particular X-ray machine (the Sensus SRT-100™), most nodular and superficial basal cell carcinomas (BCCs) can be adequately treated with a 50 kV intensity of the beam. The D ½ at 50 kV penetrates to a depth of 5.8 mm which is adequate for most nonaggressive BCCs. This same beam intensity setting is also suitable for squamous cell

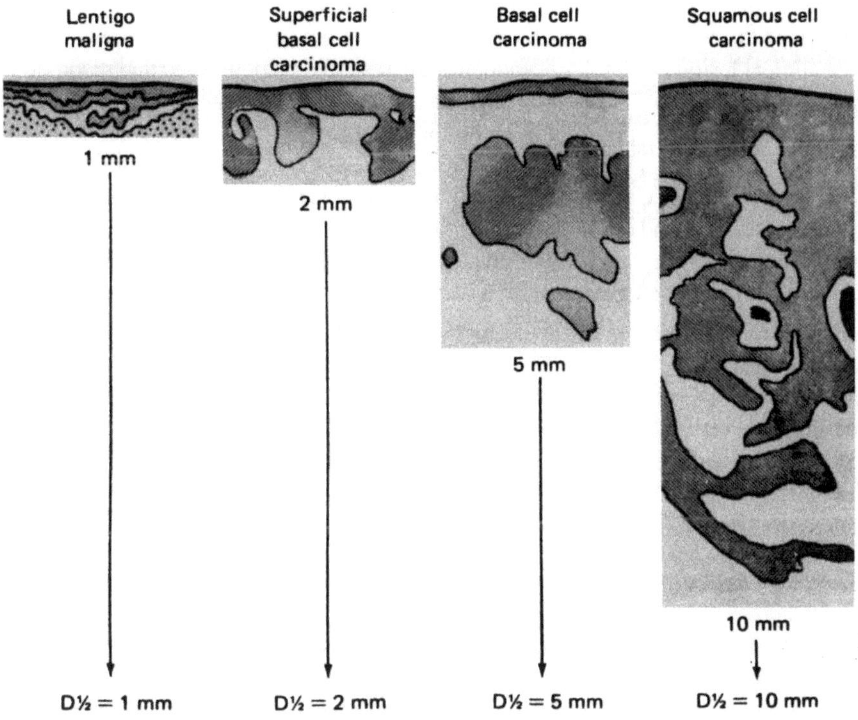

Fig. 4 Selection of D ½ for skin cancers (From H. Goldschmidt and R.G. Panizzon, *Modern Dermatologic Radiation Therapy*, 1991, Springer-Verlag: NY; p. 60. With kind permission of Springer Science+Business Media)

carcinoma in-situ (SCCIS) of the face and scalp. Occasionally, on the scalp, when there is prominent adnexal extension and there is question of superficial invasion, 70 kV may be appropriate as the D ½ is 13.9 mm. For any invasive SCC, albeit superficially invasive or more deeply invasive, we choose to select a kilovoltage of at least 70 kV with a minimum D ½ of 13.9 mm. Physicians must pay careful attention to the individual beam intensity and quality of their particular machine and select treatment parameters and D ½ values based on individual machine characteristics. Selecting the appropriate kilovoltage is crucial because although the total dose and fractionation scheme may be tailor made for the particular patient and the TDF value may be in the ideal range, if the beam undershoots the tumor depth, the overall treatment scheme is flawed from the start.

Umbra Selection

In a similar fashion, once the beam depth has been selected, the beam width must be considered. The umbra of the treatment field is directly proportional to the *clinical* margins of the lesion. Careful clinical inspection by an experienced clinician with proper illumination is the gold standard of margin delineation. If there is any question as to the borders or if it is ill-defined, scouting biopsies may be warranted. Once the clinical lesion border has been identified, it should be delineated and recorded in some fashion. Various marking techniques are available of varying degrees of permanence and visibility. One commonly employed method is to delineate the clinical lesion with a gentian violet marker or Castellani paint. A treatment margin is then selected beyond the clinically evident tumor. Five to seven millimeter margins are common and minimum recommended margins. Ill-defined and more aggressive tumors may warrant a wider margin. Lead shields are typically utilized to limit the beam to a desired treatment area. Occasionally, in some situations where a lead shield is not employed, the cone itself may serve as the desired treatment diameter.

Because there is an inherent drop-off in the beam along the edges, it is our preference to use a shield diameter smaller than the cone size to minimize the lateral edge drop-off effect. If more than one tumor is being treated concomitantly or the treatment site is to be near a previous radiation treatment site, care must be taken to prevent overlap of the treatment fields.

Dose and Fractionation Schemes

Once the kilovoltage value and umbra have been selected to match the depth and characteristics of the tumor, the dosage and fractionation scheme can be selected. The patient's age, overall health, comorbidities, travel distance, and cosmetic expectations are additional variables in determining the number of fractions to divide the dosages into. If the patient is very old, feeble, travels a long distance, and is not interested very much in cosmesis, then fewer fractions would be recommended. Similarly, if the patient is very interested in minimizing the potential for a hypopigmented patch within the treatment site and is able and willing to make more treatment sessions, then hyperfractionation may be best. Once the number of fractions is determined, the *interval* between fractions needs to be decided (i.e., 1, 2, 3, 4, or 5 fractions per week, etc.). In addition to patient demographics (i.e., age and distance to travel) and cosmetic considerations, tumor location can also be an important factor for determining the fractionation scheme.

In our experience, if the tumor is on an area with little subcutaneous tissues above underlying cartilage such as the antihelix, more fractions may be required to prevent chondritis and potentially ulceration. Similarly, tumors of the mucosal lip may best be served by increased fractions to mitigate the risk of reactive mucositis. Acute reactions will mainly depend upon overall treatment time, from the first fraction to the last. A facial area where pigment change would become a concern would substantiate a reason to expand the time [5]. Areas of low vascularity such as limbs could validate a consideration to elongate the time and also lower the dose of each fraction. Cell with low vascularity are considered stressed and their response to radiation with regard to repair is hindered.

Latent reactions are mainly dependent on total dose and dose per fraction [5]. The TDF table has a therapeutic index which is between 90 and 110. Below 90, the

Table 7 Absolute and relative contraindications for SRT

Absolute contraindications	Relative contraindications
Prior radiation—occupational or therapeutic	Aggressive histology
Radiosensitive syndromes (e.g., Gorlin's, ataxia-telangiectasia, xeroderma pigmentosum, epidermodysplasia verruciformis, etc.)	Poorly defined margins (scouting biopsies may be needed to establish margins)
Cancer arising in burn scar	Location on legs
Tumor invading bone/cartilage	Age <50 (we only consider radiation for patients >65)
	Recurrent, not previously irradiated tumors
	Highly concave or convex surfaces
	Embryological fusion planes
	Pregnancy

success rate of eradicating the lesion is lower while TDF numbers above 100, carry a higher success rate yet higher risk of adverse late skin reactions. It is important to remember that when a cell is irradiated, whether a dose of a 100 or 5,000 cGy, the membrane of the cell is permanently altered. The main culprit for the damage to the membrane is attributed to the production of hydrogen peroxide residues [6]. The cell membrane is particularly sensitive to free radical attack because its high proportion of unsaturated fatty acids. Free radicals disrupt the cell membrane's barrier function, making it vulnerable. Keeping a TDF number within a therapeutic index will maximize the quality of life for the patient and minimize the onslaught of latent reactions.

Patient Evaluation for Superficial Radiation Therapy

Not all patients are well suited for radiotherapy. Please see Table 7 for absolute and relative contraindications for radiotherapy. Absolute contraindications for radiotherapy include a history of radiotherapy in the same treatment site, a cancer arising within a burn scar, a patient with a history of a radiosensitive syndrome (e.g., Gorlin's, ataxia-telangiectasia, xeroderma pigmentosum, etc.), or tumors that invade bode or cartilage. Relative contraindications for superficial RT include tumors that exhibit aggressive histology, that have poorly defined margins, that are recurrent, that are located on highly concave or convex surfaces or along embryonic fusion planes, or that are located on the legs. Additional relative contraindications include if the patient is under 50 years old (the authors utilize RT only in patients over age 65), or if the patient is pregnant.

Similarly, not all patients are good surgical candidates. Some patients, because of age, comorbidities, and other reasons are not deemed stable enough to undergo the risks of surgery and potentially complex reconstruction of a surgical defect and would be better suited for a nonsurgical alternative if available. One common

Table 8 Eastern Cooperative Oncology Group (ECOG) score to assess patient's performance status

Grade	ECOG
0	Fully active, able to carry on all pre-disease performance without restriction
1	Restricted in physically strenuous activity but ambulatory and able to carry out work of a light or sedentary nature, e.g., light house work, office work
2	Ambulatory and capable of all self-care but unable to carry out any work activities. Up and about more than 50 % of waking hours
3	Capable of only limited self-care, confined to bed or chair more than 50 % of waking hours
4	Completely disabled. Cannot carry on any self-care. Totally confined to bed or chair
5	Dead

Source: Oken, M.M., Creech, R.H., Tormey, D.C., Horton, J., Davis, T.E., McFadden, E.T., Carbone, P.P.: Toxicity And Response Criteria Of The Eastern Cooperative Oncology Group. Am J Clin Oncol 5:649–655, 1982

example is a large SCCIS of the scalp in an elderly patient on anticoagulants who would likely have a difficult time tolerating and recovering from extensive surgery and repair. Superficial RT could potentially provide a reasonable nonsurgical option in such a patient. Finally, RT may be given special consideration for the occasional patient with a tumor amenable to either surgery or RT who refuses surgery of any kind.

Indications

It is important for all clinicians administering RT to become familiar with the local coverage determination (LCD) for radiotherapy provided by Medicare and other insurances in their respective area. General indications for radiotherapy include the following:

- Patient wishes to avoid surgery.
- Patient is on an anticoagulant (including Dabigatran or "Pradaxa," the new direct thrombin inhibitor) that cannot be reasonably discontinued prior to the procedure.
- Patient has a history of MRSA.
- The patient has a pacemaker, defibrillator, or other device or comorbidity that may add to the complexity of a surgical procedure.
- If the lesion appears to be a size or in an anatomic location where a complex closure or skin graft may be required in a patient who refuses or who is not deemed to be a good surgical candidate for extensive surgery.
- If the patient is feeble, medically unstable, or has an ECOG score of 3 or higher (see Table 8).

Part II: Practical Considerations

Radiation Positioning and Shielding

Radiation of a lesion cannot be adequately performed without proper positioning and shielding. There are several factors that must be taken into account when positioning a patient for superficial radiation therapy. These include the patient's ability to lie flat, or on their side, the mobility of the patients head and neck and the patient's ability to remain still. If the patient has good mobility it is much easier to achieve optimal treatments, if the patient has limited mobility advanced blocking techniques may be required. One must have a patient who is capable of maintaining the concentration and cooperation it requires to remain still in a darkened environment. Often our patients have some degree of dementia. This can be circumvented by a cooperative spouse or family member and by scheduling at the patients best cognitive time of day. A friendly, familiar and knowledgeable radiation tech is a tremendous asset.

Patients with good mobility can lie in the supine position and turn their head either way allowing access to the lesion. The only blocking you would require on this type of patient would be a pillow under the head and downward pressure from the SXRT machine (Fig. 5). It is helpful in these patients to place a pillow under the knees to alleviate any pressure on the lower back. This minimizes the chance of the patient moving during the treatment. The more comfortable the patient is, the less apt they are to move during treatment.

Patients with a lesion on the vertex of the scalp, or on the posterior aspect of the scalp may need to lie in the prone position for adequate treatment to be achieved.

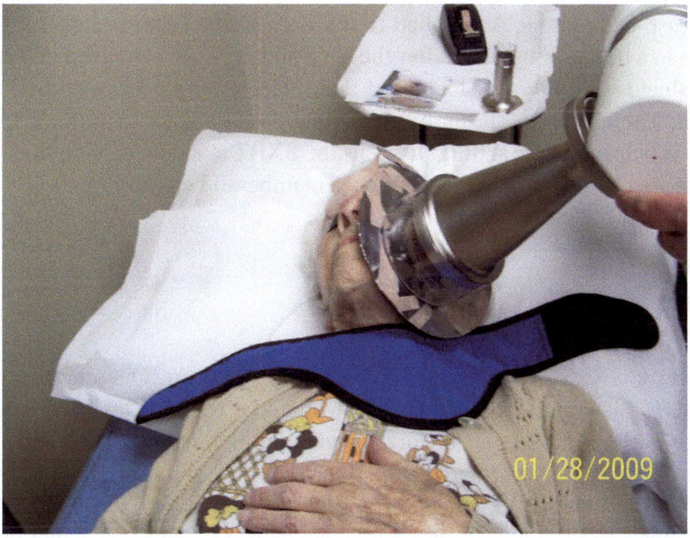

Fig. 5 Standard treatment setup for large lesion on cheek

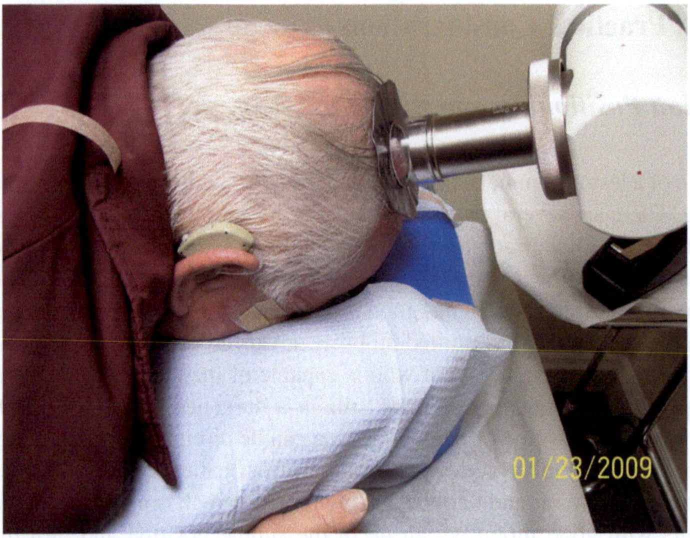

Fig. 6 Standard setup prone position for lesion on scalp

This is most easily accomplished with a prone pillow with a face cutout. With the prone pillow on the bed the patient can use a pushup-like motion to lay prone with their face in the cutout area. They can then place their hands either by their side or in front of their face (Fig. 6).

Patients who are confined to a wheelchair require very good blocking and immobilization to achieve a reliable and effective means of treatment. These patients usually require immobilization of the neck to stabilize the head. This is best achieved with the use of foam blocks applied to the neck in the same fashion as a c-collar would be in a trauma situation. After the head and neck are stabilized you can apply the eye shields and thyroid shield and then place your shield over the lesion for treatment. The use of an elastic bandage material to anchor the arm of the SXRT machine is helpful in this setting. It keeps the SXRT machine head tight against the treatment area, and also helps the patient remember to be still (Fig. 7).

Shielding

Shielding for SXRT is becoming somewhat of a lost art. One can use common hand tools to fashion the shields out of raw material which in this case is lead. It is mandatory to wear gloves when working with and shaping lead. You will also need a mask to filter out any particulates that may be inhaled during filing of the edges of the shields. The lead is available from many different radiation product companies. It comes as a roll and is very malleable (Fig. 8). Lead rolls come in varying thicknesses but at least 0.762 mm should be used at 70 kV and 1 mm at 100 kV.

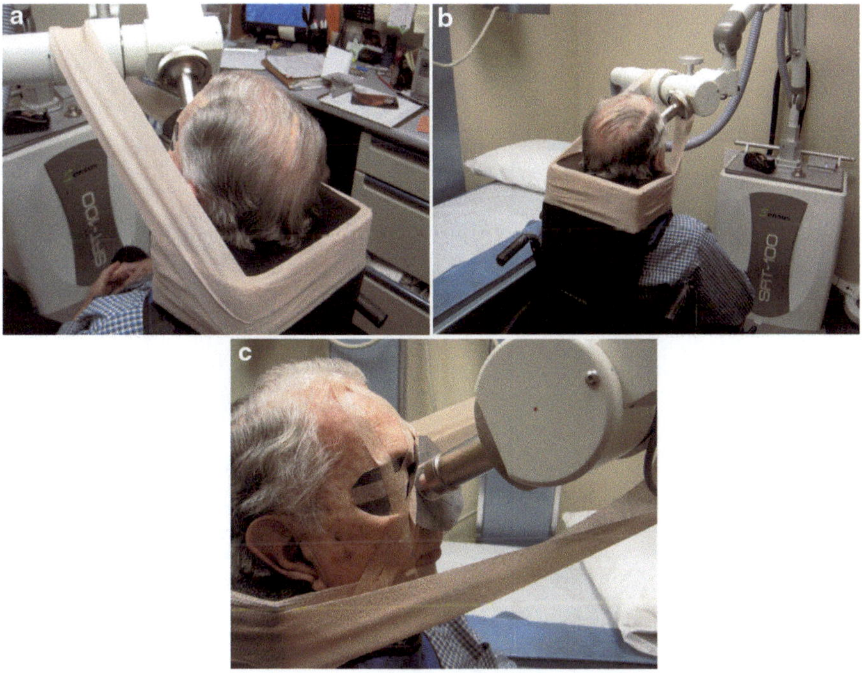

Fig. 7 (**a**) Immobilization for treatment of patient in wheelchair. (**b**) Posterior view of immobilization of head and neck. (**c**) Close-up view of treatment cone

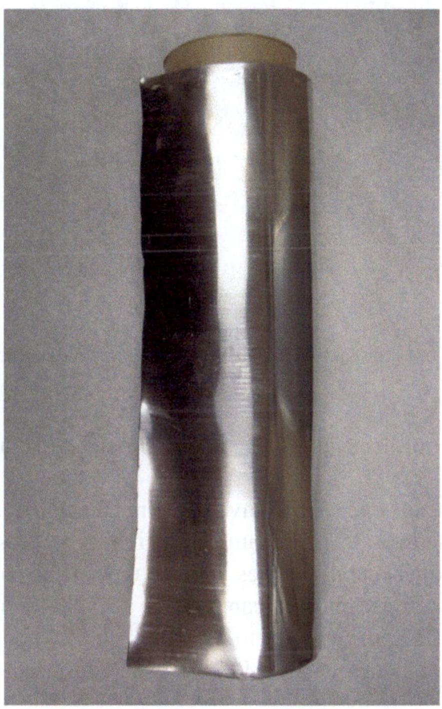

Fig. 8 Lead roll 0.762 mm thickness used to make shields

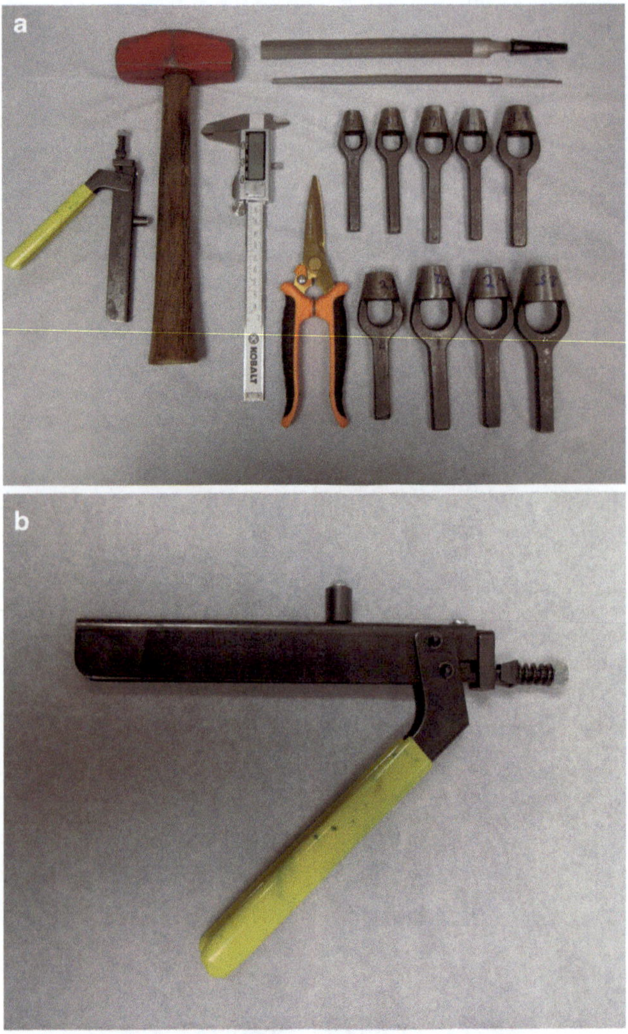

Fig. 9 (**a**) Various tools used to make shields. (**b**) Klein tools metal nibbler

All lead remnants from the making of shields should be kept in a container and disposed of properly.

There are several tools one should have in their arsenal to accomplish the task of making shields. These include a 2 lb hammer, a nibbler, metal shears, files (one flat and one round), Forstner metal punches, and a caliper (Fig. 9). These tools, when used in conjunction with one another, can produce a shield for almost any treatment scenario imaginable. It is also helpful to have a block of wood to use as a backing surface when using the metal punches. The wood will absorb the force without dulling your punches.

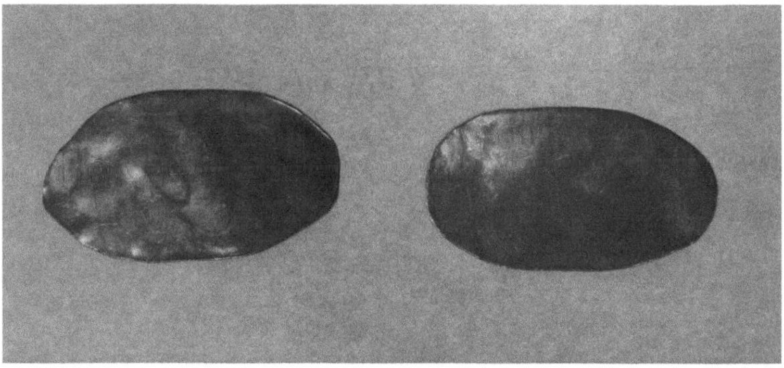

Fig. 10 Standard eye shields

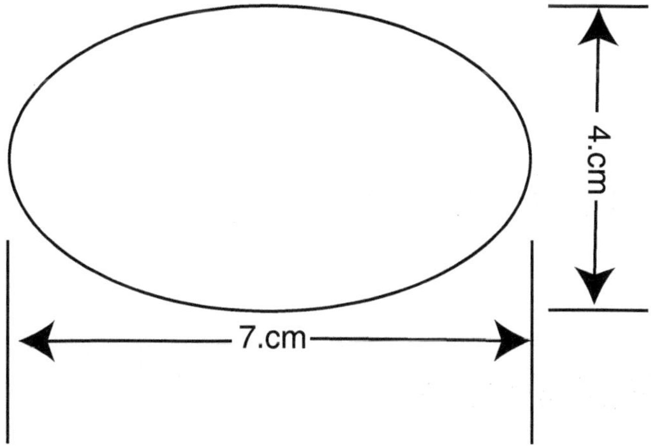

Fig. 11 Template for eye shield

The first thing you will need are eye shields, these are drawn out onto the lead roll and then cut out with the metal shears. It is helpful to find a size that works for you a good starting place is 4 cm × 7.5 cm (Figs. 10 and 11). These shields can then be smoothed on the edges by a flat file. The last step is to use a pumice stone on the edges to remove any fine burrs that may be left from the filing process. If the eye shields are not very smooth, you may cause some discomfort to the patient when they are placed over the eyes. After the shields are made, they will be flat. They then need to be placed together and bent together in a gradually arcing fashion. These may then be placed over closed eyes and taped in place first centrally like swimming goggles then in a cross-like manner starting on the contralateral forehead over the glabella contacting the eye shield midline where it is most convex and then down onto the cheek with some pressure (Fig. 12). This is repeated for the opposite side and pressure is applied to put the finishing touch on the shield to seal the orbit. If the

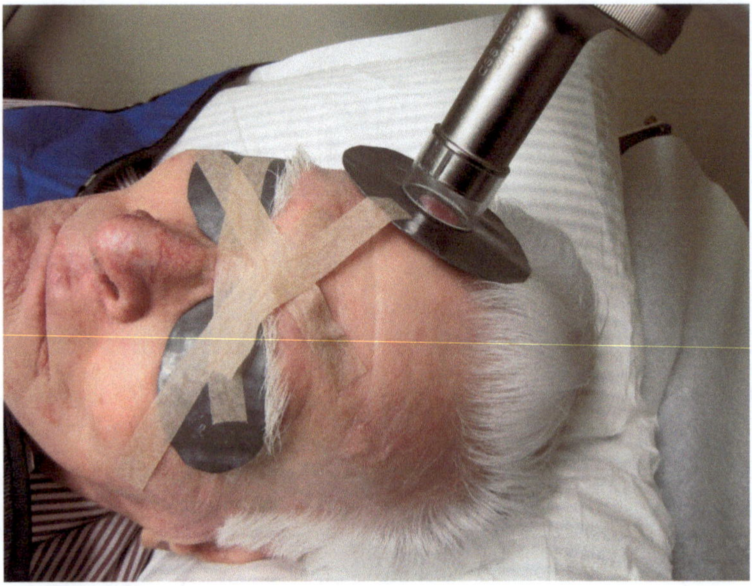

Fig. 12 Cross taping of eye shields

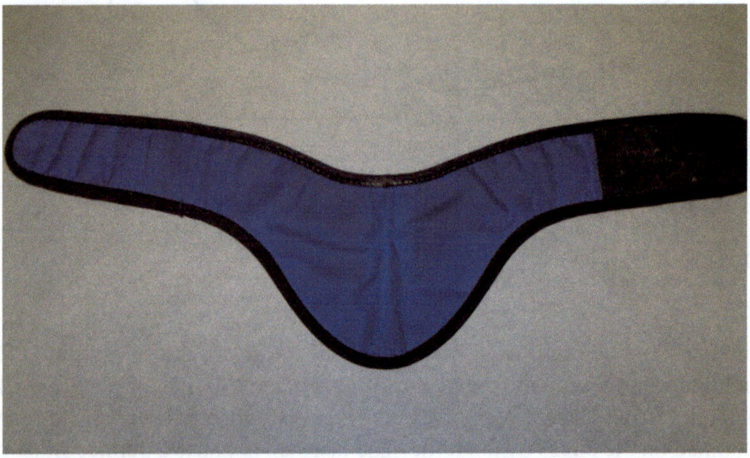

Fig. 13 Standard thyroid shield

patient can see light, they perceive that radiation may be able to affect the eye. The patient should not be able to see any light through the sides of the shields.

The next area of attention is the thyroid. It is easily covered with any commercially available thyroid shield (Fig. 13). These may be acquired from any radiation product company. They have a Velcro closure for use on sitting patients. It is simply placed over the thyroid during the treatment. One can use a larger lead apron if one is treating nonfacial lesions.

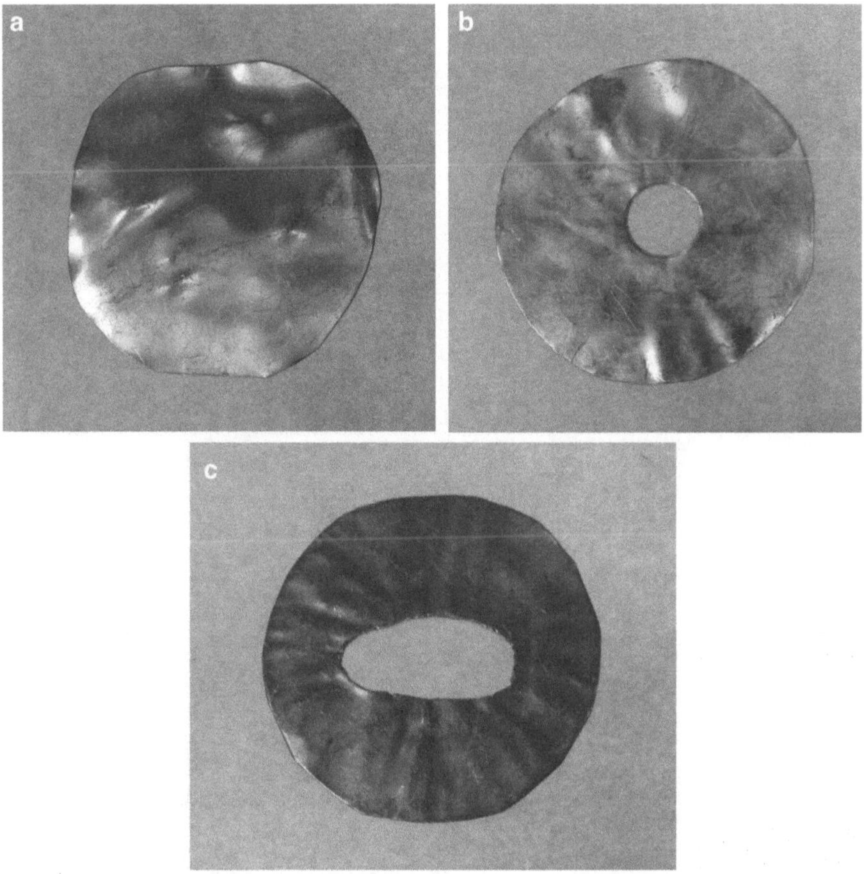

Fig. 14 (**a**) Blank shield. (**b**) Shield with round port. (**c**) Shield with elliptical port

Shielding of the lesion is accomplished by fabricating a unique shield for each treatment site. After the physician has circled the lesion to be treated, a 5–7 mm margin may be drawn around this. In most cases you will be dealing with a circular lesion, but often you will have an odd shaped area to treat. With circular lesions you will be able to measure the outer circle and establish the size of the treatment field. You can then take this measurement and choose the appropriate size punch and make your shield (Fig. 14a, b). You want to be sure you have adequate amount of shield material so that your treatment cone does not go over the edge. Most treatment shields should be 7–9 cm in width with the treatment area cut out of the center. The same approach is used if you have an elongated lesion, i.e., an elliptical excision with positive margins, you would use a punch in the center section and then use either files or metal shears or a small nibbler to elongate the sides of the treatment area out (Fig. 14c). One technique that we often use for large irregular shaped field is to

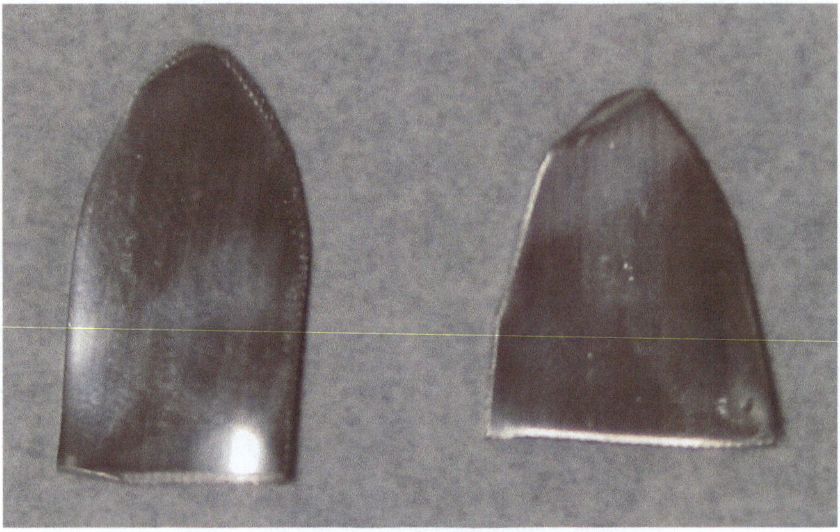

Fig. 15 Standard intranasal shields

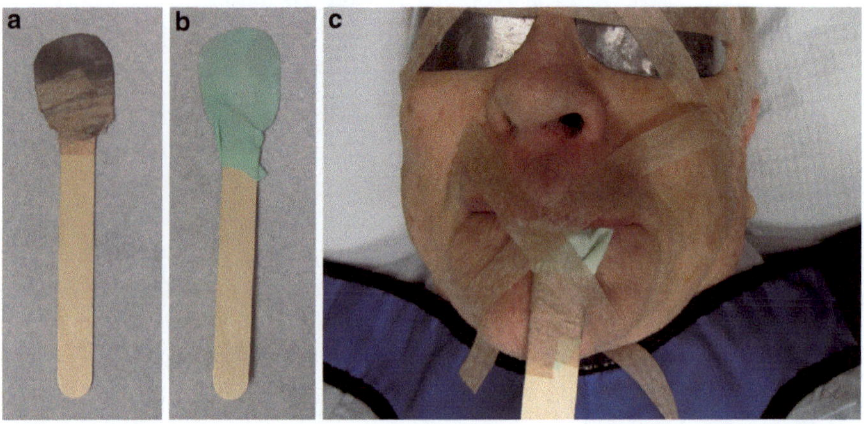

Fig. 16 (**a**) Intraoral lip shield "lollipop." (**b**) Same shield with latex glove cover. (**c**) Inserted inside lip of patient

delineate the outer treatment border with a gentian violet pen and immediately make an imprint of the field on a Telfa pad. The imprint is cut out and placed on a lead blank and the outline is traced. This simplifies the custom shield design and construction.

Lesions on the nose may require shielding inside the nose to minimize the amount of radiation-induced mucositis and to immobilize and push out the convex area to be treated. A small cutout of lead placed inside the finger of a glove and then lubricated with Vaseline can be placed inside the nostril to achieve this (Fig. 15).

When radiating the lip, a similar shielding process may be used. The "lollipop" shield can be made with an eye shield cut in half with smoothed rounded edges and the taped to a tongue depressor and then covered with the finger of a glove (Fig. 16).

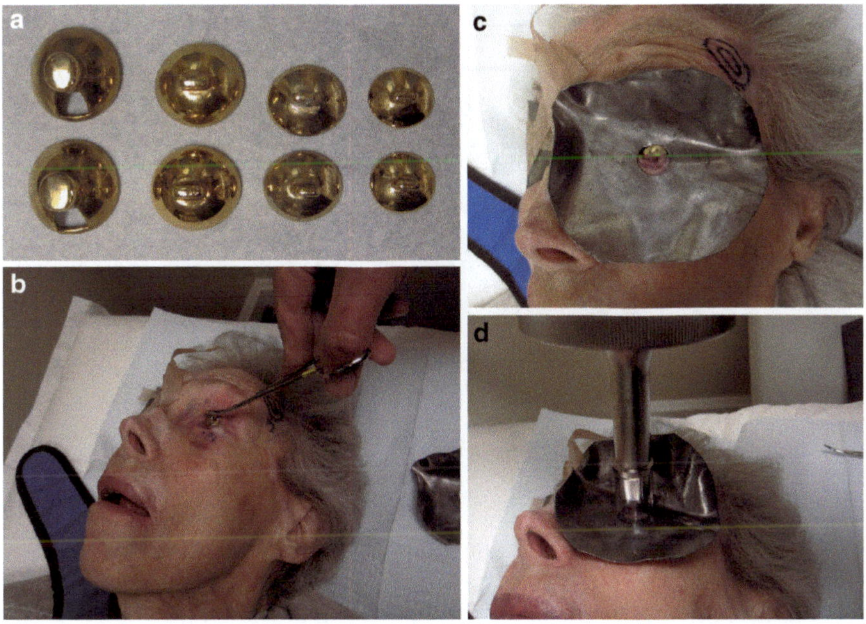

Fig. 17 (**a**) Intraocular gold-plated lead shields. (**b**) Shield being inserted with hemostats. (**c**) Intraocular shield in place with treatment shield in place. (**d**) Treatment cone applied over shield

When radiating around the eye, a gold-plated lead intraocular shield may be used (Fig. 17). The procedure for insertion of these shields is as follows: 1 drop of tetracaine ophthalmic solution is instilled into the eye. The shield is lubricated with a sterile eye lubricant. The lead shield has a tab on the top which can be grasped with a hemostat. (A curved hemostat gives you a better angle of insertion.) The superior eye lid is lifted up and the shield is placed between the upper eyelid and the globe, and then slid under the lower eyelid (Fig. 17b–d). After the shield is placed treatment of the lesion on or around the eyelid can commence. Typically a custom lead shield is used but in some cases, i.e., medial canthal concave location a treatment cone of the exact desired port can be used without a shield. The removal of the intraocular shield is the exact opposite of the insertion.

When treating the lateral canthal area, a special hybrid shield may be required. It is a combination of an eye shield and a treatment shield and may require an intraocular shield as well (Fig. 18). Proper measurement and planning is needed to accurately place the treatment aperture centered over the lesion.

When treating the ear, reflection and immobilization of the helix is paramount. You must have a stable platform to maintain the proper source to skin distance (SSD) and therefore maintain a proper D ½. If the lesion is on the flat anterior portion of the ear, you may be able to place a lead shield behind the ear to minimize any backscatter to the post auricular skin (Fig. 19a, b). In this area the treatment is the same as anywhere else. You simply make a shield that fits and place the treatment cone over the area. If the lesion is on the helix, you may need to consider some special shielding techniques. A lead taco-shaped shield may be placed behind the

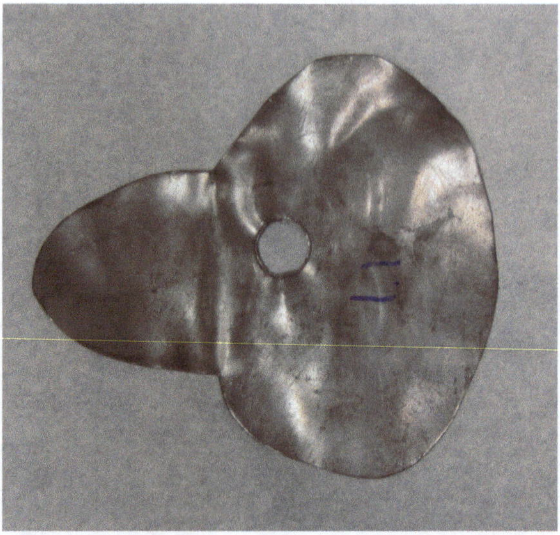

Fig. 18 Hybrid eye/treatment shield

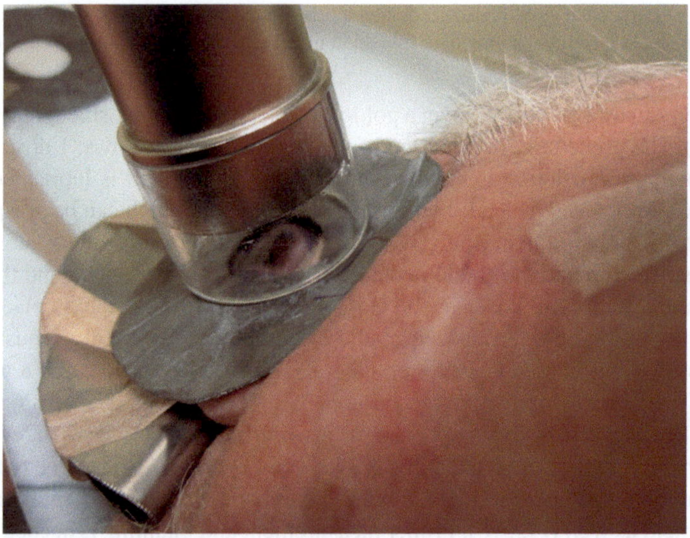

Fig. 19 Ear shield with lead "taco" bolster behind ear

ear (a rolled treatment blank works well) and then taped in place then you can make your treatment shield and treat the lesion.

Without accurate reproducible shielding and immobilization treatment cure rates will diminish and healthy noninvolved skin will be subjected to unnecessary and potentially harmful radiation. In the case of eyelid lesions damage to the lens and possibly the retina can occur. Spending time with an experienced radiation technologist in an office with a busy radiation schedule is highly recommended.

Clinical Vignette Demonstrating Treatment Planning

A 93-year-old man is referred for treatment of a nodular 8 × 8 nodular BCC on his left nasal sidewall. He is on Pradaxa, has a pacemaker, is dependent on oxygen from a nasal cannula, and refuses surgery. He is agreeable to X-ray. He can only come on Monday, Wednesday, and Friday. You decide to treat him in 5 fractions.

Review the Clinical Details

There are no evident contraindications for SRT in this patient. In fact, he actually appears to be a good candidate with many comorbidities. He is on an anticoagulant, Pradaxa, a direct thrombin inhibitor. He has a pacemaker and is on oxygen by nasal cannula, both of which could create challenge during surgery, particularly with electrocautery for hemostasis.

Review the Slides

The patient's BCC is nodular with no infiltrative component and extends to a depth of 2.5 mm. There is no clinical or histologic evidence of cartilage invasion.

Select Depth of Penetration

Kilovoltage (kV) is the main factor in terms of beam penetration. Be sure and check the machines calibration table to assess depth of penetration at different kilovoltage settings. For the SRT-100, 50 kV can be utilized for most lesions under 5.5 mm in depth, 70 kV for lesions up to 13 mm in depth, and 100 kV for lesions up to 18 mm in depth. Remember to use the D ½ philosophy. The D ½ value is the beam quality where the base of the lesion receives ½ the dose of the surface of the lesion.

In the above vignette, the nodular BCC of the nose in our patient has an approximate depth of 2.5 mm. Which kilovoltage setting would work best? At 50 kV, D ½ is 5.8 mm; at 70 kV, the D ½ is 13.3 mm; at 100 kV, the D ½ is 17.9 mm. In this example 50 kV would have ample penetrating power to the desired depth while sparing deeper structures.

Table 9 Selecting the number of fractions, interval between fractions, and fraction dosages to arrive at a desired TDF value between 90 and 110 using TDF Table 3

Total of 5 fractions

TDF # TABLE TIME DOSE FRACTION

DOSE(cGy)/ FRACTION	4	5	6	7	8	9	10	11	12
300	23	28	34	40	45	51	57	63	68
320	25	31	38	44	50	57	63	69	75
340	27	34	41	48	55	62	69	76	82
360	30	38	45	53	60	68	75	83	90
380	33	41	49	57	65	74	82	90	98
400	35	44	53	62	71	80	88	97	106
420	38	48	57	67	76	86	95	105	114
440	41	51	61	72	82	92	102	113	123
460	44	55	66	77	88	99	109	120	131
480	47	58	70	82	93	105	117	129	140
500	50	62	75	88	100	112	124	137	149
520	53	66	79	93	106	119	132	146	159
540	56	70	84	98	112	126	140	154	168
560	59	74	89	104	118	133	148	163	178
580	63	78	94	110	125	141	156		
600	66	82	99	116	132	149	165		
700	83	104	125	146	167				
800	103	128	154						
900	123	154							
1000	145	181							

700 cGy

TDF between 90 and 110

Table Modified from: Orton, C.G. and F.Ellis, *A simplification in the use of the NSD concept in practical radiotherapy.* Br J Radiol, 1973.**46**(547): p. 529-37. Please see reference

Source: Modified from Orton, C.G., and F. Ellis, A simplification in the use of the NSD concept in practical radiotherapy. Br J Radiol 1973 46(547):529–37

Select Fractionation Schedule

Factors include patient age, travel logistics, overall health of patient, location of tumor, cosmetic considerations, and tumor type and size. In this case, we opted for 5 treatment fractions on Monday, Wednesday, and Friday. Review TDF Table 3 (3 fractions/week) to obtain the dose per fraction for a 5 fraction regimen (Table 9). Remember the optimal TDF factor should be between 90 and 110.

Select Umbra, Shields, and Cone Size

The patient's lesion was 8 mm×8 mm so a clinical margin or umbra of 6 mm (5–7 mm typically recommended) may be selected or for a total of 2.0 cm. A 2.5 cm cone could then be used.

Table 10 Calibration reference table for our SRT-100 at 50 kV

Tube voltage (kV) (nominal)	SSD (cm)	Field size (cm)	HVL (mm Al)	D ½ (mm)	Output (cGy/min)	Time in min for 100 rad	500 rad	700 rad
50 kVp	15	1.0	0.44	5.8	762.3	0.13	0.66	0.92
	15	1.5	0.44	5.8	779.1	0.13	0.64	0.90
	15	2.0	0.44	5.8	791.4	0.13	0.63	0.88
	15	2.5	0.44	5.8	806.9	0.12	0.62	0.87
	15	3.0	0.44	5.8	811.7	0.12	0.62	0.86
	15	4.0	0.44	5.8	822.6	0.12	0.61	0.85
	15	5.0	0.44	5.8	824.2	0.12	0.61	0.85
	25	10.0	0.44	6.4	284.4	0.35	1.76	2.46

Select Duration by Referencing Calibration Table

We have selected the kilovoltage (based on the desired D ½), the number of fractions, the desired cGy per fraction (via referencing the TDF table), the shield size, and the cone size. The remaining variables are automatic within modern SRT machines, including mA, SSD, exposure rate. All that remains is selecting the duration of exposure. Reference the calibration table to view the automatic variables and select the appropriate duration.

Thus far we have 50 kV, 2.5 mm cone size, and a desired 700 cGy (or Rad = R) per fraction. Plug these in to determine the other variables.

At 50 kV, 10 mA, an SSD of 15 cm, and an output of 806.9 cGy/min are all standard at these settings (see calibration table in Table 10). To select the duration, refer to the calibration table for the number of minutes required. If 700 cGy is desired per treatment, then how many minutes would be needed if the exposure rate is 806.9 cGy/min? Either do the calculation or refer to the calibration table.

$$806.9 \text{ cGy/minute} \times X \text{ minutes} = 700\text{cGy}.$$
$$X = 700\text{cGy}/806.9\text{cGy/min} = 0.87\,\text{minutes}$$

The machine would calculate 806.9 cGy/min at 0.87 min for a total of 700.1 cGy per treatment. (This value would appear on the bottom right of the Sensus machine display panel as an extra confirmation that you have the correct setting.) Treatments would be repeated 3 times a week for a total of five treatments for a total of 3,500.4 cGy. Post-radiation instructions can then be given to the patient and follow-up appointment established.

Patient Eligibility

Certain types of patients might not be suited for radiation therapy and these factors should be taken into consideration. Some examples are cancer type, history of prior radiation, site of cancer, connective tissue disorders, past injury to the dermis, or unreasonable expectations for cure or cosmesis. Please see the patient eligibility form (Form 1).

Form 9.1
SRT Patient Eligibility and Treatment Selection

Name: ________________________________ DOB: _________ Field Number: _______

Pathology: BCC / SCC ____________________ Site:_______________ Size____ x ____ mm Treatment Margin:____mm

Patient Eligibility and Treatment Selection

Functional Status (check one):____ 0 (fully active) ____ 1 (ambulatory, light activity) ____ 2 (ambulatory, performs self-care)
____ 3 (limited, performs self-care) ____ 4 (completely disabled)

Relevant Functional Limitation: ____ N/A

Relevant Medical History (check all that apply):

Systemic: ____ History of MRSA infection
____ CHF
____ Cardiac Disease
____ Pacer
____ Pulmonary Disease
____ Requires O2
____ PVD
____ Bleeding Disorder
____ Anticoagulation: ________________
____ Immune suppression
____ Diabetes
____ Advanced Dementia
____ Other: ____________________

Local: ____ LE edema
____ Cutaneous Atrophy
____ Poor Local Circulation
____ Poor Tissue Mobility
____ Local Infection
____ Other: ________________________________

Indications for Superficial Radiotherapy, including Surgical Limitations:

____ NMSC, low metastatic risk ____ Advanced Age ____ Poor Wound Healing
____ Limiting Systemic / Local Disease (see above); Comments: ____
____ Tumor Size / Location; Comments:____
____ Poor Functional Status or Disabilities (see above)
____ Need for Simultaneous Treatment of Multiple Tumors
____ Inability to Perform Necessary Post-Operative Wound Care

Physician: ______________________________ Date: __________

Form 1 SRT patient eligibility and treatment selection

Patient Simulation

The simulation is the preparation of treatment with all parameters put into place without delivering the dose. The first important fact of the simulation is the patient's position. The reproducibility of the position on a day-to-day basis and the ease at which the patient can achieve it, leads to less setup error and movement. A key note in setting up a patient is to achieve as much a vertical entry a possible to eliminate angles and possible shifting during treatment.

Upon achieving a position of reproducibility, the physician needs to place the margins around the peripheral of the tumor edge (suggested 6–8 mm for basal and 7–10 mm for squamous cell). After the margin has been achieved, a customized lead cutout which best fits the margin should be placed on the skin and a photo of the patient's position and lead treatment device documented. With the completion of the lead cutout, selection of the applicator that best overlaps the outline of the aperture.

An important function of a simulation is to determine whether or not a patient will be able to handle the RT treatments. There are some patients who by virtue of a tremor, claustrophobia, dementia, or other physical limitations cannot handle lying still in a dark environment. In these cases, a close family member and empathetic, skilled tech can assist with assuring the patient, immobilizing the patient, positioning the patient, and with close monitoring of the patient. The time to determine those few individuals who cannot handle radiotherapy is simulation before any dosage is delivered.

The simulation and treatment device design form is used to document: patient's name, identification number that the facility uses. The treatment site, the lesions being treated should be assigned a number (e.g., 1, 2, 3) and a site name, such as the one used in the biopsy. Shielding to protect normal structure is then checked off with relationship to the area being treated. A general description of the patient position, lead cutout shielding size, and application size to be used during treatment are documented. Clinical photos of setup and shielding are performed. Physician's signature and the date of simulation are documented (Form 1).

Prescription and Fractionation Log

Prescription and fractionation log form assists with documentation of the fractionation scheme and daily treatments. The prescription portion of the form contains the following: the daily dose per fraction, the fractions (the number of fractions in the TDF scheme the physician has selected), the total dose (the dose the patient will receive after all fractions have been delivered, daily dose × fractions = total dose), lesion size (provided by physician based upon biopsy and measurements), shield size (measurement of the opening in the custom shield), applicator (applicator is selected that best fits the widest portion of the custom shield), energy (the selection of your energy is based upon the D ½ (or D50), if the D ½ is at a depth of the deepest portion of a lesion, then that energy is sufficient), depth (the depth should always be to the surface when using the TDF tables, normalization to a depth increases the surface

Form 9.2
SRT Simulation and Treatment Device Design

Shielding and Treatment Devices Used: A lead shield of 0.762 mm thickness is utilized to form a molded, custom shield with a
____x____cm port to correlate with the lesion size, including treatment margin. The custom lead shield is adequate to accommodate the appropriate applicator and provide adequate shielding around the treatment site. Additional shielding (as noted below) is used to protect sensitive, normal tissues.

Field Size (applicator): ___1.5cm ___2.0cm ___2.5cm ___3.0cm ___4.0cm ___5.0cm

	Shields / Treatment Devices Used	Simple / Complex Device
External:	____ Lead Apron Covering, ___Breasts, ___Abdomen, ___Pelvis/Groin, ___ Thyroid	Simple
	____ Lead External Eye Shields	Simple
	____ Head Holder	Simple
	____ Molded, Custom, Site-Specific Lead Shield	Complex
Internal:	____ Lead Ear Canal Shield	Complex
	____ Lead Intranasal Shield	Complex
	____ Lead Intraoral / Dental Shield	Complex

Total Complex Treatment Devices used:____ *Total Simple Treatment Devices used:____*

Clinical Photographs: ____ Identification ____ Lesion with Margins ____ Lesion with Shields ____ Patient positioning

Patient Positioning and Setup: ____ Prone ____ Supine ____ Sitting ____ Side-lying R/L
____ Limb Positioning or Elevation with aids ______________________________

Physician: ______________________________ Date: ____________

Form 2 SRT simulation and treatment device design

dose to the skin and in turn can exceed the 110 TDF therapeutic index that is recommended), treatment time in minutes. This portion of the prescription needs to be completed prior to the day of the first fraction. Prior predetermination and completion of this section of the form alone will limit misadministration of dosage (Form 1).

Accounting for Treatment Interruptions

When a planned treatment regimen is delayed or disrupted for some unforeseen reason, it is typically possible to complete the regimen with simple modifications. Going back to the principle noted by Strandquist, dose and time are related and there is a certain momentum gained once multiple treatments have been delivered. There is, however, a loss of biological response when treatments cease or become further spread apart and this loss of momentum is called the decay factor and must be accounted for in the TDF calculations. Below is a table presented by Orton and Ellis that can be quite useful if there is a disruption in treatment for more than 5 days (see Table 6).

Form 9.3
Superficial Radiotherapy Prescription

Name: ______________________________ DOB: _________ Field Number: _______

Pathology: BCC / SCC ______________________________
Site:______________________________

Lesion Size____ x ____ mm Treatment Margin: ____ mm

Prescription #1
Energy: ______ kV Depth: ___________ Fractionations / Week: _____
TDF: ________
Field Size (applicator):___1.5cm ___2.0cm ___2.5cm ___3.0cm ___4.0cm ___5.0cm
Custom Shielding Size: _________
Daily Fractionation Dose: _______cGyNumber of Fractionations: ______ Treatment Time / Fractionation: ________min
Total Dose: ______ cGy
Physician: ______________________ Date: _____________

Is there any interruption in treatment exceeding 5 days? N / Y
If yes, see Decay and Dose Adjustment Calculation and complete treatment under Prescription #2

Prescription #2
Energy: ______ kV Depth: ___________ Fractionations / Week: _____
TDF: ________
Field Size (applicator):___1.5cm ___2.0cm ___2.5cm ___3.0cm ___4.0cm ___5.0cm
Custom Shielding Size: _________
Daily Fractionation Dose: _______cGyNumber of Fractionations: ______ Treatment Time / Fractionation: ________min
Total Dose: ______ cGy
Physician: ______________________ Date: _____________

Fractionation Log

Fx #	Rx #	Energy (kV)	SSD (cm)	Tx Time (Min)	Dose /Tx (cGy)	Cumulative Dose (cGy)	Date	Initials (RN/MD)
1	1/ 2		15					
2	1/ 2		15					
3	1/ 2		15					
4	1/ 2		15					
5**	1/ 2		15					
6	1/ 2		15					
7	1/		15					

(continued)

	2							
8	1/2		15					
9	1/2		15					
10*	1/2		15					
11	1/2		15					
12	1/2		15					
13	1/2		15					
14	1/2		15					
15	1/2		15					
16	1/2		15					
17	1/2		15					
18	1/2		15					
19	1/2		15					
20	1/2		15					

*Treatment interruptions indicated by **bold** line following all treatments under Rx #1*

Total TDF: ______ Total Dose

Delivered: ______ cGy

Physician: ____ Date: ______________

The two main components in the decay correction factor are: total days under treatment and total days of the break. Note that the decay table does not show decay if the break is less than 5 days. Another reason for selection of a TDF scheme that is in the middle of the therapeutic index (90–110 therapeutic indexes) will have to do with a break of less than 5 day, the therapeutic change is minimal. Below there is an example of a decay calculation.

Example of a Decay Event

A patient is to receive 12 fractions, 380 cGy per fraction, 3 times a week, with a TDF number of 98. After 6 fractions patient stops treatment for 30 days. Patient's total days under treatment prior to break were 15 days. The total days of break are 30 days. Up to the time of break the TDF number that has been achieved = 49. (This is obtained by referencing Table 3 above.) Then, upon referencing the decay table for total days under treatment (15 days) and total days of rest (30 days), the resulting decay factor is 0.89. The TDF 49 multiplied by the decay factor of 0.89 = 43.61. Therefore, the new TDF number based upon decay from rest is 43.61. The 98 TDF was the therapeutic index the physician wanted to achieve. Take 98 TDF–43.61 = 54.39 and this is the remaining TDF needed.

Referring back to the 3 fractions a week TDF table (Table 3); we search for the closest TDF number to 54.39 and the options are: 400 cGy, 6 fractions = 53 TDF, 53 + 43.61 = 96.61 total TDF. Another approach could go along the line of 340 cGy, 8 fractions = 55 TDF, 55 + 43.61 = 98.61 total TDF. If one wishes to maintain the same scheme at 380 cGy, 6 fractions = 49 TDF, 49 + 43.61 = 92.61 total TDF. Note that all three examples are within the therapeutic index (90–110). If a change is made in the initial prescription, then one must correct the total dose and TDF. The second prescription site is for change in dose and change in overall TDF number.

The final portion of the form deals with the daily fraction entry. The dose is entered each day and several parameters are documented along with physician's initials. The fractionation log entries are as follows: kilovoltage (energy used), SSD (which is achieved when the applicator is contact with the skin (lead cutout) to achieve the proper dose), treatment time (time that was actually delivered), cGy per fraction (dose delivered per treatment fraction), total cGy (dose per fraction is added together in this column for a total accumulated dose), date (dose are dated each time they are delivered), and initialed (initialed by physician or state authorized personnel).

Second Check Calculations for Patients' Dose Delivery

A check of the consoles treatment time is performed with an independent calculation. This is confirmed with the output sheet that was provided by the physicist after the superficial radiation therapy machine is calibrated. The output sheet will have several columns of information: the tube voltage (energy in kVp), SSD, field size (defined by the applicator), HVL (in mm of Al), the D ½ or D50 (depth of the 50 % isodose line), output in cGy/min (used in the second check calculation), and time in minutes for cGy (reference to three dose entries of 100, 500, and 700 cGy and the treatment times they would yield).

The second check calculation is performed by taking the dose per fraction divided by the output in cGy/min for a specific energy and applicator used in treatment (Form 4).

Example of a Second Check Calculation

Patient is to be treated with 50 kV using a 2.0 applicator. Treatment fractionation dose came out to be 382.6 cGy per fraction, 12 fractions, 98 TDF. Calculation is the dose of 382.6 cGy divided by 725.5 cGy/min = 0.53 min (Representing the ramp-up of current + seconds of calculated treatment time in seconds = total increments used to treat in a minute).

Form 9.4

SRT Treatment Time Calculation with Decay and Dose Adjustment Calculation

Name: ______________________________ DOB: _________ Field Number: ______

Site:______________________________________

Field Size (applicator): _______cm Energy: ________ kV

Dose per Fractionation: _________ cGy = Treatment Time: ______ Min
Energy Output: cGy/min

Calculated Treatment Time: ______ Min Computed Treatment Time: ______ Min.

Physician: ______________________________ Date: __________

Decay and Dose Adjustment Calculation

Reason for Treatment Interruption:
____

Dates Treated: __/__/__ to __/__/__ Interruption: __/__/__ to __/__/__ Treatment Resumed: __/__/__

Number of Treatment Days: _______ Number of Days Off Treatment: ________

TDF of Fractionations Delivered: _____ X Decay Factor: _______ = Adjusted TDF: ________

Original TDF: ______ - Adjusted TDF: ______= Remaining TDF: ______ New Total TDF: ______

Comments:
____

Treatment to be completed under Prescription #2 parameters

Physician: ______________________________ Date: __________

Form 4 SRT treatment time calculation with decay and dose adjustment calculation

Weekly Management of Patient's Dose Response

During treatment, review of the treatment area should be performed weekly. A weekly management form assists in reviewing, documenting, and verifying the fraction number, dose per fraction, total dose at the point of evaluation, dose delivery parameters (note if changes in delivery have changed since previous fraction), eacth site's reaction to treatment up to this point, any systemic or constitutional complaints or concerns as well as the general constitutional and cognitive state of the patient. Based on this inventory, recommendations or modifications can be made if necessary (Form 5).

Form 9.5

Weekly Evaluation and Management for Superficial Radiotherapy

Name: ________________________________ DOB: _________ Field Number: _______

Pathology: BCC / SCC ________________________ Site:________________________________ Dose / Fx: _______cGy

	Fx #	**5**	**10**	**Final Treatment #**
	Date			
Subjective	None			
(√=present)	Redness			
	Pruritus			
	Pain			
	Drainage			
	Fatigue			
	Other			
Objective	Erythema			
(√=present)	Atrophy			
	Scaling			
	Crusting			
	Erosion			
	Ulceration			
	Edema			
	Purpura			
	Tenderness			
	Warmth			
	Drainage			
	Other			
	Cumulative Dose (cGy)			
Assessment	Appropriate rxn			
(√ one only)	Excessive rxn			
	Insufficient rxn			
	Other			
Plan	Dose Reviewed			
(√=complete)	Dosimetry Reviewed			
	Simulation Reviewed			
	Clinical set-up Reviewed			
	External Shields Reviewed			
	Internal Shields Reviewed			
	Continue Current Tx?	Y / N *(see comments)*	Y / N *(see comments)*	NA
	Alter Tx?	N / Y *(see comments)*	N / Y *(see comments)*	NA
	Special care			
	Comments			
MD				

Additional Comments:
____
____
____
____

Post-SRT Follow up:__________________________
Physician:________________________________

Form 5 Weekly evaluation and management for superficial radiotherapy

Upon completion of the treatment, the reaction in the biological sense continues for 1–2 weeks after the final fraction [7]. From previous chapters we learn that radiation goes from a physical to a chemical reaction. The final phase is a biological one that continues after the final treatment. Usually healing is completed 3–4 weeks after final treatment.

Conclusion

Treatment planning for superficial X-ray delivery is paramount to safe and successful outcomes. Consider the words of Dr. George MacKee, one of the early pioneers in the field, "Unfortunately they (X-rays and radium) are dangerous agents in unskilled hands. Every physician who employs X-rays and radium should have a thorough training and should possess modern knowledge and equipment." Know your machine well; keep it calibrated, select beam quality that will match the depth of the tumor adequately, check and double check treatment parameters and regimens so that the D ½ and TDF are in the optimal range, use proper shielding and safety precautions, and with appropriate use, this modality with continue to serve as a tremendous tool in the dermatologist's armamentarium.

References

1. Wang CC, editor. Clinical radiation oncology, introduction, techniques, and results. New York: Wiley-Liss; 2000. p. 9–10.
2. Hall EJ. Radiobiology for the radiologist. 5th ed. Philadelphia: Lippincott Williams & Wilkins; 2000. p. 400–398.
3. Goldschmidt H. Ionizing radiation therapy in dermatology. J Am Acad Dermatol. 1994;30 (2 Pt 1):159–60.
4. Hall EJ. Radiobiology for the radiologist. 5th ed. Philadelphia: Lippincott Williams & Wilkins; 2000. p. 409–10.
5. Giusti AM, Raimond M, Ravagnan G, Supora O, Parasassi T. Human cell membrane oxidative damage induced by single and fractionated dose of ionizing radiation. Int J Radiat Biol. 1998;74(5):595–605.
6. Goldschmidt H. Ionizing radiation therapy in dermatology. J Am Acad Dermatol. 1994;30 (2 Pt 1):166–7.

Current Use of Dermatologic Radiotherapy in the United States

Christopher M. Wolfe and Armand B. Cognetta Jr.

Introduction

There has been a notable decline in the use of radiotherapy in dermatology beginning with Goldschmidt's observations published in 1975 [1]. Since that time period surveys into the ongoing use of radiotherapy by dermatologists have documented the continued decline of the use of this modality and a de facto relinquishment of the use of radiotherapy to treat non-melanoma skin cancer (NMSC) to radiation oncologists.

In the fall of 1974 a comprehensive survey of the Task Force on Ionizing Radiation of the National Program for Dermatology of the American Academy of Dermatology was conducted with the results reported by Herbert Goldschmidt [1]. A detailed questionnaire was sent to 4,560 dermatologists in the United States and Canada; of 2,444 replies 44 % of respondents reported using radiotherapy weekly. Superficial X-ray or Grenz-ray equipment was reported to be available in 55.5 % of dermatologic offices. In 1981 Goldschmidt in an editorial for the Archives of Dermatology makes an important observation that statistics for that time period showed that radiotherapy had been used routinely in the treatment of 10–20 % of skin cancers in leading dermatologic institutions where all other forms of therapy were also available [2]. Goldschmidt notes that at that time (1981) 400,000 new cases of skin cancer were occurring each year in the United States; if dermatologists were to cease using ionizing radiation, 40,000–80,000 patients would have to be treated with other modalities that may not have been the treatment of choice. He goes on to say that such patients would have to be referred to radiation oncologists

C.M. Wolfe (✉)
Lake Erie College of Osteopathic Medicine, 1858 West Grandview Boulevard, Erie, PA 16509-1025, USA
e-mail: wolfe1pa@gmail.com

A.B. Cognetta Jr.
Dermatology Associates of Tallahassee, Chief, Division of Dermatology, Florida State University College of Medicine, 1707 Riggins Road, Tallahassee, FL 32308, USA
e-mail: acognetta@gmail.com

A.B. Cognetta and W.M. Mendenhall (eds.), *Radiation Therapy for Skin Cancer*, DOI 10.1007/978-1-4614-6986-5_10, © Springer Science+Business Media New York 2013

who have less experience in the treatment of skin cancers than qualified skin specialists [2]. Goldschmidt held the belief that dermatologists were the only specialists with special training in differential diagnosis, histopathologic diagnosis, and various treatment modalities available and were the best qualified to perform and select the most appropriate modality.

Extensive dermatopathology training aids the dermatologist in estimating the depth, aggressiveness, and extent of a skin cancer which is paramount in determining the most suitable form of radiotherapy, whether it is superficial radiotherapy in the dermatology office setting or megavoltage modalities through the use of linear accelerators by radiation oncologists for deeply seated tumors or as adjuvant treatment for perineural invasion. As such, dermatologists formally trained in Mohs micrographic surgery may be ideally suited to institute the use of radiotherapy in their practice settings, offering a full range of skin cancer treatment modalities at one site. In our practice setting we currently utilize Mohs surgery and reserve radiotherapy for patients over the age of 65 if the appropriate indications exist and it is deemed the best option during informed consent. Our current indications are listed in a separate chapter. Our selection process involves examining the pathology slide of every lesion considered for superficial radiotherapy. Possible options for those that do not regularly review histopathological specimens for depth assessment, tumor type, and aggression could include requesting that maximum thickness of the tumor be reported as well as tumor subtype and aggressive factors within the pathology report. Clinical correlation with the patient at consult or treatment day for the presence of comorbidities, frailty, ECOG status, anticoagulant use, and the clinical extent of tumor border enables a thorough assessment of suitability for superficial radiotherapy.

Superficial radiotherapy in the dermatologic setting will become an increasingly important modality as the over 65 and over 85 population swell over the next 4 decades. Factors that may warrant cost-effective and efficacious nonsurgical modalities in the future include a larger patient population with multiple comorbidities, the increasing use of anticoagulant medications, and longer life spans. Currently the reported median age for NMSC is 68 [3] and it is estimated that between 40 and 50 % of Americans who live to age 65 will develop NMSC [4]. According to the U.S. Census Bureau population projections, the over 65 age group will more than double between 2010 and 2050 and triple for the over 85 population in the same time frame (Fig. 1).

In the United States in 2006 there were an estimated 3.5 million new cases of NMSC diagnosed, with the over 65 population responsible for 62 % of these new diagnoses [5]. Rogers et al. [5] using Medicare and U.S. Census Bureau data, in what was perhaps the most complete evaluation to date of the skin cancer epidemic in the United States, noted an increase in the total number of procedures for NMSC from 1,158,298 to 2,048,517 from 1992 to 2006. The authors conclude that the increase was due mainly to an increase in the number of affected individuals (Medicare patients over the age of 65). Comparing this increase over the 1992–2006 time period to the U.S. Census Bureau population projections in Fig. 1, there will be a dramatic surge in the number of new skin cancers within the United States over the next few decades. Due to the aforementioned patient factors, there will be an

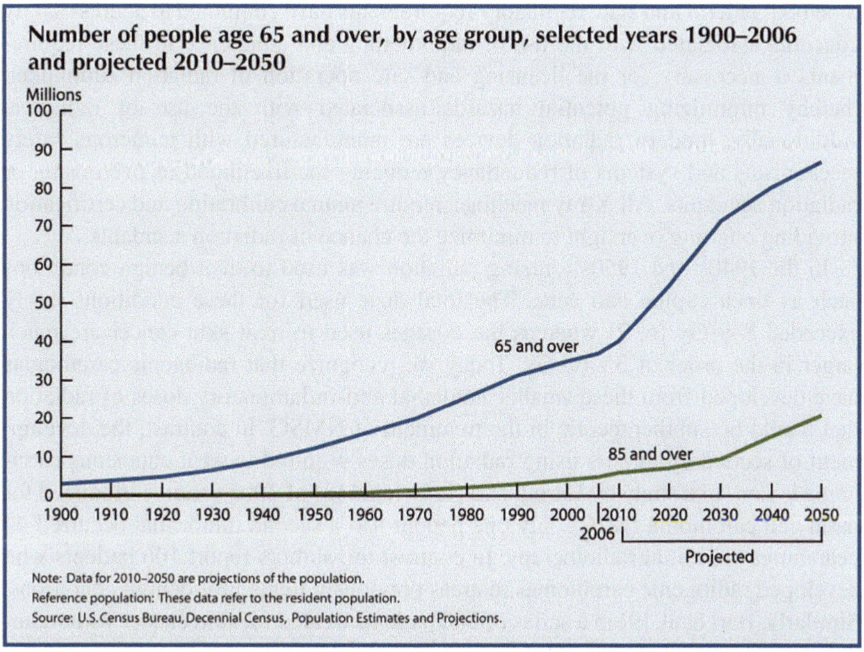

Fig. 1 Number of people age 65 and over, by age group, selected years 1900–2006 and projected 2010–2050

increasing need for the use of radiation in the treatment of skin cancer, including superficial radiotherapy by dermatologists as well as orthovoltage and electron beam radiotherapy by radiation oncologists, now and in the future. Dermatologists and radiation oncologists are uniquely situated to meet that need and to work with other specialists such as Mohs and reconstructive surgeons.

Reasons that have been cited by dermatologists who do not utilize radiotherapy include safety issues, licensing regulations, maintenance, start-up costs, and a lack of teaching on the practical application and use of superficial radiotherapy. In the next few sections we will explore these areas in greater detail and present possible solutions when needed.

Safety Issues/Radiogenic Carcinomas

Safety issues were once a concern as indiscriminate use resulted in many mishaps early after the discovery of radiation as a potential treatment for various ailments. The government recognizing the need to protect the public and the environment from unrestricted and unlicensed sources of ionizing radiation created the Atomic Energy Act of 1954 and later the Energy Reorganization Act of 1974. Since that time both federal and state regulatory requirements have continued to address safety concerns associated with the use of radiotherapy and adherence to these requirements is necessary for the licensing and safe operation of radiation equipment, thereby minimizing potential hazards associated with the use of radiation. Additionally, modern radiation devices are manufactured with numerous safety mechanisms and systems of redundancy reducing the likelihood of overdosing or radiation accidents. All X-ray machines require annual calibration and certification providing ongoing oversight to minimize the chance of radiation accidents.

In the 1940s and 1950s ionizing radiation was used to treat benign conditions such as tinea capitis and acne. The total dose used for these conditions rarely exceeded 8–9 Gy [6, 7] whereas the dosages used to treat skin cancer are much larger in the order of 35–60 Gy. Today we recognize that radiogenic carcinomas have developed from these smaller nonlethal anti-inflammatory doses of radiation that would be subtherapeutic in the treatment of NMSC. In contrast, the development of secondary tumors using radiation doses required to treat cutaneous carcinoma is rare. In a study by Ehring and Gattwinkel [8] of 2005 patients irradiated for basal cell carcinoma (BCC) only one patient had a second tumor that occurred 40 years after the initial radiotherapy. In contrast the authors report 106 patients who developed radiogenic carcinomas in areas previously treated for benign conditions. Similarly, Bart et al. [9] in a series of 500 patients treated for skin cancer with radiotherapy report only three possible radiogenic carcinomas. The risk of radiation-induced carcinogenesis appears to peak at small doses and declines at doses required to treat skin cancer [10]. It appears that small doses, insufficient to cause cell killing, are able to induce mutagenic alterations leading to skin cancer. Halpern [11] reports that the incidence of radiation therapy-related cancers has been reduced to less than 0.3 % due to refinement of calibration techniques and the availability of more efficacious radiation modalities [12, 13].

Licensing Regulations and Maintenance

Modern radiation equipment is manufactured to comply with federal and state licensing regulations. Facility design requirements are dictated by state health boards and for most states are accessible online. These facility design requirements are intended to protect individuals from unintended radiation exposure and for the safety of the patient being treated. More stringent requirements are necessary for machines operating at higher peak kilovoltages (kVp) usually above 150 kVp. As most radiation equipment used by dermatologists who treat skin cancer operates below 100 kVp the requirements are less stringent. Common requirements include two-way communication between the patient and physician during treatment, direct visualization of the patient during the treatment delivery, and lead shielding of the treatment area. The amount of lead lining required for dermatologists operating at 150 kVp or less is 1/16 of an inch to protect from the direct beam and 1/32 of an inch to protect from scatter, with the requirement that walls be lined up to 7 ft high [14]. Computation of the lead barrier requirements and which walls require shielding is based on occupancy in adjacent rooms, location of the treatment area, and the amount of scatter to adjacent areas. A radiation physicist can determine the amount of scatter and leakage in the treatment area and adjacent rooms to determine which walls, floors, and ceilings require lead lining as well as optimal placement of equipment to minimize radiation exposure to operator and non-radiation workers.

The cost for maintenance of radiation equipment varies by manufacturer. Most will provide tiered levels of maintenance coverage. With our current radiation unit maintenance coverage includes a guaranteed response time of 48 h for an engineer to be on-site with all tiers of service and can vary from $6,950 to $21,900 annually. It is wise to consider the service coverage and promptness of on-site coverage for any radiation machine that is considered for purchase as fraction schedules used to treat skin cancer are often on an every other day schedule. We maintain an older fully calibrated and well-maintained older backup X-ray unit to assure uninterrupted treatment courses.

Start-up Costs

In the next few decades there will be an ever-increasing number of patients in whom dermatologic office-based radiotherapy may be an important modality. In our own Mohs referral-based practice we presently treat 300–400 skin cancers annually with radiotherapy (up from 200 annually 1 decade ago), many of whom were referred for Mohs surgery. The growing over 65 population and the availability of efficient modern dermatologic radiation equipment have likely contributed to the increased use of this modality within our own practice. Viewing the U.S. Census population projections of patients over age 65, which will increase from 39 to 57 million by 2020 and to 79 million by the year 2030, it is feasible to assume that the patient base requiring dermatologic radiotherapy will expand in a similar fashion. Depending on the number of patients and the fractionation schedule and lease/purchase option utilized, it may take several years to recoup the initial investment in radiation equipment. The current cost for new modern equipment is in the $200,000 range. Used or refurbished X-ray machines are available often for a fraction of this cost, often from older retiring clinicians who want to keep the art of dermatologic radiotherapy alive. Another viable option to reduce start-up costs is to arrange a cooperative agreement between 2 and 3 local dermatologists interested in providing dermatologic radiotherapy services to their patients in a fixed location or via mobile unit that is able to serve a greater geographical area.

Other costs include state licensing and radiation physicist site commissioning. The state licensing fees vary by state, most are less than $200 annually and vary between $30 and $120. A radiation physicist site commissioning is required upon installation of the radiation equipment with annual recertification and calibration of equipment. The radiation physicist can conduct the annual state inspection at the same time the radiation equipment is calibrated. The annual radiation physicist certification and calibration cost approximately $700 nationwide.

The cost for lead lining a treatment area depends on multiple factors and has been estimated to cost between $2,700 and $4,200 [14]. Treatment rooms on a one-story building with concrete floors will cost less as no shielding is typically required for the floor or ceiling. Leaded sheetrock is available for new construction and lead lining can also be retrofitted for use in an existing room.

Lack of Teaching on the Practical Application and Use of Superficial Radiotherapy

The American Academy of Dermatology and its approved residency programs are the stewards of educational programs for current and future dermatologists. In 1975 Goldschmidt reporting on the use of radiation by practicing dermatologists in the United States and Canada found that 44.3 % of 2,500 survey participants utilized radiotherapy [1]. Goldschmidt reported in his 1975 article that there had been a noticeable decline during the previous 30 years in the use of radiotherapy by dermatologist as well as a decline and de-emphasis on the teaching of radiation techniques in many dermatologic training programs. Proof of the de-emphasis of radiotherapy in dermatology residencies came in 1986 when Kingery surveyed program directors of dermatologic training centers [15]. Ninety-eight of 105 program directors responded, only 12 % ($n=12$) had and used X-ray machines, 58 % ($n=57$) had no X-ray equipment, 22 % ($n=22$) had Grenz ray equipment, and 81 % ($n=79$) included didactic instruction on the theory and practice of radiation therapy. More recently in 2005, Schalock et al. [16] in a survey of 111 program directors (87 respondents) noted that only 10 % have and use radiation equipment and similar to Kingery's findings 80 % included instruction on theory and practice of radiation theory in their curriculum.

Solutions to the lack of practical instruction have been presented previously. In 1981 Goldschmidt noted that most departments that do not provide practical instruction lack the financial means or space for the equipment [2]. He proposed three possible solutions that would not add any additional burden to training programs. The first would be an optional 3- to 6-month training program in dermatologic radiotherapy offered at nationally known dermatology departments with expertise in dermatologic radiotherapy. The second solution would be the designation of official preceptors in this field which include experienced practicing dermatologists with expertise in radiotherapy. Dermatology residents could spend 3–6 months (full or half time) to gain practical experience. The third he deemed less desirable which included dermatology residents attending radiation oncology clinics, he felt the number of skin cancers treated would be too limited to be useful.

Practical instruction in dermatologic radiotherapy is currently carried out via two modes within our practice. First we provide practical training and instruction on all aspects of dermatologic radiotherapy as part of our Procedural Dermatology (Mohs)

Fellowship. Fellows first observe, then assist, and as they demonstrate competence in delivering superficial radiotherapy they are able to perform treatments. Annually, approximately 300–400 NMSCs are treated with radiotherapy in our practice. Though our Procedural Dermatology Fellowship is 1 year in length the learning curve is relatively quick as modern radiotherapy machines deliver treatments more efficiently. After patient setup and shielding it takes approximately 40 seconds to deliver one treatment. The second model we have utilized to help practicing dermatologist gain practical experience is in line with Goldschmidt's solution to identify preceptors. Dermatologists that are interested in gaining such experience are instructed in the operation of our machine, patient setup, the use of lead shielding, fractionation schedules, and informed consent for radiotherapy during a 2- to 3-day visit. All skin cancers treated within our practice undergo histological review to select possible treatment options based on patient and tumor characteristics such as location of the skin cancer, anticoagulant use, the presence or absence of aggressive features, and patient age. Visiting dermatologists and their staff witness radiation consultation, informed consent, initial treatments, and the process whereby we preselect skin cancers suitable for radiotherapy from the pool of patients referred to us for surgery. Training includes lesion identification, delineation of the tumor and treatment field, the creation of treatment devices (custom shielding), patient positioning, radiotherapy planning, weekly management of ongoing patients, long-term follow-up of patients treated with radiotherapy in selected lesions, and how we log and document all aspects of treatment.

Cost Analysis of RT in Dermatology Setting Versus Radiation Oncology Setting and Mohs Surgery

Prior cost-analysis reports of radiation treatment for skin cancer in dermatologic literature did not differentiate between dermatologic office-based radiotherapy and radiation delivered by radiation oncologist in a hospital setting. Rogers and Coldiron [17] report the cost of radiation therapy for a BCC on the cheek to be $2,591–$3,460; however, specific Current Procedural Technology (CPT) codes and facility fees used in this calculation are not available within the manuscript. We assume these are based on radiation treatments delivered by radiation oncologists in a hospital setting. The main drivers for cost of radiation treatments are the setting in which treatment is delivered (office vs. hospital), the voltage/modality used, and the number of fractions used. We will compare the cost for office-based dermatologic radiotherapy based on the fractionation schedule we have used for the past 28 years (5 fractions) and a 10-fraction schedule that many dermatologists use, the cost to have the same lesion treated by radiation oncologists in the hospital setting, and the cost for Mohs surgery of the same lesion. Our long-term recurrence rate with superficial radiotherapy is 5 % for all tumor types [18] using liberal criteria for recurrence. Any tumor which arose contiguous to a radiation treatment field (which extended 5–10 mm beyond the clinical tumor) was counted as a recurrence, despite the fact that the patient population of north Florida and south Georgia/Alabama area have multicentric disease.

Historically the long-term recurrence rate for Mohs surgery is reported to be 1 %, we will therefore use recurrence rates of 5 % for superficial radiotherapy and 1 % for Mohs surgery for quantifying the costs to treat recurrences. All projected recurrences are assumed to be treated with Mohs surgery and a full-thickness skin graft which will be added to the total cost of treatment. For example, Mohs surgery cost is projected at $1,760.79, if the recurrence rate is 5 % then 1,760.79 × 0.05 = $88.04 will be added to the cost of treatment with radiotherapy.

The calculations are for treatment for a 1 cm BCC on the nasal tip or ala as this is one of the most common, and valuable, anatomic locations for dermatologic radiotherapy. In 2012, Cognetta et al. report 48 % ($n=821$) of 1,715 treatments over a 10-year period using superficial radiotherapy were on the nose [18]. Similarly, in 2005 Schulte et al. report 38 % ($n=489$) of 1,259 treatment locations as being on the nose [19].

Rogers and Coldiron [17] reported 1.76 stages as the national average for Mohs surgery which includes all sites. More recently Alam et al. [20] conducted a study using the case logs of 20 Mohs surgeons across the United States and analyzed 2,000 Mohs cases in which they report number of stages by site. The nose required an average of 2.01 stages. The authors note that surgeons in different parts of the country did not differ in terms of the number of stages per case. Additionally, sites such as the nose, ear, and eyelid account for the majority of cases that require more stages. For the cost of Mohs surgery we calculated the cost of 1.76 stages and 2 stages of Mohs and repair with a full-thickness skin graft, flap, and complex repair. Multiple surgery reduction rules were applied.

Dermatologic office-based radiotherapy is calculated based on the 5-fraction schedule we use at a 50, 70, or 100 kVp setting (superficial/soft X-ray) and a 10-fraction schedule. Fees include treatment planning, treatment delivery, and weekly management. Hospital-based radiation is based on a common fractionation schedule used by many institutions of 50 Gy in 20 fractions using a 250 kVp setting (orthovoltage X-ray) [21]. Megavoltage electron beam and megavoltage photon radiation are also used to treat skin cancer typically with 6 or 9 MeV (6,000–9,000 keV) linear accelerator machines, which we will also calculate for comparison using the same 20-fraction treatment schedule. All fees are calculated according to the 2012 resource-based relative value scale (RBRVS) Medicare physician fee schedule for the geographical area "Rest of Florida." Hospital fees are calculated according to Medicare's Outpatient Prospective Payment System (OPPS) using the Ambulatory Payment Classification (APC) codes for the same geographic area (Table 1).

From this cost analysis it is apparent that office-based dermatologic radiotherapy costs less than both Mohs micrographic surgery and hospital-based radiotherapy for skin cancers on the nose amenable to radiotherapy. It is important to note that recurrence rates and associated costs will be higher if office-based dermatologic radiotherapy is used nonselectively, without careful and reproducible delineation of adequate margins beyond the tumor (treatment field), or without evaluating lesions histologically to determine suitability for office-based radiotherapy. The cost and

Table 1 Cost analysis to treat a 1-cm basal cell carcinoma on the nasal tip or ala

Method	CPT codes	Total cost/total cost + cost of treating recurrences
Mohs micrographic surgery (2.0 stages)	17311, 17312, 15260 (graft)	1760.79/1778.40
	17311, 17312, 14060 (flap)	1525.50/1543.10
	17311, 17312, 13151 (complex)	1268.46/1286.06
Mohs micrographic surgery (1.76 stages)	17311, 17312, 15260 (graft)	1665.65/1683.26
	17311, 17312, 14060 (flap)	1430.31/1447.91
	17311, 17312, 13151 (complex)	1173.32/1190.92
Dermatologic office-based radiation (5 fractions)	77261, 77300, 77332, 77427, 77401 × 5	504.07/592.11
Dermatologic office-based superficial radiation (10 fractions)	77261, 77300, 77332, 77427 × 2, 77401 × 10	792.55/880.59
Hospital-based orthovoltage radiation (20 fractions)	77261, 77300, 77332, 77427 × 4, 77401 × 20	3359.71/3447.75
Hospital-based megavoltage electron beam radiation (20 fractions)	77261, 77300, 77332, 77280, 77427 × 4, 77403 × 20	5704.21/5792.25

difficulty to re-treat lesions previously irradiated are significant (see the chapter "Treatment Selection for Superficial Radiotherapy (SRT)"). Superficial radiotherapy is not intended to take the place of Mohs surgery or hospital-based radiotherapy. If, however, superficial radiotherapy is not available for lesions amenable to this method a more expensive form of treatment will most likely be utilized. From a cost containment and patient choice perspective it is therefore important that office-based dermatologic radiotherapy continues to be available and selectively utilized in light of the financial constraints on the healthcare system today, especially in light of the rapidly expanding elderly, and feeble, population.

References

1. Goldschmidt H. Ionizing radiation therapy in dermatology. Current use in the United States and Canada. Arch Dermatol. 1975;111(11):1511–7.
2. Goldschmidt H. Dermatologic radiotherapy 1981. Arch Dermatol. 1981;117(11):685–8.
3. Whaley JT. Non-melanoma skin cancers. The Abramson Cancer Center of the University of Pennsylvania: OncoLink; 2011. http://www.oncolink.org/types/article.cfm?c=18&s=88&ss=866&id=9624&CFID=52640767&CFTOKEN=91975169. Accessed 19 May 2012.
4. Marchetti M, Salmaso R, Polonio S, Perin D, Salviato T, Onnis A. Ki-67 expression in vulvar carcinoma. Preliminary results. Eur J Gynaecol Oncol. 1996;17(5):361–4.
5. Rogers HW, Weinstock MA, Harris AR, Hinckley MR, Feldman SR, Fleischer AB, et al. Incidence estimate of nonmelanoma skin cancer in the United States, 2006. Arch Dermatol. 2010;146(3):283–7.
6. Shore RE, Albert RE, Reed M, Harley N, Pasternack BS. Skin cancer incidence among children irradiated for ringworm of the scalp. Radiat Res. 1984;100(1):192–204.

7. Epstein E. Thyroid cancer due to X-ray treatment of acne. JAMA. 1969;209(10):1529–30.
8. Ehring F, Gattwinkel U. Radiotherapy of upper lip basalioma. Hautarzt. 1974;25(8):368–72.
9. Bart RS, Kopf AW, Petratos MA. X-ray therapy of skin cancer: evaluation of a "standardized" method for treating basal-cell epitheliomas. Proc Natl Cancer Conf. 1970;6:559–69.
10. Goldschmidt H, Breneman JC, Breneman DL. Ionizing radiation therapy in dermatology. J Am Acad Dermatol. 1994;30(2 Pt 1):157–82; quiz 83–6.
11. Halpern JN. Radiation therapy in skin cancer. A historical perspective and current applications. Dermatol Surg. 1997;23(11):1089–93.
12. Upton AC. Radiation carcinogenesis. In: Bush H, editor. Methods in cancer research. New York: Academic; 1967.
13. Karapurkar AP, Pandya SK, Desai AP. Radiation induced sarcoma. Surg Neurol. 1980; 13(6):419–22.
14. Bodian AB. Equipment and financial aspects in an office setting. In: Panizzon RG, Cooper JS, editors. Radiation treatment and radiation reactions in dermatology. New York: Springer; 2004. p. 25–31.
15. Kingery FA. Radiation therapy in dermatologic training centers. J Am Acad Dermatol. 1986;14(6):1108–10.
16. Schalock PC, Carter J, Zug KA. Use of ionizing radiation in dermatologic training centers. J Am Acad Dermatol. 2006;55(5):912–3.
17. Rogers HW, Coldiron BM. A relative value unit-based cost comparison of treatment modalities for nonmelanoma skin cancer: effect of the loss of the Mohs multiple surgery reduction exemption. J Am Acad Dermatol. 2009;61(1):96–103.
18. Cognetta AB, Howard B, Heaton H, Stoddard E, Hong HG, Green WH. Superficial X-ray in the treatment of basal and squamous cell carcinomas: a viable option in select patients. J Am Acad Dermatol. 2012;67(6):1235–41.
19. Schulte KW, Lippold A, Auras C, Bramkamp G, Breitkopf C, Elsmann HJ, et al. Soft X-ray therapy for cutaneous basal cell and squamous cell carcinomas. J Am Acad Dermatol. 2005;53(6):993–1001.
20. Alam M, Berg D, Bhatia A, Cohen JL, Hale EK, Herman AR, et al. Association between number of stages in Mohs micrographic surgery and surgeon-, patient-, and tumor-specific features: a cross-sectional study of practice patterns of 20 early- and mid-career Mohs surgeons. Dermatol Surg. 2010;36(12):1915–20.
21. Solan JM, Brady LW. Skin cancer. In: Halperin EC, Perez CA, Brady LW, editors. Principles and practice of radiation oncology. 5th ed. Philadelphia, PA: Lippincott Williams & Wilkins; 2008. p. 690–700.

Grenz Ray Therapy

Armand B. Cognetta Jr. and Kerry M.W. Fike

History

The history of grenz ray can be traced back to experiments by F. Shulz in 1910. He utilized an X-ray tube with a very thin glass window at 15 kV and termed the resultant radiation "over soft X-ray." In 1911, Lindemann constructed an X-ray tube with a lithium-borate glass window to further minimize the tube's intrinsic filtration and allow the passage of even longer wavelength X-rays. Following in these footsteps, Bucky modified a water-cooled Muller tube with a chromium iron anode and thin Lindemann glass window and produced what he termed grenz ray. They were named because of his recognition that these wavelengths which range from 1 to 4 Å straddled the electromagnetic spectrum between ultraviolet and X-ray. Bucky felt that he was dealing with a new form of X-ray, while many of his contemporaries thought that the properties of grenz ray were at the very edge of the X-ray spectrum.

Physical Characteristics of Grenz Ray

The quality of grenz ray is dependent on the same parameters of ordinary photon X-rays other than the inverse square rule, which is negated by the fact that these beams are so soft that they are filtered by air. Listed below are some of the central parameters:

kV (kilovolt)—typically, grenz rays are generated by tube energies between 10 and 20 kV.

A.B. Cognetta Jr. (✉)
Dermatology Associates of Tallahassee, Chief, Division of Dermatology, Florida State University College of Medicine, 1707 Riggins Road, Tallahassee, FL 32308, USA
e-mail: acognetta@gmail.com

K.M.W. Fike
Dermatology Associates of Tallahassee, 1707 Riggins Road, Tallahassee, FL 32308, USA

A.B. Cognetta and W.M. Mendenhall (eds.), *Radiation Therapy for Skin Cancer*,
DOI 10.1007/978-1-4614-6986-5_11,

Filtration—while more powerful X-rays typically utilize aluminum filters to harden the beam, filtration is rarely used with grenz ray. When filtration is utilized, much lower atomic weight material such as cellulose may be used to remove the ineffective part of the spectrum. Alternatively, very thin aluminum foils may be utilized to achieve a D ½ of 0.5–1 mm. The tube window itself must be thin and of a low molecular weight substance such as beryllium which is used in modern machines. Pyrex windows which were used in conventional superficial units effectively filter out all grenz rays. Grenz ray is so soft that clinicians utilizing it must take care to remove all traces of makeup and moisturizers because they can harden or attenuate the beam.

TSD—The target skin distance of grenz ray is one of the most important variables. As mentioned, grenz ray is absorbed by air so the standard inverse square rule cannot be utilized to make dosage or calibration calculations (vide infra). Exact measurements and patient positioning are necessary and treatment should not be done without cones or cylinders to fix the distance and field.

HVL—As with superficial photon radiotherapy, the thickness of aluminum to attenuate the beam to 50 % of its D_{max} is termed the half value layer and is used to define the beam quality. Historically, grenz ray has been divided into three ranges based on HVL:

Beam quality	HVL (mm Al)
Soft	0.020–0.022
Medium	0.023–0.029
Hard	0.030–0.036

D½—The D ½ philosophy which is discussed elsewhere in this treatise requires that the chosen beam penetrates and is not attenuated more than 50 % to the base of the tumor or condition.

Beam quality	D ½ (mm)
Soft	~0.5
Hard	~ 1.0

Wavelength—Bucky and others have defined grenz ray by their wavelength which ranges from 1 to 4 Å. The correlation between tube kV and wavelength has been described by the formula:

$$\text{Wavelength (min)} = 12.354/\text{kV}$$

Other Physical Properties

In the grenz ray region, backscatter is not significant and absorption curves are essentially equivalent to depth dose curves. The depth dose increases very slowly between soft and medium and more so between medium and hard. Above 0.036 mm Al HVL the depth dose and quality as one gets into the region of superficial radiation escalates much quicker [1]. For this reason, Bucky set the upper limit of grenz ray at 0.036 mm Al HVL. In deference to him, the Council for the Study of Grenz Ray Therapy set the upper limit of the grenz ray range at HVL 0.035 mm Al on March 17, 1950 [2].

Calibration

Most radiation physicists are not familiar with or equipped to calibrate a grenz ray unit. Many therapy physicists do not possess the thin window chamber and thin aluminum sheets required for the calibration of these units. Chambers with Mylar windows work well and one example is the Capintec PS-033. This chamber has an ultrathin Mylar 0.5 mg/cm^2 window. Not all Accredited Dosimetry Calibration Laboratories (ADCLs) can calibrate these chambers at grenz ray kVs; however, at the time of the printing of this text, K&S Associates of Nashville, Tennessee provides this service. Dermatologists employing grenz ray should employ a physicist experienced with this modality. Although the present protocol by the American Association of Physicists in Medicine (AAPM) for X-ray therapy calibration Report 76 by Task Group #61 does not address X-ray therapy below 40 kV X-ray beams, it can be used as a general guide to the calibration of grenz ray machines. The British Journal of Radiology supplement 25 is another good source of information, because it contains percent depth dose and backscatter information for beams with HVLs as thin as 0.01 mm Al. It has been the experience of the authors that our grenz ray unit, which is infrequently used, takes more time, effort, and cost to calibrate than our standard 50/70/100 kV unit or our backup 80 kV unit.

The cone's circumference is generally limited to ¾ of the TSD. There is a significant drop off at the shoulder of the field, due to the fact that because of air absorption, the TSD is significantly longer at the perimeter than that of the central beam. Hollander, in his classic 1952 treatise on grenz ray [2], relates that the measured beam reduction when one goes from a TSD of 10–20 cm is 78 % of that calculated by the inverse square law. This falls to a 44 % reduction of the calculated beam when one goes from a TSD of 10–50 cm. This drop-off diminishes to 88 % of the calculated beam from a TSD of 10–20 cm with a 20 kV beam. Accurate calibration is vital and far more complex with grenz ray than any other modality. This is in order to reduce the chance of under or over treatment of in situ malignancies or inflammatory disease, both of which can have serious consequences and constitute mistreatment.

We recently contacted our physicist to help us produce a beam which had a D ½ of 1 mm. We needed to treat atypical junctional melanocytic proliferation in elderly patients with equivocal slow Mohs margins or be able to recreate the Miescher technique as a primary therapy for elderly or feeble patients with facial lentigo maligna. This process required the HVL of the unit to be increased from 0.038 to 0.06 mm Al. This was accomplished by adding a 0.08 mm Al filter to the beam. The consequence of using this filter is a drastic reduction in dose output.

Radiobiological Effect of Grenz Ray

In his classic 1928 book, Gustav Bucky states that "the employment of electromagnetic oscillations from about 2 Å units produces unique clinical and biological manifestations" [3].

Grenz ray photons are absorbed mainly by the photoelectric effect. The resulting photoelectrons have a short path, because their energy is equal to that of the initiating photon minus the binding energy of the electron shell. Previous studies have shown that when looking at the range from 3 to1000 kV, the coefficient of chromosome breakage peaks at 4.1 Å [4]. Comparative studies of the biologic effect of X-rays and neutrons to other ionizing radiation have been performed. The low energy photons of grenz ray are comparable to higher energy gamma rays based on the dominance of photoelectric absorption at low energies. The relative biologic effectiveness (RBE) increases as the energy of photons and the energy of the secondary electrons emitted decreases. This translates into an increase in linear energy transfer (LET) or stopping power, with a D_{max} at the skin surface (as with all photon radiotherapy) where the majority of energy is absorbed within the epidermis and upper dermis.

Several studies have shown a marked and sustained reduction in Langerhan cells at 1 and 3 weeks [5–9]. The deposition of the majority of its modest energy in the epidermis, and its effect on Langerhan cells may explain why grenz ray has been used successfully for inflammatory disease such as contact dermatitis, eczema, and psoriasis and in situ/superficial/precancerous neoplasms including lentigo maligna, squamous cell carcinoma in situ (SCCIS), superficial basal cell carcinoma (sBCC), and actinic keratosis [10].

Physical Effects of Grenz Ray

Early on, grenz ray dosages and therapeutic treatment were prescribed in increments and multiples of the clinically observed and measured erythema dose. This was similar to ultraviolet therapy. The erythema dose of grenz ray appears earlier and can be more intense than that of superficial radiotherapy and has been measured at between 250 and 400 cGy. At higher single or cumulative dosages, this erythema can be quite intense and is not a contraindication for continued or further treatments. In fact, in its extreme (i.e., the Miescher technique), one expects and strives for a brisk desquamative response which occurs between a cumulative dose of 3,000–10,000 cGy over a 1–2 week period, in fractions of 1,000–2,000 cGy. Clinicians look for and carefully document the erythema seen after one or two 200–300 cGy treatment fractions as evidence and clinical assurance that the tube is functioning well and is well-calibrated.

Cosmesis

Pigmentation often occurs and can be longstanding. This can be especially significant and disconcerting when treating lentigo maligna, where the pigmentation may persist and take 6–12 months to resolve. Pigmentation is accentuated when lead shields are used because the line of demarcation is sharp. However, pigmentation is diffuse when open cones are used and the central field fades into the peripheral field. This is because of the difference in the TSD centrally vs. peripherally. Epilation has been reported to rarely occur. Hollander calculated that to achieve a reversible epilating dose of 350 cGy to the hair bulb, one must give a 5,000 cGy surface dose of grenz ray with a HVL of 0 0.034 mm Al where 7 % reaches the bulb. Long-term sequellae such as telangiectasias and atrophy have been described by early workers in the field and in clinicians who did not take care to protect themselves or their patients from chronic cumulative large doses. Secondary basal cell carcinomas (BCCs) and squamous cell carcinomas (SCCs) have been reported at doses over 100 Gy (vide infra).

Grenz Ray for In Situ Malignancies and Precancers

Grenz Ray for Lentigo Maligna

In the Miescher technique, a beryllium-window tube at 12 kV was used with an additional 1 mm thick filter of tissue-equivalent material (Cellon). 10,000 cGy in 5 fractions of 2,000 cGy were given every 3–4 days [11]. In 1971 Kopf et al. reported on the use of the Miescher technique in eight patients with lentigo maligna, using 12 kV and a D ½ of 1.3 mm [12]. In 1976 they published follow up data on the original eight patients, as well as eight subsequent patients treated in the interim between 1971 and 1976 [13]. Of these original 16 patients, five had recurrences or residual disease and three developed metastatic disease. This brought an abrupt end to the use of grenz ray in their department, and had a dampening effect on the use of grenz ray for lentigo maligna in the United States. One postulated downfall in the original study by Kopf et al. had been that patients who developed metastases had probably progressed to LMM with dermal invasion prior to treatment with the Miescher technique.

Despite this honest display of failure, others before and after have utilized grenz ray, superficial X-ray, and even electrons for lentigo maligna. Desquamative dosage/fractionation plans have been used in patients who were poor surgical candidates or had diffuse/non-resectable disease.

The D ½ philosophy for the treatment of malignancies suggests that radiation quality for a given lesion should deliver at least 50 % of the surface dose to the deepest part of the tumor. Under this concept, most in situ neoplasms can be treated with grenz ray using a D ½ between 0.5 and 1 mm.

In a retrospective study, Farshad et al. included 150 patients with lentigo maligna (LM) and lentigo maligna melanoma (LMM). Ninety-three had LM, 54 had LMM, and 3 had both (Farshad et al. calculated that 96 had LM and 57 had LMM). They employed the use of grenz ray (12 kV, 100–120 Gy at 3–4 day intervals for 10–12 fractions with a D ½ of 1 mm) in 96 patients with LM and 11 with LMM. Fifty-seven patients also received deeper penetrating X-rays (20 or 30 kV). Forty-six patients with LMM received 42–54 Gy (20–50 kV) at 3–4 day intervals over 7–9 fractions. There was a 7 % recurrence rate in 101 of 150 patients available for 2-year follow up [14]. They recommended using a safety margin around the visible lesion of at least 10 mm, in order to prevent recurrences at the edge of the radiotherapy field.

In another study, Schmid-Wendtner et al. excised the nodular portions of LMM before irradiation of the lentiginous part of the lesion [15]. They found that once LM transitions into LMM, superficial X-ray is less effective than in LM. They treated 64 patients (42 had LM and 22 had LMM) with a total dose of 100 Gy applied in 10 fractions (5 fractions per week over 2 weeks at 14.5 kV, D ½ of 1.1 mm). No patients with LM had recurrence, but 2 of 22 patients with LMM needed surgical excision for local recurrence.

Over a 30-year period, physicians at the Princess Margaret Hospital in Ontario, Canada treated patients with orthovoltage radiotherapy for LM and LMM. The following three studies highlight their experience. They give reference to the Miescher technique despite the fact that all three studies utilized deeper penetrating X-rays.

In the first of the three studies, Dancuart et al. looked at the fact that only one third of all histologically proven LMM show nodule formation clinically [16]. In their study they avoided the Miescher technique because of the difficulty in determining dermal extension. Using this as a reference point, they utilized conventional orthovoltage radiotherapy to treat eight patients with LM and 15 patients with LMM. Their patients were treated with either 100 kV (HVL 0.7 mm Al), 140 kV (HVL 3.6 mm Al), or 280 kV (HVL 1.25 or 3 mm Cu). The authors felt that they avoided "geographic miss" of dermal extension in LM and LMM by using a minimum irradiation energy of 100 kV with a D ½ of 6 mm. 1 of the 8 patients with LM had a recurrence on the edge of the previously treated irradiated zone 12 months after initial irradiation. The patient was treated with further radiation and did well. 6 of the 8 patients with LM achieved remission for 1–4½ years following radiotherapy. 1 of the 8 patients with LM had residual pigmentation on the cheek. 14 of the 15 patients treated from LMM went into remission. Two of those 14 had some residual pigmentation. 1 of the 15 patients with LMM had a central recurrence, but was treated with salvage excision and did well. In general, doses ranged between 3,500 cGy in 5 fractions and 4,500–5,000 cGy in 10–15 fractions.

In the second of the three studies that utilized orthovoltage radiotherapy, Harwood published similarly successful results using 100 kV (HVL 0.7 mm Al) for LM (23 patients) and 125–175 kV for LMM (28 patients) [17]. Patients were treated with 3,500 cGy for 5 fractions in 1 week, 4,500 cGy for 10 fractions in 2 weeks, or 5,000 cGy for 15–20 fractions in 3–4 weeks. 18 of 23 patients with LM had no recurrence. Two patients with LM failed irradiation. 1 of those 2 patients refused conventional irradiation and was treated with a single exposure of 2,000 cGy, but the lesion persisted and was excised. The second patient had an edge recurrence and was doing well after he was re-irradiated. The final three patients could not be evaluated because of short follow-up time. 23 of 28 patients with LMM were locally controlled for 6 months to 8 years. Two of 28 patients with LMM developed local recurrence treated with salvage excision. 3 of the 28 patients were not assessable because of short follow-up time. 1 of those 3 had a level five LMM that arose in a preexisting LM. Harwood noted that lesions may take up to 2 years to completely regress following treatment.

Although surgical excision remains the treatment of choice for small lesions of LM, in the last of the three studies, Tsang et al. demonstrated that orthovoltage radiotherapy was a good alternative for large lesions in facial areas. They demonstrated that radiotherapy was also a cost-effective treatment strategy, on par with excisional surgery. They looked at 54 patients with LM. There were 18 younger patients treated with excision, and 36 older patients with larger lesions treated with radiotherapy. 1 of the 18 younger patients had a recurrence treated with salvage excision. 3 of the 36 older patients' disease not controlled by irradiation alone were successfully treated with salvage excision. The excision revealed invasive melanoma in 2 of the 3 patients (no papules or nodules present clinically). One patient with residual pigmentation was unavailable for follow up [18].

Gaspar et al. pointed out the fact that the major drawback with radiotherapy treatment of LM is the lack of histopathologic confirmation that there is no LMM present. They looked at treatments for LM. After reviewing many of the studies done, they concluded that radiotherapy is an acceptable treatment for LM if used by experienced clinicians [19].

A recent well-done study from Sweden published by Hedblad et al., looked at grenz ray treatment of LM and early LMM over almost 20 years. Five hundred and ninety-three patients were treated with grenz rays in three groups [20]. The grenz ray unit delivered a HVL of 0.02 mm Al with a D ½ of 0.5 mm. Treatment doses ranged from 100 to 160 Gy twice weekly over 3 weeks. Grenz ray was curative in 520 of 593 patients (88 %) overall in all three groups, after one fractionated treatment. Complete clearance was seen in 290 of 350 patients (83 %) in the group receiving primary treatment with grenz ray alone. The complete clearance rate in the group of patients who received partial excision followed by grenz ray was 64 of 71 (90 %). Lastly, the complete clearance rate in the group of patients who received prophylactic grenz ray after radical excision was 166 of 172 (97 %).

Hedblad et al. reported that 73 of 593 patients (12 %) did not clear in one fractionated treatment. Within the group that did not clear in one fractionated treatment, 15 of 73 (21 %) had a weak radiation dermatitis with residual lesions, and 36 of 73 patients (49 %) had recurrence. Skin folds and residual "field effects" contributed to the recurrences due to the application of insufficient safety margins. The remaining 22 of 73 patients who did not clear in one fractionated treatment (30 %) showed histological changes consistent with proliferation of atypical melanocytes in adnexal structures.

Hedblad et al. treated 46 of 73 (63 %) patients who had recurrent or persistent lesions with additional fractionated grenz ray treatment. Three additional grenz ray treatments were combined with shave excision, and eight additional grenz ray treatments were combined with surgical excision. Several teaching points were highlighted by the authors. The first lesson was that high risk relapse sites are often seen in areas with hyperplastic adnexal structures such as the ala nasi, beard area, and scalp. In order to reduce recurrences, they recommended distending deep skin folds and wrinkles near the forehead and eyes when the cone is applied. In addition, the authors encouraged the use of a Woods light to help demarcate the clinical borders of the lesion so that sufficient safety margins of at least 1 cm can be used.

Grenz Ray for Bowen's Disease

There are a variety of treatment options for Bowen's disease or SCCIS depending on the histological characteristics of the lesion. As with LM and LMM, surgical removal offers the highest cure rate, but there are topical chemotherapeutic drugs, photodynamic therapy, and local destructive modalities that can successfully treat this tumor. In addition, various X-ray treatments have been used against SCCIS.

In 1977, Stevens et al. published a report of 19 lesions of SCCIS treated 2–3 times a week using 12–14 kV and 500 cGy over 10 fractions for a total dose of 5,000 Gy [21]. The HVL was 0.030–0.034 mm Al, and the D ½ was 0.7–0.9 mm. Of the 19 lesions treated, 17 had good cosmesis with successful treatment. One lesion persisted and was found to be superficially invasive SCC after excision. One lesion recurred 4 months after grenz ray treatment was completed. The depth of the overlying scale combined with the depth of the lesion exceeded the D ½, explaining why treatment with grenz ray failed.

Renato G. Panizzon, former editor of this book and a renowned expert on grenz ray and photon radiation therapy, recommended a dosage of 6 Gy twice weekly for 12 fractions using a D ½ of 1 mm [22]. In the event that there is significant adnexal involvement, then superficial radiotherapy or orthovoltage may be a better choice of treatment.

Herbert Goldschmidt, the editor of this textbook in the 1970s and a true expert and champion of radiation in dermatology, also edited the book "Physical Modalities in Dermatologic Therapy, Radiotherapy, Electrosurgery, Phototherapy, Cryosurgery" in which Lewis recommends 3,000 cGy for two doses 2 weeks apart for Bowen's disease and superficial SCC. For very inflamed lesions, the regimen can be reduced to 2,000 cGy on alternate weeks for three doses [23].

In another reference, Panizzon discourages the use of grenz ray for SCCs that extend into cartilage, bone, mucous membranes, or chronic scars [24].

Dupree et al. looked at the use of radiotherapy for the treatment of Bowen's disease of the lower extremity. They did not use grenz ray. They concluded that the use

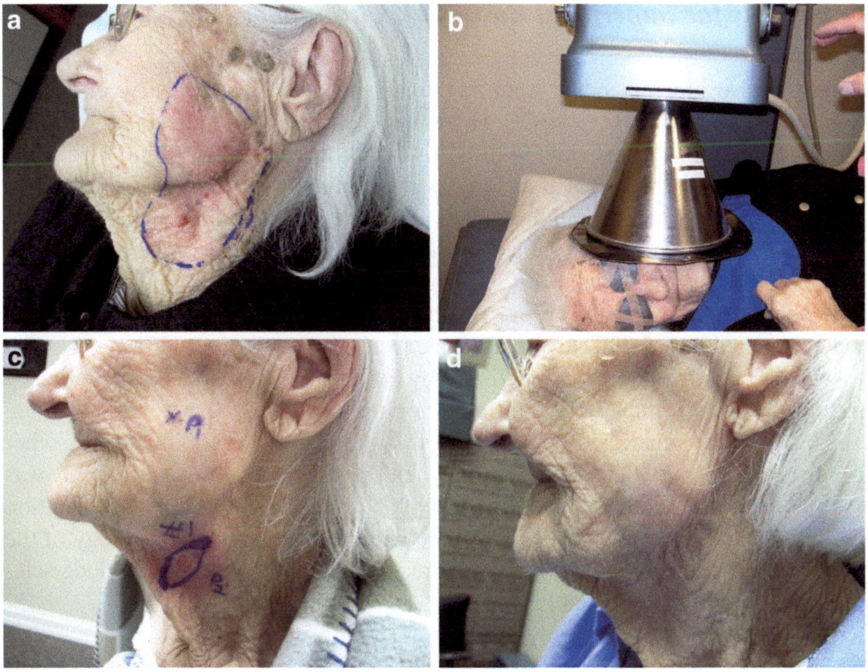

Fig. 1 SCCIS extending from the left cheek to the left neck (**a**) before treatment with grenz ray, (**b**) during treatment with grenz ray, (**c**) 8 months post-grenz ray treatment at elliptical excision of invasive SCC, and (**d**) 16 months after grenz ray treatment

of superficial and orthovoltage radiotherapy for the lower extremities may be problematic. Although the lesions are successfully treated, many lesions may become nonhealing ulcers after these types of radiotherapy. The tendency to ulcerate may be due to peripheral vascular disease and nutritional deficiencies [25]. This may be a reason to consider grenz ray therapy, due to its more superficial penetration and lower risk of causing nonhealing ulcers.

We treated a patient with a large (7.5 × 11.5 cm) SCCIS extending from the left cheek to the left neck with grenz ray (15 kV, D ½ = 0.42 mm, at 1,000 cGy once per week for 3 fractions). She responded to the treatment well (see Fig. 1). She subsequently developed two invasive SCCs, one of which was excised and the other which was not treated after biopsy (per patient request) due to no visible residual tumor. This case illustrates the fact that grenz rays do not penetrate deeply enough to treat invasive skin cancers. In addition, a large skin cancer which has only been partially biopsied may harbor subclinical invasive tumor which does not manifest clinically until after successful treatment of the in situ portion. Therefore, grenz ray treated skin cancers need close clinical follow up after treatment. Patients should be instructed to return to the office for evaluation of any new growths or recurrences in the treated field.

Grenz Ray for Superficial Basal Cell Carcinoma

Panizzon also recommended grenz ray treatment at 6 Gy twice a week for 12 fractions in the treatment of sBCC. He notes only modest side effects such as pigmentary alterations in the skin, with no risk of posttreatment alopecia. Therefore, the treatments can be repeated as long as the lifetime total dosage is not reached (100 Gy), and a 6-month minimal interval between treatment series is preserved [22]. Lewis recommends the same dosage of grenz ray for superficial multicentric BCC, SCCIS, and superficial SCC. A non-inflamed or minimally inflamed lesion may be treated with 3,000 cGy for two doses, 2 weeks apart. An inflamed lesion may be treated with 2,000 cGy on alternate weeks for three doses [23].

Another treatment regimen published by Ford and Prazak, found equal efficacy in three different regimens. The different regimens were 3,000 cGy in one sitting, 1,500 cGy every other day for three doses (4,500 cGy), or 3,000 cGy every other day for three doses (9,000 cGy) [26]. They felt that the single dose of 3,000 cGy was "simple, expedient and highly satisfactory," but cautioned against late radiation atrophy. In another reference, Panizzon recommends checking the histology of the tumor before proceeding with grenz ray treatment. It is important to exclude sclerosing tumors from treatment [24].

Grenz Ray for Actinic Keratosis

Disseminated actinic keratosis is a very widespread precancerous condition that can represent an extreme therapeutic dilemma. On the one hand, these lesions are at risk of transitioning into invasive SCC. On the other hand, the surface area that can be covered by these often coalescing, contiguous papules, and plaques may become unmanageable to treat. Current therapeutic modalities may be ineffective in reaching the adnexal structures where these lesions often make their transition to early skin cancer. Recurrences are common and may require combination treatment with several modalities being used together.

Several regimens have been described. At the Denver Skin Clinic they administered more than 40,000 grenz ray treatments for actinic keratoses. For facial AKs, a dose of 1,300–2,000 cGy in 1 fraction may be used, depending on the "transparency" of the patient's skin [23]. According to Lewis, there is no discernible pigmentary alteration, and treatment of eyelids is safe. Patients should be counseled to expect some posttreatment erythema for 1–2 days. During the 7–11th day posttreatment, the author noticed a more lasting reaction that peaked between day 17 and 22, before leaving normal appearing skin by posttreatment day 50. The gradual onset of erythema seemed to cause less discomfort than 5-fluorouracil treatment. Hand and forearm lesions may be treated with a single fraction of 1,500–2,000 cGy. There is a recurrence rate of approximately 5 % after 3 years.

Cipollaro, also a former editor of this textbook, recommends a total dose of 3,000 cGy given over a period of 1–2 weeks in fractions of 1,000 cGy. This regimen

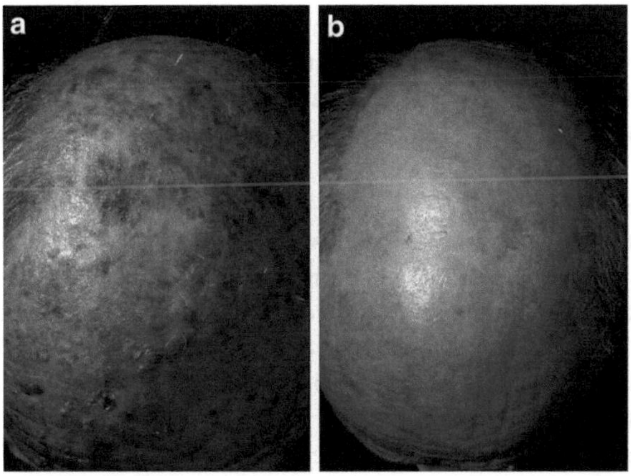

Fig. 2 (**a**) Before and (**b**) 6 months after treatment of disseminated AK on the scalp with grenz ray at 6 Gy twice weekly for 6 fractions (reprinted from Panizzon, R.G., Basal Cell and Squamous Cell Carcinoma—Radiotherapeutic Approaches. In Sternemann M, Wiegel T, Geilen CC, Orfanos CE, Hinkelbein W (eds), Controversies in the Treatment of Skin Neoplasias. Front Radiat Ther Oncol. Basel, Karger, 2006, vol. 39, pp. 38–49, with copyright permission from S. Karger AG, Basel)

is effective for the thicker lesions that are often present [27]. More recently, Pannizon recommended a regimen consisting of 6 Gy times six sessions twice weekly for disseminated AK. Of note, they mention that only rare subsequent doses are required years later. A photograph of dramatic improvement is pictured on the scalp (see Fig. 2) [24].

We are currently developing a protocol which will stack grenz ray with red light PDT for use in diffuse hypertrophic actinic keratosis on the arms and hands. We plan to optimize the PDT by utilizing fractional CO_2 laser pretreatment as described by Dr. R. Rox Anderson [28].

Grenz Ray for Inflammatory Skin Diseases

Decades before the introduction of potent topical anti-inflammatory medications, dermatologists utilized and depended on grenz ray to treat a wide variety of chronic superficial dermatoses [29]. Although some dermatoses responded better than others, the Bucky ray provided many dermatologists with a tool in their armamentarium that could be calibrated, fractionated, and controlled [30]. Immediate and long-term side effects were generally well-accepted [31]. Treatment parameters, contraindications, and dosages for specific inflammatory conditions were outlined for the practitioner [32, 33]. Even after the introduction of potent topical corticosteroids, grenz ray was proven in numerous studies to be a very useful addition to the treatment regimens of many patients suffering from chronic, refractory eczema, and psoriasis [34]. Although superficial radiotherapy has been shown to be more effective than grenz ray in the treatment of chronic eczema, grenz ray carries a lower risk of carcinogenesis. However the lack of long-term follow up and the relapsing nature of this condition limit the long-term potential usefulness of grenz ray in this setting. A multitude of inflammatory diseases have been treated with grenz ray since its discovery in the 1920s. We will focus on several of these which have been studied.

In a review article by Warner and Cruz, five studies were summarized looking at the treatment of eczema with grenz ray [34]. In the first study by Lindelöf et al., six subjects were treated with 3 Gy 3 times weekly. The results showed that grenz ray could suppress allergic contact nickel dermatitis in sensitive patients. In the second study by Lindelöf and Lindberg, there were 11 subjects also treated with 3 Gy 3 times weekly. Subjects were exposed to serial dilution sodium lauryl sulfate patch tests. Results showed that there was no significant improvement in irritant contact dermatitis treated with grenz ray.

The three remaining studies cited looked at grenz ray in chronic hand dermatitis. In the first study by Fairris et al., 25 subjects were treated with 1 Gy superficial X-ray on the one hand and 3 Gy grenz ray on the other hand. Superficial X-ray was better at improving the symptoms; however, grenz ray was also effective. In the second study by Cartwright and Rowell, 30 subjects were treated with 3 Gy on the one hand and sham therapy on the other hand. Patients continued tar paste or corticosteroid ointment during the grenz ray treatment. The authors concluded that grenz ray was no better than placebo against refractory hand eczema. In the third study by Lindelöf et al., 24 patients were treated on the one hand with six weekly treatments of 3 Gy after topical steroids. The other hand was treated with sham therapy after topical steroids. The conclusion was that grenz ray is a useful adjunctive treatment to steroids in the management of chronic hand eczema.

Psoriasis is another chronic skin condition that responds to grenz rays. Six studies were summarized in the article by Warner and Cruz [34]. In the first study by Harber, 76 subjects were treated with three different regimens on the trunk and extremities. The first regimen used 2 Gy of grenz ray 4 times a week, the second regimen was 160 cGy of X-rays 4 times a week, and the third regimen was an untreated control. In 80 % of cases, either type of radiation treatment produced more clinical improvement in psoriasis than nonirradiated control sites. In 70 % of cases there was no statistical difference between the two types of radiation. However, in 20 % of cases, grenz ray treated lesions were significantly more improved than X-ray treated lesions. In 8 % of cases, X-ray treated lesions were significantly more improved.

Warner and Cruz reviewed a second study, by Broderson and Reymann, in which 20 subjects with trunk and extremity psoriasis had half of their bodies treated with 12 kV of grenz ray 3 times a week after betamethasone ointment. The other half of the body received sham therapy after betamethasone ointment. Patients felt that the addition of grenz ray to their treatment regimen improved their psoriasis compared to topical steroids alone.

In the next three studies reviewed by Warner and Cruz, Johannesson and Lindelöf looked at scalp psoriasis. In the first study, 16 subjects had half the scalp treated with six weekly 4 Gy doses of grenz ray, while the other half of the scalp received sham therapy. 87.5 % of patients had complete healing of the scalp psoriasis on the treated side. In the second study, 17 subjects underwent the same treatment as above, after pretreatment with betamethasone solution to the entire scalp. The addition of topical steroid pretreatment increased the complete healing to 88.2 % in this study. In addition, the combination of grenz ray and topical steroids gave a longer remission time than with grenz ray alone. In the third study, there were 40 subjects enrolled. Half the subjects were treated with six weekly whole scalp grenz ray treatments at 4 Gy. The other half of subjects received the same grenz ray treatment, plus betamethasone solution. This study found no statistical difference in healing rates between subjects treated with grenz ray vs. grenz ray and topical steroids.

In the last study, Lindelöf treated psoriatic nails with ten weekly 10 kV doses of grenz ray on the one hand while the other hand received sham therapy. He found that grenz ray is useful in treating psoriatic nails when applied to nails of normal thickness.

Histiocytosis X is a clonal proliferative disorder that is very challenging to treat [35]. It is thought to be related to a local proliferation and dissemination of Langerhans cells. Current treatment is based on whether the presentation is single system or multisystem disease. In single system skin disease, grenz ray may be useful when systemic involvement has been ruled out [7]. Lindelöf treated a 29 year-old woman who had histiocytosis X concentrated in the scalp, axilla, and inguinal regions. She had unsatisfactory response to PUVA, especially in the scalp. He treated her with five courses of grenz ray over 2 years. She was treated with 10 kV, at a D ½ of 0.5 mm. The scalp received 4 Gy and the axillary and inguinal regions received 1–2 Gy per week for 6–10 weeks. The patient had marked improvement of the scalp. However, the axillary and inguinal regions were no better than after PUVA treatment. When histiocytosis X is confined to the skin, grenz ray is a convenient treatment that is capable of producing a reduction in Langerhans cells.

Grenz ray treatment provides patients with relief from disabling benign conditions, with only a small risk of cutaneous malignancy in the event that the treatment dose exceeds well-established upper limits (100 Gy) [36]. Reports began to surface which highlighted the potential for grenz ray therapy to induce squamous cell carcinoma [37]. Unfortunately, some practitioners adopted mistaken beliefs that overestimated and confused the risk of carcinogenesis due to these super soft X-rays [38]. As a result, administration by dermatologists and training of dermatology residents in the use of this most superficial cutaneous radiation modality suffered tremendously [39]. Due to confounders encountered in a study looking at skin tumors resulting from grenz ray treatments, it was difficult to conclude whether a causal relationship existed between grenz ray and squamous cell carcinoma [40]. Bucky himself asserted that "In contradistinction to Roentgen rays, in which the dangerous and therapeutic doses are narrowly separated, the margin in Grenz rays is distinctly wide. Nevertheless, since the Grenz rays are an effective agent, ill-advised and repeated overdosage may provoke injury, either atrophy, or with higher tension, possibly telangiectasias" [3]. Patients' response to grenz ray therapy was favorable, and did not depend on disease duration or previous treatment modalities used [41]. Dr. Goldschmidt advocated for radiotherapy training so that skin specialists could expertly select the best methods of treatment for cutaneous neoplasms and other resistant skin problems [42].

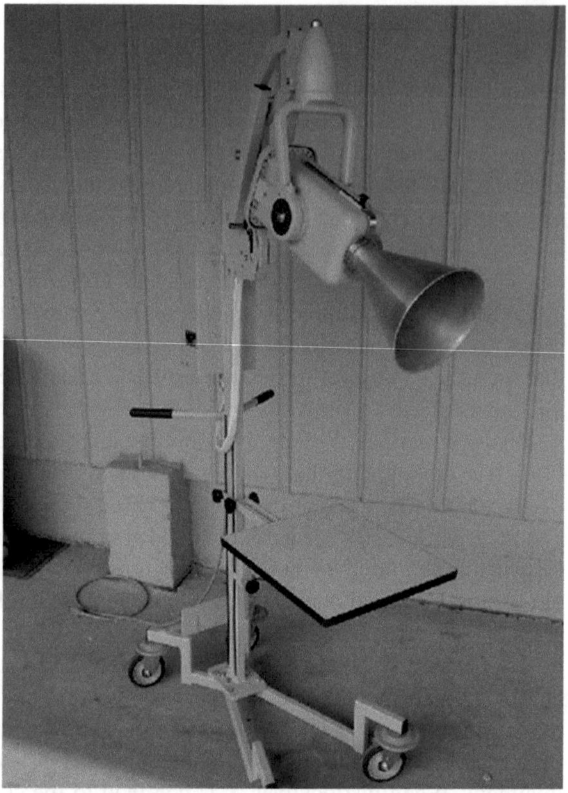

Fig. 3 Portable grenz ray unit by X-Cel X-Ray Corporation

As specialists in the diagnosis and treatment of diseases involving the skin, mucous membranes, hair, and nails, dermatologists should be able to design cutaneous treatment plans using the best combination of medical therapy, surgical therapy, and radiotherapy available. In most instances, radiotherapy is best reserved for difficult cases in which other treatment modalities have failed. In other situations, radiotherapy may be best for patients who are poor surgical candidates due to existing comorbidities or functional limitations.

Due to its unique characteristics, grenz ray treatment is well-suited to resistant superficial neoplasms and inflammatory conditions. Effective results can be obtained with low total dosages (50 Gy per field per lifetime) that are below those potentially associated with increasing the risk of skin cancer [43]. These low dosages in combination with other treatment modalities represent the best adjunctive therapies against chronic skin diseases. It has been our experience that patients with recalcitrant inflammatory dermatoses have traveled long distances in order to obtain the unique and long-lasting effectiveness of grenz ray treatment in our office, where we have the only unit available in our area. There is only one supplier of grenz ray machines in the United States. This is the X-Cel X-Ray Corporation in Crystal Lake, Illinois (http://www.xcelxray.com; Fig. 3). In Europe, the Progressus Medica AB in Stockholm, Sweden (http://www.progressusmedica.se) is a supplier of grenz ray machines. In the past there were several suppliers, and older refurbished grenz ray units were often available from retiring practitioners. Dual machines which administer grenz ray and deeper penetrating X-rays have also been built. Our mentors have avoided these machines because they can pose a safety hazard. Although we do not have first-hand experience with these dual machines, we maintain respect for their potential danger based on the wisdom of our predecessors, which we will not challenge here. It is the responsibility of anyone who purchases a grenz ray machine to have it registered, maintained and calibrated periodically. Physicians treating patients with grenz ray therapy must utilize it with the same prudence and precaution as any ionizing radiation source. As further studies emerge, we anticipate a renaissance in its use due to the unique properties, safety profile, cumulative experience, and published data supporting it.

Acknowledgments We would like to express our deepest gratitude to Ken Morse and Jeffrey Long for personal communications regarding the content of this chapter. Their invaluable contributions to the radiobiology and calibration of our equipment allow us to treat the patients in our practice who benefit from grenz ray therapy.

References

1. Ebbehøj E. Ultraweiche Röntgenstrahlen. Copenhagen: NYT Nordisk Forlag, Arnold Busck; 1937.
2. Hollander MB. Grenz rays. J Invest Dermatol. 1953;21(1):15–25.
3. Bucky G, Combes F. Grenz ray therapy: principles, methods, clinical applications. New York: Springer; 1954. p. 1, 83.
4. Catcheside DG, Lea DE. The effect of ionization distribution on chromosome breakage by x-rays. J Genet. 1943;45(2):186–96.
5. Lindelöf B, Forslind B. Electron microscopic observations of Langerhans' cells in human epidermis irradiated with grenz rays. Photodermatology. 1985;2(6):367–71.
6. Lindelöf B, Liden S, Ros AM. Effect of grenz rays on Langerhans' cells in human epidermis. Acta Derm Venereol. 1984;64(5):436–8.
7. Lindelöf B. Histiocytosis X, in an adult: treatment of skin lesions with Grenz rays. J Am Acad Dermatol. 1988;19:426–7.
8. Ek L, Lindelöf B, Liden S. The duration of Grenz ray-induced suppression of allergic contact dermatitis and its correlation with the density of Langerhans cells in human epidermis. Clin Exp Dermatol. 1989;14(3):206–9.
9. Beitner H, Nakatani T, Lindelöf B. An ultrastructural study of human epidermal Langerhans cells irradiated with grenz rays and ultraviolet A. Photodermatol Photoimmunol Photomed. 1990;7(6):266–8.
10. Lindelöf B. Grenz ray therapy in dermatology. An experimental, clinical and epidemiological study. Acta Derm Venereol Suppl (Stockh). 1987;132:1–67.
11. Miescher G. Über melanotische Präcancerose. Oncologia. 1954;7:92–4.
12. Petratos M, Kopf A, Bart R, Grisewood E, Gladstein A. Treatment of melanotic freckle with x-rays. Arch Dermatol. 1972;106(2):189–94.
13. Kopf A, Bart R, Gladstein A. Treatment of melanotic freckle with x-rays. Arch Dermatol. 1976;112:801–7.
14. Farshad A, Burg G, Panizzon R, Dummer R. A retrospective study of 150 patients with lentigo maligna and lentigo maligna melanoma and the efficacy of radiotherapy using Grenz or soft x-rays. Br J Dermatol. 2002;146:1042–6.

15. Schmid-Wendtner MH, Brunner B, Konz B, Kaudewitz P, Wendtner CM, Peter RU, et al. Fractionated radiotherapy of lentigo maligna and lentigo maligna melanoma in 64 patients. J Am Acad Dermatol. 2000;43:477–82.
16. Dancuart F, Harwood A, Fitzpatrick P. The radiotherapy of lentigo maligna and lentigo maligna melanoma of the head and neck. Cancer. 1980;45:2279–83.
17. Harwood A. Conventional fractionated radiotherapy for 51 patients with lentigo maligna and lentigo maligna melanoma. Int J Radiat Oncol Biol Phys. 1983;9:1019–21.
18. Tsang R, Liu F, Wells W, Payne D. Lentigo maligna of the head and neck. Results of treatment by radiotherapy. Arch Dermatol. 1994;130:1008–12.
19. Gaspar Z, Dawber R. Treatment of lentigo maligna. Australas J Dermatol. 1997;38:1–8.
20. Hedblad M, Mallbris L. Grenz ray treatment of lentigo maligna and early lentigo maligna melanoma. J Am Acad Dermatol. 2012;67:60–8.
21. Stevens D, Kopf A, Gladstein A, Bart R. Treatment of Bowen's disease with grenz rays. Int J Dermatol. 1977;16:329–39.
22. Panizzon R. Grenz rays: an alternative treatment for superficial skin cancers in elderly patients. Aging Health. 2009;5(4):495–6.
23. Lewis H. Grenz-ray therapy: regimens and results, chapter 15. In: Goldschmidt H, editor. Physical modalities in dermatologic therapy, radiotherapy, electrosurgery, phototherapy, cryosurgery. New York: Springer; 1978. p. 173–84.
24. Panizzon R. Basal cell and squamous cell carcinoma—radiotherapeutic approaches. In: Sternemann M, Wiegel T, Geilen C, Orfanos C, Hinkelbein W, editors. Controversies in the treatment of skin neoplasias. Frontiers of radiation therapy and oncology, vol. 39. Basel: Karger; 2006. p. 38–49.
25. Dupree M, Kitely R, Weismantle K, Panos R, Johnstone P. Radiation therapy for Bowen's disease: lessons for lesions of the lower extremity. J Am Acad Dermatol. 2001;45(3):401–4.
26. Ford S, Prazak G. Superficial epitheliomatosis treatment by grenz ray. Bull Assoc Mil Dermatologists. 1962;2(2):6–14.
27. Cipollaro A, Crossland P. Grenz rays. Chapter 12. In: X rays and radium in the treatment of diseases of the skin. 5th ed. Philadelphia: Lea & Febiger; 1967. p. 183–195.
28. Hædersdal M, Katsnelson J, Sakamoto F, Farinelli W, Doukas A, Tam J, et al. Enhanced uptake and photoactivation of topical methyl aminolevulinate after fractional CO_2 laser pretreatment. Lasers Surg Med. 2011;43:804–13.
29. Eller J, Bucky G. The use of the "grenz" (infra-roentgen) rays in dermatologic conditions: preliminary report of clinical and biologic observations. Arch Dermatol. 1928;17(2):221–38.
30. Scholtz M. Grenz rays: their therapeutic value in dermatology. Arch Dermatol. 1932;26(5): 802–15.
31. Bucky G. Actual superficial therapy by "grenz" (infra-roentgen) rays: its correlation with internal organs. Arch Dermatol. 1927;15(6):672–7.
32. Kalz F. Theoretic considerations and clinical use of grenz rays in dermatology. Arch Dermatol Syph. 1941;43(3):447–72.
33. Hanfling S. Grenz ray (supersoft roentgen ray) therapy of cutaneous diseases. Arch Dermatol. 1948;58(4):390–7.
34. Warner JA, Cruz P. Grenz ray therapy in the new millenium: still a valid treatment option? Dermatitis. 2008;19(2):73–80.
35. Taverna J, Stefanato C, Wax F, Demierre M. Adult cutaneous Langerhans cell histiocytosis responsive to topical imiquimod. J Am Acad Dermatol. 2006;54(5):911–3.
36. Kingery F, Russell P, Larsen W. Safety of grenz ray therapy. Arch Dermatol. 1990;126(1):119–20.
37. Brodkin R, Bleiberg J. Neoplasia resulting from grenz radiation. Arch Dermatol. 1968;97(3): 307–9.
38. Gladstein A. Dermatologic radiation and cancer. Arch Dermatol. 1990;126(1):120–1.
39. Kingery FA. Radiation therapy in dermatologic training centers. J Am Acad Dermatol. 1986; 14:1108–10.

40. Lindelöf B, Eklund G. Incidence of malignant skin tumors in 14,140 patients after grenz-ray treatment for benign skin disorders. Arch Dermatol. 1986;122(12):1391–5.
41. Schalock P, Zug K, Carter J, Dhar D, MacKenzie T. Efficacy and patient perception of Grenz ray therapy in the treatment of dermatoses refractory to other medical therapy. Dermatitis. 2008;19(2):90–4.
42. Goldschmidt H. Dermatologic radiotherapy: the risk-benefit ratio. Arch Dermatol. 1986; 122(12):1385–8.
43. Panizzon R. Radiation therapy of benign dermatoses. Chapter 4. In: Panizzon R, Cooper J, editors. Radiation treatment and radiation reactions in dermatology. Berlin: Springer; 2004. p. 33–40.

Radiotherapy for Cutaneous Squamous and Basal Cell Carcinomas

William M. Mendenhall

Introduction

Skin cancer is relatively common and is usually treated surgically. Although radiotherapy (RT) has been used frequently in the past, advances in surgical techniques and reconstructive procedures have led to a decline in the use of this modality. Nevertheless, RT is still frequently used to optimize the likelihood of cure, function, and/or cosmesis. This especially is true for patients with head and neck lesions where these goals are often more difficult to achieve [1–10]. The goal of this paper is to discuss the role of RT in the management of patients with cutaneous squamous cell carcinomas (SCCs), basal cell carcinomas (BCCs), and metatypical basal cell (basosquamous) carcinomas with an emphasis on cancers arising on the head and neck. RT may generally be stratified into two categories: (1) superficial orthovoltage RT with beam energies less than 100 kVp that may be administered for superficial lesions using a hypofractionated schedule by a dermatologist or a radiation oncologist; and (2) higher energy photon and electron beams administered by a radiation oncologist for more advanced lesions. This chapter will discuss the latter category.

Staging

Optimally, a staging system should be employed when evaluating outcomes data. Unfortunately, much of the outcomes data pertaining to SCCs and BCCs are not stratified by stage. The 2010 staging system described by the American Joint Committee on Cancer (AJCC) is depicted in Table 1 [11]. Staging of the primary lesions depends on size and extension into adjacent structures, such as bone, cartilage,

W.M. Mendenhall (✉)
Department of Radiation Oncology, College of Medicine, University of Florida, 2000 SW Archer Road, Gainesville, FL 32610, USA
e-mail: mendwm@shands.ufl.edu

A.B. Cognetta and W.M. Mendenhall (eds.), *Radiation Therapy for Skin Cancer*, DOI 10.1007/978-1-4614-6986-5_12, © Springer Science+Business Media New York 2013

Table 1 The American Joint Committee on Cancer—definition of TNM [11]

Primary tumor (T)[a]	
TX	Primary tumor cannot be assessed
T0	No evidence of primary tumor
Tis	Carcinoma in situ
T1	Tumor 2 cm or less in greater dimension with less than two high-risk features[b]
T2	Tumor greater than 2 cm in greatest dimension or tumor of any size with two or more high-risk features[a]
T3	Tumor with invasion of maxilla, mandible, orbit, or temporal bone
T4	Tumor with invasion of skeleton (axial or appendicular) or perineural invasion of skull base
Regional lymph nodes (N)	
NX	Regional lymph nodes cannot be assessed
N0	No regional lymph node metastasis
N1	Metastasis in a single ipsilateral lymph node, 3 cm or less in greatest dimension
N2	Metastasis in a single ipsilateral lymph node, more than 3 cm but not more than 6 cm in greatest dimension; or in multiple ipsilateral lymph nodes, none more than 6 cm in greatest dimension; or in bilateral or contralateral lymph nodes, none more than 6 cm in greatest dimension
N2a	Metastasis in a single ipsilateral lymph node, more than 3 cm but not more than 6 cm in greatest dimension
N2b	Metastasis in multiple ipsilateral lymph nodes, none more than 6 cm in greatest dimension
N2c	Metastasis in bilateral or contralateral lymph nodes, none more than 6 cm in greatest dimension
N3	Metastasis in a lymph node, more than 6 cm in greatest dimension
Distant metastasis (M)	
M0	No distant metastasis
M1	Distant metastasis
Depth/invasion	>2 mm thickness
	Clark level ≥ IV
	Perineural invasion
Anatomic location	Primary site ear
	Primary site non-hair bearing tip
Differentiation	Poorly differentiated or undifferentiated

Source: Used with the permission of the American Joint Committee on Cancer (AJCC), Chicago, IL. The original source for this material is the AJCC Cancer Staging Handbook, Seventh Edition (2010) published by Springer Science and Business Media LLC, www.springerlink.com

[a]Excludes cSCC of the eyelid

[b]High-risk features for the primary tumor (T) staging

and nerves. It is important to specify whether the tumor is clinically or pathologically staged. By definition, patients treated with RT alone must be clinically staged and this tends to result in underestimation of the extent of disease [12]. The outcomes of patients who are pathologically staged should not be compared to those clinically staged because the comparison will be biased. Additionally, because the staging system is modified every few years, it is important to note the edition of the AJCC system that was employed when assessing outcomes data.

Table 2 Clinical staging system for metastatic cutaneous squamous cell carcinoma to the parotid and/or neck [13]

Parotid	
P0	No clinical disease in the parotid
P1	Metastatic node up to 3 cm in diameter
P2	Metastatic node >3 cm and up to 6 cm in diameter or multiple nodes
P3	Metastatic node >6 cm in diameter or disease involving the facial nerve or skull base
Neck	
N0	No clinical disease
N1	Single ipsilateral neck node up to 3 cm in diameter
N2	Single node >3 cm in diameter or multiple nodes or contralateral nodes

Source: Data from Andruchow JL, Veness MJ, Morgan GJ et al. Implications for clinical staging of metastatic cutaneous squamous carcinoma of the head and neck based on a multicenter study of treatment outcomes. *Cancer* 2006;106(5):1078–1083

Although the probability of regional and/or distant metastases is low, the likelihood increases with lesions that are extensive, poorly differentiated, and/or recurrent after prior treatment. Patients with SCC and perineural invasion (PNI) exhibit an increased risk of regional metastases [12]. Lymph nodes most often involved are in the parotid and/or neck. Andruchow and colleagues [13] have proposed a modification of the staging system for patients with positive nodes in these sites (Table 2).

Selection of Treatment Modality

The probability of cure for early-stage lesions is similar after surgery or RT. Therefore, the decision of which modality to employ depends on other factors, including function, cosmesis, patient age, cost, medical condition of the patient, treatment availability, and the wishes of the patient. Patients with advanced cancers are often best treated with surgery and adjuvant RT, if the functional and cosmetic outcomes are acceptable. In young patients, it is desirable to avoid RT because the late effects of irradiation progress gradually with time and, with very long-term follow-up, may be associated with a suboptimal cosmetic result.

Radiotherapy Alone

Resection of a relatively early-stage lesion of the eyelid, external ear, or nose may result in a significant cosmetic defect that would require a complex reconstruction. Patients with lesions in these locations are often better treated with RT, particularly if they are older and/or have a limited life expectancy. Advanced unresectable cancers, such as those with PNI with gross disease in the cavernous sinus, are treated with RT alone. Patients with advanced resectable cancers may be treated with RT alone depending on other factors, such as medical comorbidities.

Lesions on the scalp and anterior aspect of the lower leg over the tibia are located in areas where there is little tissue between the skin and underlying bone and are at increased risk for a bone exposure or necrosis after RT. Skin cancer in these locations is preferably treated surgically. Similarly the hands and feet generally do not tolerate high-dose RT well and skin cancers in these locations are better treated with an operation. Patients with connective tissue disorders, such as scleroderma, are at increased risk for a late complication after RT and, thus, this modality is best avoided.

Adjuvant Radiotherapy

Postoperative RT is added in situations where the likelihood of residual disease is relatively high, particularly if the probability of salvage of a local recurrence is relatively modest. Indications for postoperative RT include positive margins, PNI (particularly if it is symptomatic), multiple recurrences, and bone invasion. Some indications for postoperative RT are stronger than others, such as positive margins in patients with SCCs. Others, such as focal cartilage invasion with widely negative margins, are not strong indications in the absence of other adverse findings. Patients with BCCs on free skin that have been resected with a focally positive margin may be followed and treated only in the event of a subsequent recurrence.

Management of Regional Lymph Node Metastases

Patients who present with clinically negative regional nodes (cNo) and who receive definitive RT to the primary lesion receive elective nodal RT (ENI) if the risk of occult metastases is thought to be 15–20 % or higher. Patients with SCC and asymptomatic (incidental) PNI are in this category and would receive ENI. Patients with lower lip SCCs that involve the midline may have an unpredictable spread pattern to bilateral level I lymph nodes and would require bilateral ENI.

Skin cancer metastatic to the parotid nodes is managed in the same way that one would manage a high-grade parotid malignancy with superficial or total parotidectomy followed by postoperative RT [14, 15]. The facial nerve is preserved, unless it is necessary to resect it to achieve a gross total resection [16]. Although the risk of subclinical disease in the clinically negative nodes is probably 20 % or higher, the ipsilateral neck may be electively irradiated when the parotid is treated postoperatively. Preoperative RT is used for patients with borderline resectable metastases. RT alone is used for patients with unresectable disease and for those who are medically inoperable.

Cervical node metastases are managed in the same way that metastatic nodes are managed for primary mucosal carcinomas [17]. Neck dissection alone is sufficient for the patient with a solitary node with no extracapsular extension. Patients with more advanced disease receive postoperative RT. Depending on the location of the primary tumor and involved nodes, the probability of subclinical disease in the clinically negative parotid may be high and the parotid nodes should be considered for elective treatment.

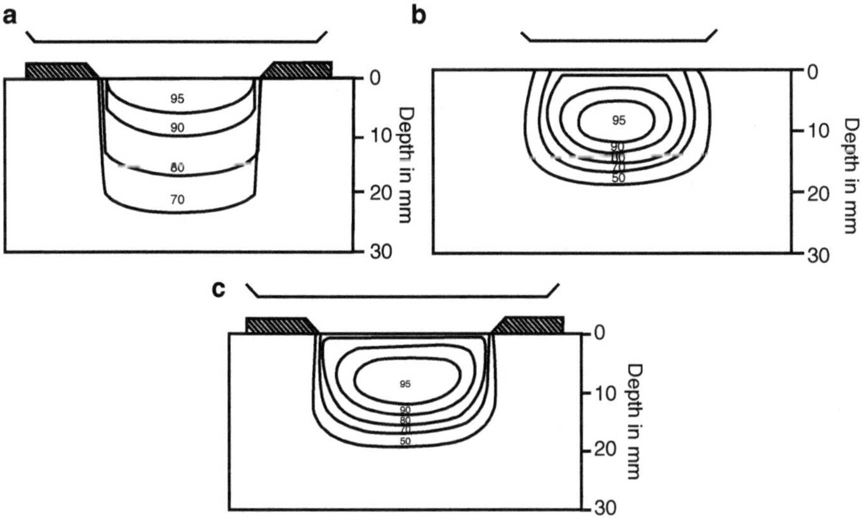

Fig. 1 (**a**) X-rays of 250-kVp (HVL 1.4 mm Cu) with secondary collimation of the phantom surface, source-to-surface distance (SSD) = 50 cm. Isodose %: 95, 90, 80, 70. (**b**) Electron beam of 6-MeV with secondary collimation 5 cm above the phantom surface (at the level of the electron cone). Source of collimator distance (SCD) = 95 cm. SSD = 100 cm. Isodose %: 95, 90, 80, 70, 50. (**c**) Electron beam of 6-MeV with tertiary collimation on the phantom surface. SSD = SCD = 100 cm. Isodose %: 95, 90, 80, 70, 50. *Source*: Mendenhall WM, Amdur RJ, Hinerman RW, Cognetta AB, Mendenhall NP. Radiotherapy for cutaneous squamous and basal cell carcinomas of the head and neck. Laryngoscope. 2009 Oct;119(10):1994–9

Treatment Techniques

Primary tumor: The major RT techniques are as follows: (1) orthovoltage RT; (2) electron beam; (3) high-energy photons; (4) proton beam; and (5) interstitial brachytherapy. The majority of skin cancers are optimally treated with orthovoltage RT, such as 250 kVp X-rays. A customized lead shield is constructed to fit on the skin surface to collimate the beam. The advantages of orthovoltage RT compared with electrons are as follows: (1) the maximum dose is at the skin surface; (2) there is less beam constriction, both at the surface and at depth, so that smaller fields may be used; (3) the dose distribution is less likely to be adversely impacted by irregular surface contours, such as the nose and external ear; and (4) it is easier to shield the eye because there is less penetration through eyeshields, particularly at higher electron energies (see Fig. 1 and Table 3) [18]. Disadvantages of orthovoltage RT are that it has a higher exit dose compared with electrons, and there is a higher differential dose absorbed in bone and cartilage vs. soft tissue. Another disadvantage of orthovoltage RT is that most radiation oncology departments do not have orthovoltage equipment.

Table 3 Ocular protection: dose beneath the eye shield [18]

Structure (depth)	250-kVp X-ray (HVL 1.4 mm Cu) (%)	Electron-beam energy (MeV) (%) 6	8	10	12	14	17	20
Cornea (1 mm)	10	18	37	64	75	93	98	102
Lens (8 mm)	9	9	19	36	46	61	70	87
Retina (23 mm)	10	19	22	22	21	23	25	29

Source: Data from Amdur RJ, Kalbaugh KJ, Ewald LM et al. Radiation therapy for skin cancer near the eye: Kilovoltage x-rays versus electrons. *Int J Radiat Oncol Biol Phys* 1992; 23(4):769–779
kVp kilovolt peak; *HVL* half-value layer

Table 4 Guidelines for selection of external-beam dose [21]

Orthovoltage dose (cGy)	Examples
6,500 over 7 weeks	Large untreated lesion with bone/cartilage invasion or large recurrent tumor
6,000 over 7 weeks	Large untreated lesion with minimal or suspected bone/cartilage invasion
5,500 over 6 weeks	Moderate to large inner canthus, eyelid, nasal, or pinna lesions (20–30 cm^2 area)
5,000 over 4 weeks	Small, thin lesion (less than 1.5 cm) around eye, nose, or ear (10 cm^2 area)
4,500 over 3 weeks	Moderate-sized lesion on "free" skin or postoperative treatment of moderate-sized cancer on "free" skin with positive margins
4,000 over 2 weeks or 3,000 over 1 week	Small lesions (1 cm) on "free" skin
The following schemes are used when the late cosmetic result is not important and travel for the patient is difficult	
4,000 in 10 fractions or 3,000 in 5 fractions or 2,000 in 1 fraction	Rapid fractionations schemes produce a high cure rate for small lesions, but the cosmetic result may be less than optimal after 5 years

Doses are increased by 10 % when using megavoltage beams to account for differences in radiobiological effectiveness (RBE)
Source: Data from Mendenhall WM, Kalbaugh KJ, Mendenhall NP, Parsons JT. Radiotherapy as definitive treatment and as a surgical adjunct. In: Weber RS, Miller MJ, Goepfert H, editors. *Basal and Squamous Cell Skin Cancers of the Head and Neck*. Baltimore: Williams & Wilkins, 1996: 331–350

Additional differences between photon beams and electron beams are that, for photons, as beam energy increases, surface dose decreases and exit dose increases. In contrast, for electrons, as beam energy increases, surface dose increases and exit dose increases. However, even for high energy electron beams, such as 20 MeV, one can only treat to a target depth of 4–5 cm before the dose falls off to a point where the tumor would be underdosed. Most skin cancers, if treated with electrons, are irradiated with 6–9 MeV beams, depending on the thickness of the lesion, with 0.5–1.0 cm of tissue equivalent material to assure an adequate surface dose. Our bias is to treat most skin cancers with orthovoltage RT except for scalp lesions where electron beam is employed to decrease the exit dose to the brain.

Regardless of whether electrons or orthovoltage irradiation are used, a lead mask is usually required to collimate the beam on the surface to obtain a sharp beam edge. Guidelines for selection of the dose-fractionation schedule are depicted in Table 4.

These doses are increased by 10 % to account for the difference in radiobiological effectiveness (RBE) when used for megavoltage beams. The maximum suggested skin doses for palliation are shown in Table 5. Although fractionation schedules that include a small number of fractions are more likely to result in a suboptimal cosmetic outcome, these schedules are useful for treating elderly, infirm patients where more protracted schedules are not possible.

Megavoltage photons are useful for treating advanced cancers, such as those that exhibit PNI extending towards the skull base. Depending on the situation, intensity-modulated radiotherapy (IMRT) may be used to produce a more conformal dose distribution to decrease the dose to surrounding normal tissues and diminish the probability of late complications. Proton beam is especially useful for tumor extending to the skull base in close proximity to the visual apparatus and central nervous system (CNS). Because of the absence of an exit dose, protons may be used to achieve very tight dose distributions with steep dose gradients, thus lowering the doses received by normal tissues more effectively than that can be obtained with IMRT. Another strategy that may be used to reduce the risk of late complications, when large volumes adjacent to and/or including the skull base are irradiated, is hyperfractionation. Bhandare et al. have shown that a hyperfractionated schedule delivering 1.2 Gy per twice-daily fraction resulted in a lower risk of optic neuropathy compared with once-daily fractionation [19].

Regional node metastases: Parotid nodes are irradiated with either an appositional mixed photon–electron beam or photons alone using either a "wedge pair" technique or IMRT to reduce the dose to the adjacent cerebellum and temporal lobe. We prefer the latter technique because of the lower risk of CNS injury. Dose fractionation schedules include 60 Gy in 30 once-daily fractions for negative margins and 66–70 at 2 Gy per once-daily fraction or 74.4 Gy at 1.2 Gy per twice-daily fraction for positive margins.

Patients with axillary lymph nodes are treated with anterior and posterior megavoltage beams. Patients with ilioinguinal lymph node metastases are irradiated with IMRT to create a cylindrical dose distribution to reduce the dose to the bowel. Patients are treated to 45 Gy in 25 fractions followed by a reduction and boost to 55–65 Gy depending on the amount of suspected residual disease. The total dose is less than that employed in the head and neck because the risk of morbidity is higher, particularly edema of the involved extremity.

Results

Primary lesion: The outcomes of a series of patients treated at Washington University (St. Louis) are shown in Tables 6 and 7. Patients treated with superficial X-rays (i.e., orthovoltage RT) tended to have local control rates that were as good, or better than, those achieved with electron beam, probably because it is easier to make a mistake and underdose the tumor with the latter. Schulte and coworkers reported on 1,113 patients treated with orthovoltage RT for 1,267 skin cancers and followed for a

Table 5 Suggested maximum skin doses for palliation with 250 kVp X-rays (below moist desquamation level for the average patient) [22]

	Total dose (cGy)						
Field size (area in cm^2)	One dose (1 exposure)	2 doses (2 exposures)	4 doses (4 exposures)	5 doses (5 exposures)	2 weeks (10 exposures)	3 weeks (15 exposures)	5 weeks (25 exposures)
Small fields							
10	2,000	2,750	3,500	3,750	5,000	5,500	6,000
50	1,750	2,500	3,250	3,500	4,500	5,000	5,500
Medium fields							
100	1,500	2,000	2,500	2,750	3,750	4,250	5,000
150	1,250	1,750	2,250	2,500	3,250	3,750	4,500
Large fields							
200	1,000	1,500	2,000	2,250	3,000	3,500	4,250
300	Not recommended	Not recommended	Not recommended	2,000	2,750	3,250	4,000

Source: Data from Mendenhall WM, Million RR, Mancuso AA, Cassisi NJ, Flowers FP. Carcinoma of the skin. In: Million RR, Cassis NJ, editors. *Management of Head and Neck Cancer: A Multidisciplinary Approach*. Philadelphia: J.B. Lippincott Company, 1994: 643–691

The total doses listed are administered over a treatment course of the indicated length, divided into the indicated number of fractional treatments

Table 6 Local tumor control with radiotherapy according to size, cell type, and presentation [23]

Size (cm)	Basal cell, previously untreated (%)	Basal cell, recurrent (%)	Squamous cell, previously untreated (%)	Squamous cell, recurrent (%)
≤1	64/66 (97)	22/23 (96)	11/11 (100)	10/12 (83)
1.1–3	71/75 (95)	27/36 (75)	19/21 (90)	7/13 (54)
3.1–5	11/13 (85)	7/9 (78)	7/8 (88)	6/9 (67)
>5	12/13 (92)	1/2 (50)	3/5 (60)	6/11 (55)
Size not specified	4/4 (100)	1/1 (100)	0/1 (0)	4/6 (67)
Total	162/171 (95)	58/71 (82)	40/46 (87)	33/51 (65)

From Mallinckrodt Institute of Radiology, St. Louis, Mo. Data from Lovett RD, Perez CA, Shapiro DL, Garcia DM. External irradiation of epithelial skin cancer. *Int J Radiat Oncol Biol Phys* 1990; 19:235–42

Table 7 Local control rates according to external-beam technique (339 patients) [23][a,b]

	Size			
Modality	≤1 cm (%)	1.1–5 cm (%)	>5 cm (%)	Not specified (%)
Basal cell carcinoma				
Superficial X-ray	69/71 (97)	84/90 (93)	4/4 (100)	3/3 (100)
Electron beam	11/12 (92)	16/22 (73)	4/5 (80)	1/1 (100)
Combination	5/5 (100)	13/16 (81)	5/6 (83)	0/0
Photons (1.2–4 MV)	1/1 (100)	3/5 (60)	0/0	1/1 (100)
Squamous cell carcinoma				
Superficial X-ray	12/12 (100)	10/11 (91)	1/1 (100)	0/0
Electron beam	3/4 (75)	7/10 (70)	3/4 (75)	0/1 (0)
Combination	4/5 (80)	19/26 (73)	4/8 (50)	2/4 (50)
Photons (1.2–4 MV)	2/2 (100)	3/4 (75)	1/3 (33)	2/2 (100)

[a]From Mallinckrodt Institute of Radiology, St. Louis, MO. Data from Lovett RD, Perez CA, Shapiro DL, Garcia DM. External irradiation of epithelial skin cancer. *Int J Radiat Oncol Biol Phys* 1990; 19:235–242

[b]Significance levels: basal cell carcinoma, 1.1–5 cm, superficial X-ray (84/90) vs. electron beam/combination (29/38), $P = 0.013$; squamous cell carcinoma ≤1 cm, superficial X-ray (12/12) vs. electron beam/combination (7/9), $P = 0.17$; squamous cell carcinoma, 1.1–5 cm, superficial X-ray (10/11) vs. electron beam/combination (26/36), $P = 0.41$

median of 82 months (Table 8) [20]. Patients were usually treated at 5 Gy per fraction. The incidence of soft-tissue necrosis was 6.3 %; 83 % healed with conservative treatment.

Al-Othman et al. [1] reported on 85 patients with 88 clinical T4 SCCs (37), BCCs (41), and metatypical BCCs (10) treated with definitive RT at the University of Florida between 1964 and 1997. Forty-three lesions were previously untreated and 45 cancers were recurrent after prior surgery. The 5-year outcomes were as follows: local control, 53 %; ultimate local control, 90 %; regional control, 93 %; ultimate regional control, 100 %; distant metastasis-free survival, 95 %; cause-specific survival, 76 %; and overall survival, 56 %. Thirteen (15 %) of 85 patients developed a severe treatment-related complication.

The results of treatment for patients with PNI are described in another chapter.

Table 8 Raw and cumulative recurrence rates of BCCs and SCCs after soft X-ray therapy [20]

	Recurrence rates (%)				
			Cumulative after		
Tumor	Number	Raw	5 years	10 years	15 years
BCCs and SCCs, total[a]	1,267	5.1	4.7	6.9	7.4
BCCs, total	1,019	4.5	4.2	6.1	6.1
T1[b]	615	2.4[c]	3.9	4.7	4.7
T2[b]	366	5.2[c]	4.2	8.6	8.6
T3[b]	22	9.1[c]	11.4	11.4	
Previously untreated (primary)	964	4.4	4.2	5.7	5.7
Previously treated and recurrent	55	7.3	4.3	13.2	13.2
SCCs, total	245	6.9	6.0	10.5	12.8
Tis[b]	13	7.7[d]	11.1		
T1[b]	79	1.3[d]	1.7	1.7	1.7
T2[b]	138	8.7[d]	7.4	14.2	19.0
T3[b]	14	21.4[d]	25.9	25.9	
Previously untreated (primary)	233	6.4	5.8	9.6	12.0
Previously untreated and recurrent	12	16.7	30.0	30.0	

Source: Data from Schulte KW, Lippold A, Auras C et al. Soft x-ray therapy for cutaneous basal cell and squamous cell carcinomas. *J Am Acad Dermatol* 2005; 53(6):993–1001

[a]Including three patients with combinations of BCCs and SCCs

[b]Multiple (>1) tumors in same irradiated field were excluded

[c]Differences of the raw recurrence rate of BCCs Tis-T3 were statistically significant (X^2, 6.99; $P<0.05$)

[d]Differences of the raw recurrence rate of SCCs Tis-T3 were statistically significant (X^2, 9.13; $P<0.05$)

Regional Nodes

Veness and colleagues [15] reported on 167 patients treated at Westmead Hospital (Sydney, Australia) between 1980 and 2000 for cutaneous SCCs metastatic to the parotid and/or cervical nodes. Twenty-one patients (13 %) were treated with surgery alone and the remainder received surgery and adjuvant RT. The median time to recurrence after treatment was 8 months. The 5-year local-regional recurrence and disease-free survival rates were as follows: surgery and RT, 20 % and 73 %; and surgery alone, 43 % and 54 %, respectively. Multivariate analysis revealed that multiple positive nodes and treatment with surgery alone were significantly associated with decreased survival.

Hinerman et al. [14] reported on 117 patients with 121 clinically positive parotids treated at the University of Florida between 1969 and 2005. Patients were treated with preoperative RT and surgery (17 parotids), surgery and postoperative RT (87 parotids), and RT alone (17 parotids). The 5-year outcomes were as follows: local (parotid) control, 78 %; local-regional control, 74 %; distant metastasis-free survival, 92 %; disease-free survival, 70 %; and overall survival, 54 %. The 5-year local-regional control rate was 83 % after surgery and postoperative RT vs. 59 % after preoperative RT and surgery, and 47 % after RT alone. Three (3 %) patients developed severe complications.

Conclusion

Definitive RT is useful for treating early-stage skin cancers in locations where resection would result in a significant cosmetic and/or functional deficit. Postoperative RT is indicated for patients in which the probability of residual disease after surgery is high, and the likelihood of successful salvage is modest. Patients with parotid-node metastases are optimally treated with surgery and adjuvant RT. In general, it is desirable to avoid irradiating young patients because the late effects of RT progress with time and may, over the course of several years, result in a suboptimal cosmetic outcome. The likelihood of an irradiation-induced malignancy is likely less than 1 % with a latency period of 7–10 years or more. Nevertheless, this is an additional reason to select surgery rather than RT, depending upon the situation.

References

1. Al-Othman MO, Mendenhall WM, Amdur RJ. Radiotherapy alone for clinical T4 skin carcinoma of the head and neck with surgery reserved for salvage. Am J Otolaryngol. 2001;22(6):387–90.
2. Petsuksiri J, Frank SJ, Garden AS, Ang KK, Morrison WH, Chao KS, et al. Outcomes after radiotherapy for squamous cell carcinoma of the eyelid. Cancer. 2008;112(1):111–8.
3. Schlienger P, Brunin F, Desjardins L, Laurent M, Haye C, Vilcoq JR. External radiotherapy for carcinoma of the eyelid: report of 850 cases treated. Int J Radiat Oncol Biol Phys. 1996;34(2):277–87.
4. Griep C, Davelaar J, Scholten AN, Chin A, Leer JW. Electron beam therapy is not inferior to superficial x-ray therapy in the treatment of skin carcinoma. Int J Radiat Oncol Biol Phys. 1995;32(5):1347–50.
5. Kwan W, Wilson D, Moravan V. Radiotherapy for locally advanced basal cell and squamous cell carcinomas of the skin. Int J Radiat Oncol Biol Phys. 2004;60(2):406–11.
6. Caccialanza M, Piccinno R, Kolesnikova L, Gnecchi L. Radiotherapy of skin carcinomas of the pinna: a study of 115 lesions in 108 patients. Int J Dermatol. 2005;44(6):513–7.
7. Rio E, Bardet E, Ferron C, Peuvrel P, Supiot S, Campion L, et al. Interstitial brachytherapy of periorificial skin carcinomas of the face: a retrospective study of 97 cases. Int J Radiat Oncol Biol Phys. 2005;63(3):753–7.
8. Hernandez-Machin B, Borrego L, Gil-Garcia M, Hernandez BH. Office-based radiation therapy for cutaneous carcinoma: evaluation of 710 treatments. Int J Dermatol. 2007;46(5):453–9.
9. Ashby MA, Smith J, Ainslie J, McEwan L. Treatment of nonmelanoma skin cancer at a large Australian center. Cancer. 1989;63(9):1863–71.
10. Silva JJ, Tsang RW, Panzarella T, Levin W, Wells W. Results of radiotherapy for epithelial skin cancer of the pinna: the Princess Margaret Hospital experience, 1982–1993. Int J Radiat Oncol Biol Phys. 2000;47(2):451–9.
11. American Joint Committee on Cancer, editor. Cutaneous squamous cell carcinoma and other cutaneous carcinomas. In: AJCC cancer staging manual. 7th ed. Chicago, IL: Springer; 2010. p. 371–2.
12. Mendenhall WM, Amdur RJ, Hinerman RW, Werning JW, Malyapa RS, Villaret DB, et al. Skin cancer of the head and neck with perineural invasion. Am J Clin Oncol. 2007;30(1):93–6.
13. Andruchow JL, Veness MJ, Morgan GJ, Gao K, Clifford A, Shannon KF, et al. Implications for clinical staging of metastatic cutaneous squamous carcinoma of the head and neck based on a multicenter study of treatment outcomes. Cancer. 2006;106(5):1078–83.

14. Hinerman RW, Indelicato DJ, Amdur RJ, Morris CG, Werning JW, Vaysberg M, et al. Cutaneous squamous cell carcinoma metastatic to parotid-area lymph nodes. Laryngoscope. 2008;118(11):1989–96.
15. Veness MJ, Morgan GJ, Palme CE, Gebski V. Surgery and adjuvant radiotherapy in patients with cutaneous head and neck squamous cell carcinoma metastatic to lymph nodes: combined treatment should be considered best practice. Laryngoscope. 2005;115(5):870–5.
16. Iyer NG, Clark JR, Murali R, Gao K, O'Brien CJ. Outcomes following parotidectomy for metastatic squamous cell carcinoma with microscopic residual disease: implications for facial nerve preservation. Head Neck. 2009;31(1):21–7.
17. Ch'ng S, Maitra A, Allison RS, Chaplin JM, Gregor RT, Lea R, et al. Parotid and cervical nodal status predict prognosis for patients with head and neck metastatic cutaneous squamous cell carcinoma. J Surg Oncol. 2008;98(2):101–5.
18. Amdur RJ, Kalbaugh KJ, Ewald LM, Parsons JT, Mendenhall WM, Bova FJ, et al. Radiation therapy for skin cancer near the eye: kilovoltage x-rays versus electrons. Int J Radiat Oncol Biol Phys. 1992;23(4):769–79.
19. Bhandare N, Monroe AT, Morris CG, Bhatti MT, Mendenhall WM. Does altered fractionation influence the risk of radiation-induced optic neuropathy? Int J Radiat Oncol Biol Phys. 2005;62(4):1070–7.
20. Schulte KW, Lippold A, Auras C, Bramkamp G, Breitkopf C, Elsmann HJ, et al. Soft x-ray therapy for cutaneous basal cell and squamous cell carcinomas. J Am Acad Dermatol. 2005;53(6):993–1001.
21. Mendenhall WM, Kalbaugh KJ, Mendenhall NP, Parsons JT. Radiotherapy as definitive treatment and as a surgical adjunct. In: Weber RS, Miller MJ, Goepfert H, editors. Basal and squamous cell skin cancers of the head and neck. Baltimore: Williams & Wilkins; 1996. p. 331–50.
22. Mendenhall WM, Million RR, Mancuso AA, Cassisi NJ, Flowers FP. Carcinoma of the skin. In: Million RR, Cassisi NJ, editors. Management of head and neck cancer: a multidisciplinary approach. Philadelphia: J. B. Lippincott; 1994. p. 643–91.
23. Lovett RD, Perez CA, Shapiro SJ, Garcia DM. External irradiation of epithelial skin cancer. Int J Radiat Oncol Biol Phys. 1990;19(2):235–42.

Brachytherapy

Rosalind Sandell and Murad Alam

Abbreviations

BCC	Basal cell carcinoma
Cs	Cesium
HDR	High-dose rate
I	Iodine
Ir	Iridium
LDR	Low-dose rate
MDR	Medium-dose rate
NMSC	Nonmelanoma skin cancer
SCC	Squamous cell carcinoma

Introduction

Brachytherapy, derived from the Greek word "brachy" or short distance, involves placement of radioactive sources directly onto or into target tissues [1]. The origins of this treatment modality, which dates back to the discovery of radium, are dermatological, as initial experiments occurred on human skin with the goal of treating various skin diseases and malignancies [2, 3]. Although brachytherapy fell out of favor as a modality for the treatment of skin lesions by the mid-1940s, it has continued to serve as an important alternative for skin cancer management despite

R. Sandell, BA
Loyola University Chicago Stritch School of Medicine, Maywood, IL, USA

M. Alam, MD, MSCI (✉)
Department of Dermatology, Northwestern University Feinberg School of Medicine, Chicago, IL, USA
e-mail: m-alam@northwestern.edu

A.B. Cognetta and W.M. Mendenhall (eds.), *Radiation Therapy for Skin Cancer*, DOI 10.1007/978-1-4614-6986-5_13, © Springer Science+Business Media New York 2013

challenges to its survival from surgery and other treatment modalities. Today, brachytherapy remains an appropriate and effective option for selected patients with specific skin cancer lesions, most notably nonmelanoma skin cancers (NMSCs) that are not better served by surgical removal or non-radiotherapy local destruction [1]. The following chapter will review the historical use of brachytherapy in dermatology, technical aspects of administration, and current use, including efficacy, cosmesis, and adverse events.

Historical Use in Dermatology

Brachytherapy has been used to treat skin conditions since the discovery of radium by French physicists Marie and Pierre Curie in 1898 [1, 4]. The first described self-exposure experiments involving close contact between radium and human skin occurred in 1900, initially by two Germans, Friedrich Walkoff and Friedrich Giesel, and then by Pierre Curie and his associate Henri Becquerel. Curie wrapped a sample of radium salts in a thin rubber covering and applied this to an area of his forearm for 10 h. He studied the wound, which resembled a burn, for weeks, and after 52 days a permanent gray scar remained [3].

The results of this and other self-exposure experiments amongst himself and colleagues led Curie to loan radium to Henri Danlos, a dermatologist at the Hôpital St-Louis in Paris [3]. Danlos and Bloch subsequently performed the first medical radium treatment on a patient in 1901, which involved local application of a sealed radium source to the nonmalignant skin condition cutaneous lupus erythematosus. In St. Petersburg in 1903, the first histologically confirmed skin cancers were successfully treated using the same approach. In 1909, Forssel noted that a short single application of beta-emitting radium directly on a cavernous hemangioma initiated a healing process similar to that of spontaneous regression without leaving a visible scar, and the use of Forssel's technique for the treatment of cavernous hemangiomas was subsequently documented into the late 1950s [5]. Implantation of radium tubes directly into sarcomas and carcinomas was first used in 1910 by Abbe, heralding the advent of what is now known as interstitial brachytherapy [2].

Of the various dermatologic applications for brachytherapy that were attempted at the turn of the twentieth century, the area that received the most focus over time was treatment of skin cancer. Early on, use of radium was limited to a few major institutions and relatively few specialists in private practice due to a lack of access to radium and prohibitive costs. However, by the late 1920s it became possible for any practitioner to either rent or purchase both radium and radon for in-office use. Dermatologists and radiologists had the ability to order any amount of radium salt or radon in applicators of various sizes, shapes, and forms, including plaques, tubes, needles, and seeds, which were then delivered directly to the physician's office. Despite its increased cost, radon gas was often preferred over radium element due to the smaller size of radon emanation tubes and the increased versatility of radon applicators; however, both radon and radium were used frequently [6].

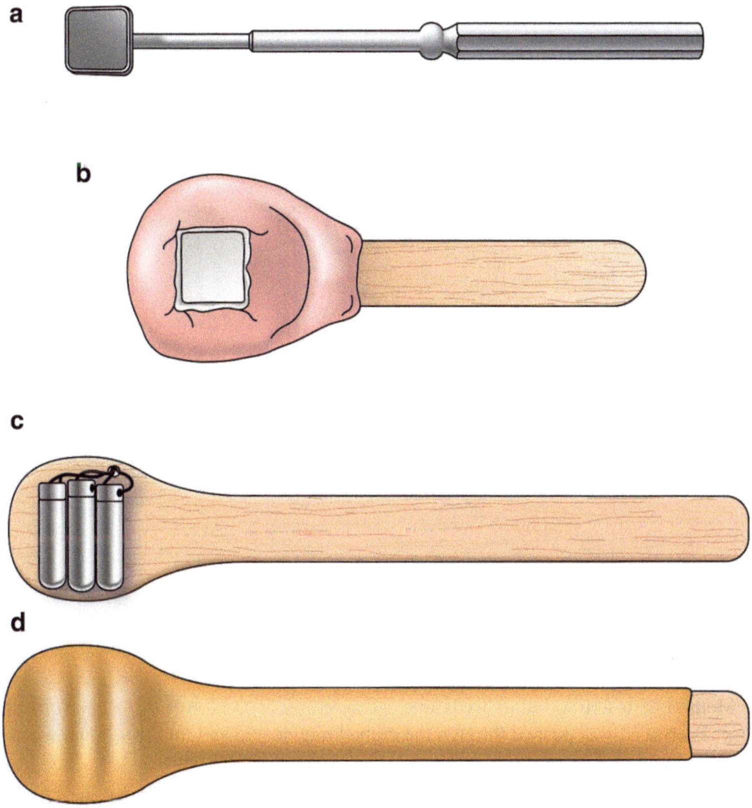

Fig. 1 Several devices used to create a plane radiating surface for cutaneous and mucosal lesions. Each type of applicator could differ in size, shape, and radium content depending on the lesion being treated [6]. (**a**) Flat radium applicator with removable handle attached to a radium plaque. (**b**) Flat radium applicator embedded in dental compound and arranged for treatment of a lesion on the dorsal surface of the tongue. (**c**) Three tubular applicators attached to a flat wooden device. Tubular applicators could be filled with radium or radon gas. (**d**) Same as part (**c**), covered in heavy rubber. Filtration of this device was achieved by applying a thin metallic screen to the tubes and then covering the device with rubber to remove secondary rays

Filtration, or screening, of the very "soft" beta rays emitted from all applicators was standard practice in order to avoid severe superficial tissue reactions. Very thin screens of various metals and rubber were employed for this purpose (Fig. 1c, d). Special techniques and instruments were also developed to enhance operator safety and avoid direct contact between practitioners' hands and the radioactive applicators, since the potential adverse effects of handling radium were well known by this time [6].

Modern interstitial and surface-mold brachytherapy techniques, which will be discussed in a later section, have been modeled after techniques that were developed and used successfully during this period. For easily accessible lesions that

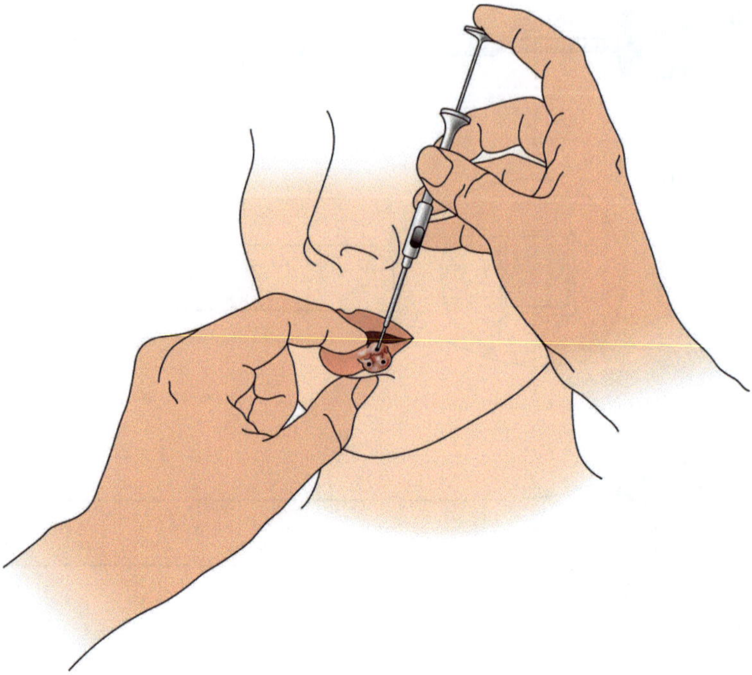

Fig. 2 Method of inserting radon seeds into a carcinoma of the lower lip, as performed in the 1920s [6]. Each seed was pushed through the embedding needle and into the tissue, where it was left permanently in situ

warranted superficial therapy, radium plaques, radium tubes, or radon tubes were applied directly to the tumor or a short distance from it using a variety of devices. For irregular or inaccessible cutaneous or mucosal lesions, it was customary to make a mold or cast of the tumor lesion using dental compound. Either radium element applicators or radon emanation tubes were then applied to this mold, creating a plane radiating surface directly over the tumor (Fig. 1). Where intralesional (interstitial) therapy was indicated, tiny glass or gold radon seeds were most often permanently implanted into malignant tissue (Fig. 2) [6]. After about 1930 radium puncture became the preferred technique, in which 2–7 radium needles loaded with 5–10 mg of radium were applied to the surface of the tumor at intervals of 5 mm for 4–5 h. At that time, the 10-year control rates with direct contact therapy and radium puncture were reported to be 73.8 % and 84 %, respectively [1].

However, despite the growth and advancement of brachytherapy techniques during this period, by the mid-1940s the popularity of brachytherapy as a modality for the treatment of skin lesions began to decline as it was gradually replaced by X-ray therapy [7, 8]. X-rays had become easier and more convenient to employ and at least as equally efficient as radium in the majority of cases. In the following decades, brachytherapy continued to be utilized in dermatology, but the indications became much more limited. It remained the treatment of choice for areas that poorly tolerate irradiation such as the dorsum of the hand and foot, as well as for patients who were unable to leave their homes for treatment, but it lost ground in most other areas [8].

Notably though, the field of brachytherapy has continued to advance, primarily because it has remained a preferred treatment modality for other types of malignancies [9]. After World War II, many new artificial radionuclides became available, most notably cesium-137 (^{137}Cs), iridium-192 (^{192}Ir), and iodine-125 (^{125}I), which carried certain advantages over radium [2, 10]. In addition, since the mid-1960s, radioactive sources are no longer implanted directly into the patient for safety reasons. This practice exposed the radiation oncologist and staff to unacceptable levels of irradiation, so instead nonradioactive applicators such as tubes or catheters are first implanted into the target site, and then radioactive sources are "afterloaded" into this apparatus. In the 1970s, manual afterloading was replaced by remote afterloading, which allows the operator to remain in a shielded site and eliminates all exposure for medical personnel [1, 10]. Later, high-dose-rate (HDR) units were introduced as opposed to the already widely used low-dose-rate (LDR) units. HDR permits the radioactive source to be removed between treatments, making short sessions of irradiation possible on an outpatient basis, without any undue risk of irradiation to the patient or medical staff [2]. More recently, brachytherapy has significantly benefited from further studies regarding dosimetry as well as the use of advanced imaging technologies, which have enabled optimization of treatment planning, dose distribution, and clinical outcomes [9, 10].

Today, brachytherapy is a mainstay of treatment for prostate, breast, cervical, endometrial, and certain head and neck cancers [1, 9]. Teletherapy, also called external beam radiation (see Chap. 12), remains the most commonly used radiation modality for skin cancer in the United States [11, 12], but brachytherapy continues to be a widely accepted treatment option for specific nonmelanoma skin cancer lesions. Furthermore, due to the important recent advances in the field mentioned above, brachytherapy has been gaining popularity again [13], and use for skin cancers is gradually increasing worldwide [14].

Technical Aspects

Brachytherapy has consistently provided a highly conformal radiation therapy modality vs. other radiation methods [9]. Because all brachytherapy techniques involve placement into or onto the target tissue, the normal tissue outside the radiation zone receives a negligible radiation dose. This minimizes unwanted dose delivery to nearby radiation-sensitive tissues such as the brain or bone, and ensures the best chance of prompt healing and the smallest chance of late radiation morbidity. Thus, brachytherapy can be performed on the scalp and other areas of the body where traditional external radiotherapy may be less safe [1].

Modes of Administration

In modern brachytherapy, placement of the radioactive source may be on the body surface (surface-mold technique), into body tissues (interstitial), into a body cavity (intracavity), or across a tissue boundary into a contained space (transluminal) [1]. Both the surface-mold technique and interstitial brachytherapy have been used in the treatment of skin cancer.

The surface-mold technique utilizes custom molds that are created from impressions of the tumor surface. Molds are constructed from pliable materials, such as silicone or polymethyl-methacrylate, and are then fitted with radioactive isotopes and applied directly to the tumor [15]. Radioactive sources are loaded into the mold in such a way as to distribute uniform dosage throughout the tumor volume. Surface-mold brachytherapy is most often used for the treatment of well-circumscribed, superficial tumors [1].

Interstitial brachytherapy constitutes an invasive means of internal radiation therapy in which radioactive wires or seeds are placed directly within the tissue at the target site. Interstitial brachytherapy is well suited for certain areas, such as the eyelid, where the creation of the precise surface mold required for surface-mold brachytherapy is technically unfeasible [1].

Radiation Source and Dose Delivery

Interstitial brachytherapy implants may be permanent or temporary [16]. Permanent brachytherapy implants emit radiation at very-LDR that is equivalent to less than 0.4 Gy/h for the lifetime of the radioactive isotope. Typically, ^{125}I is utilized in permanent implants because of its emission of relatively low mean energies [1].

On the other hand, temporary implants are associated with greater variation in dose rates (Table 1). LDR implants deliver 0.4–2 Gy/h over durations from 24 to 144 h in an inpatient setting. Medium-dose-rate (MDR) devices deliver 2–12 Gy/h and HDR devices deliver greater than 12 Gy/h [17]. The most commonly used isotope for temporary implantation is ^{192}Ir. ^{192}Ir has a half-life of 74.2 days and emits γ rays with a mean energy of 380 keV. Other γ-emitting isotopes used for temporary implantation include cobalt and cesium, especially in the past [1].

Surface-mold brachytherapy is often delivered using HDR units, but has also been studied using LDR units. ^{125}I has been used for LDR surface-mold brachytherapy, while most studies on HDR surface-mold brachytherapy have evaluated the use of the γ-emitting ^{192}Ir [1]. Notably, at least two studies on surface-mold brachytherapy have explored the use of a mixed β-γ isotope, either rhenium-188 or holmium-166 [18, 19].

A single treatment of LDR brachytherapy can span 3–5 days, requiring hospitalization for the patient and radiation protection for individuals who are in contact with the patient for the duration of treatment. Alternatively, a HDR brachytherapy treatment can be completed in 1–30 min, usually in the outpatient setting. However,

Table 1 Comparison of dose delivery with common brachytherapy techniques

	LDR ^{192}Ir	MDR	HDR
Dose rate	Low	Medium	High
Duration per treatment	2–6 days	1 day	Minutes
Duration of treatment course	2–6 days	1 day	3–5 weeks
Availability (internationally)	++	–	–
Ease of optimization	–	–	+
Dose per treatment, Gy	60	40	0.18–0.7[a]
No. of fractions	1	1	7–35
Total dose as sole modality, Gy	60	40	35–50[a]

Adapted from J Am Acad Dermatol, 65(2), Alam M, Nanda S, Mittal BB, Kim NA, Yoo S, The use of brachytherapy in the treatment of nonmelanoma skin cancer: A review, 377–88, Copyright 2011, with permission from Elsevier

HDR high-dose rate; *Ir* iridium; *LDR* low-dose rate; *MDR* medium-dose rate

[a]Common regimens may include 20–35 fractions of 180–200 cGy each in daily or twice-daily treatments; 5 fractions of 700 cGy for total dose of 35 Gy; or 10 fractions of 500 cGy for total dose of 50 Gy

HDR brachytherapy is more likely to cause damage to surrounding healthy tissue than is LDR therapy. To prevent such complications, the total dose of HDR brachytherapy is commonly divided into a few or as many as 30–40 sessions, occurring every 1–28 days [1].

Operator Safety

As with all radiotherapy techniques, brachytherapy involves potential risks of radiation exposure to medical personnel involved in treatment. LDR is associated with secondary radiation risk because the duration of treatment is extended for days, and HDR is associated with radiation risk because the radiation source is of high intensity. As mentioned above, remote afterloading techniques are often used to enhance operator safety. Afterloading allows nonradioactive implantation devices, such as flexible plastic or stiff guiding metal tubes, to be placed within the tumor first, and then radioactive sources can be mechanically loaded through these tubes or catheters remotely [1, 2, 10].

Selected Studies Regarding the Use of Brachytherapy

Surface-Mold Brachytherapy

LDR surface-mold brachytherapy has been studied in retrospective studies and case series evaluating the treatment of NMSCs of the face and eyelid (Table 2). In one retrospective case–control study, the cosmetic outcome was compared for 15

Table 2 Summary of previous studies of brachytherapy for nonmelanoma skin cancer

Study	Site studied	Lesion type	Modality	Treatment time	Dosage (cGy)/ fractions	Follow-up (mo)	Recurrence rate
Avril et al. [27]	Face	BCC (347)	LDR interstitial	165 h	5,700–9,600/1	48	8/95
Berridge and Morgan [20]	Face	BCC (30/30)	LDR surface mold	168 h	6,000–6,500/1	120 (minimum)	Unknown
Conill et al. [30]	Eyelid	SCC (4/24) BCC (19/24) Adenocarcinoma (1/24)	LDR interstitial	54–55 h (total)	4,000	43 (mean)	2/24
Conill et al. [29]	Lip	SCC (52/54) BCC (2/54)	LDR interstitial	86 h	6,000–6,500/1	96 (mean)	2/54
Debois [24]	Nose	Epidermoid (60/370) BCC (300/370) Other (10/370)	HDR surface mold	48 h (total)	2,400	>36	11/368
Guix et al. [22]	Face	SCC (34/136)	HDR surface mold (117/136)	3–8 min/ session	6,000–6,500/33–36 (<4 cm)	60	3/136
		BCC (102/136)	HDR Brock applicator (19/136)		7,500–8,000/10 (>4 cm)		
Lee et al. [19]	Various	SCC (3/5) BCC (1/5) Bowen (1/5)	HDR surface patch	30 min–1 h (total)	5,000	8–20	0/5
Ozyar and Gurdalli [26]	Scalp	BCC (1/1)	HDR surface mold	Not stated	4,050/multiple	72	0
Rio et al. [28]	Face	SCC (88/97) BCC (9/97)	LDR interstitial	74–79 h	5,000–6,500	55 (median)	10/97
Rudoltz et al. [25]	Forearm, back of hand	SCC (1/1)	HDR surface mold	30 min/ session	6,000/30	7	0
Sedda et al. [18]	Various	SCC (37/53) BCC (16/53)	HDR surface resin	15 min–2 h/ session	4,000–6,000/1–3	51 (mean)	0/53

Semrau et al. [34]	Scalp	SCC (1/1)	HDR surface mold	Not stated	6,600/>33	24	0
Shields et al. [21]	Eyelid	BCC (2/8) Adenoid cystic carcinoma (4/8) Conjunctival melanoma (1/8) Metastatic carcinoma (1/8)	LDR plaque	96 h	5,000/1	24 (BCC only)	0/2
Somanchi et al. [32]	Back of hand, fingers	SCC (25/25)	HDR surface mold	Not stated	4,000–4,500/8	60 (mean)	1/25
Svoboda et al. [23]	Various	Metastases (10/106) Bowen (9/106) SCC (11/106) BCC (76/106)	HDR surface mold	Up to 5 min/session	1,200–5,000/1–15	9.6 (mean)	4/106

Adapted from J Am Acad Dermatol, 65(2), Alam M, Nanda S, Mittal BB, Kim NA, Yoo S, The use of brachytherapy in the treatment of nonmelanoma skin cancer: A review, 377–88, Copyright 2011, with permission from Elsevier

BCC basal cell carcinoma; *HDR* high-dose rate; *LDR* low-dose rate; *SCC* squamous cell carcinoma patients treated for basal cell carcinoma (BCC) of the face using gold grain Elastoplast molds (Beiersdorf, Birmingham, England) and 15 patients treated for the same indication using fractionated superficial X-ray [20]. The brachytherapy arm tumors received total doses of 60–65 Gy during a 7-day application, and all of the case and control tumors had been treated over 10 years prior. Long-term cosmesis was observed to be superior in the brachytherapy group. This result was attributed to the rapid decrease in brachytherapy radiation dose beyond the superficial tissues. It was also hypothesized that X-ray treatment may be relatively more likely to induce very late skin and subcutis adverse effects than brachytherapy [1]. One case series described the treatment of several eyelid tumors, including two neglected BCCs on the verge of orbital invasion [21]. LDR brachytherapy was applied using a 15-mm diameter gold shield to which an ^{125}I plaque was affixed on the exterior (eyelid side). The shield served to protect the globe while permitting irradiation of the target eyelid lesion with 50 Gy to a 5 mm depth.

High-dose rate surface-mold brachytherapy has been studied in prospective and retrospective cohort studies and case reports investigating its use on NMSCs located in areas such as the nose, eyelid, ear, and back of the hands. These areas were chosen either because they are difficult to treat surgically or because they would benefit from the ability of brachytherapy to confine radiation to a superficial treatment area [1]. A series of prospective cohort studies evaluating the efficacy of NMSC treatment with ^{192}Ir HDR surface-mold brachytherapy demonstrated good posttreatment cosmesis and low recurrence rates up to 5 years later. Relatively smaller lesions were associated with higher rates of tumor control and more favorable cosmesis compared to larger lesions. Furthermore, Guix et al. [22] used HDR surface-mold brachytherapy to irradiate 136 patients with primary and recurrent facial NMSCs, noting a 5-year remission rate of 99 % for primary tumors ($n=73$) and 87 % for recurrent lesions ($n=63$). Notably, serial biopsies and skin examinations were not performed to confirm these remission rates. Additionally, this study reported adequate dose distribution to depths of 5 mm, although these results have not been replicated. Cosmesis was assessed by subjective and objective measurements, including the absence of edema, alopecia, hypopigmentation, hyperpigmentation, fibrosis, scars, telangiectasia, and late effects on normal tissue, at 6 and 12 months. Out of 136 patients, 133 were reported to have favorable cosmetic outcomes, defined as minimal to no treatment sequelae at the 6-month follow-up visit. The remaining 3 patients, all of whom had initial cancer lesions larger than 4 cm, experienced radiation necrosis in normal tissue [1]. The extent to which normal tissue had been damaged was not specified [1, 22]. In a study by Svoboda et al. [23], 96 primary skin neoplasms (9 Bowen disease, 11 squamous cell carcinomas (SCCs), 76 BCCs) at various locations were treated using HDR surface-mold brachytherapy. Results indicated tumor regression without recurrence in all but four cases. Each of the four recurrent cases was a BCC with initial diameter greater than 2 cm and a depth greater than 3 mm.

HDR surface-mold brachytherapy has also been associated with low rates of recurrence and good cosmesis in studies of NMSC at functionally and cosmetically important anatomic sites, such as the nose and hand. Debois [24] used ^{137}Cs surface-mold brachytherapy on 370 primary lesions, the vast majority of which were BCC, of the nose. The reported recurrence rate at 3 years was 3 % (11/368), although this may have been an underestimate due to possible ascertainment bias and lack of additional follow-up [1]. In contrast to most other studies, this study reported more recurrences in tumors of smaller diameter (<2 cm) [22, 23]. This atypical outcome may have been a result of the overwhelming preponderance of small tumors (87 %) included in the study rather than any inherent increased risk of recurrence for the smaller tumors. Also, the authors did not characterize the subtype of treated BCCs, therefore it is not clear to what extent recurrence may have been associated with tumor subtype rather than size. Another site-specific study used HDR surface-mold brachytherapy to treat 25 patients for SCC on the back of the hand. There were one case of recurrence and one case of radiation necrosis, the latter resulting from treatment of a large tumor. Functional outcomes including grip strength, joint mobility, fine touch, and two-point discrimination were not found to be significantly different between treated and nontreated hands. As with previously discussed studies, these suggest that HDR brachytherapy can induce prolonged remission with few peripheral tissue effects in relatively small, well-demarcated NMSC, although long-term cure was not shown and objective or unbiased measures of cosmesis remain lacking [1, 22].

Another application for which HDR surface-mold brachytherapy has been utilized is for multiple, recurrent NMSC tumors with extensive and irregular surface areas. One case report demonstrated successful treatment without recurrence of multiple recurrent SCCs on the forearm of a patient [25], and two case reports successfully utilized surface-mold helmets for SCCs [16] and BCCs [26] on the scalp. Erythema, ulceration, moist desquamation, or bleeding were reported, but follow-up revealed no short-term recurrence, providing some evidence for the efficacy of HDR brachytherapy on extensive, recurrent lesions [1].

Lastly, at least two studies have evaluated HDR brachytherapy using β-emitting isotopes, which may pose less risk to neighboring normal tissue [21] and usually requires only 1–3 treatment visits vs. many more with γ-emitters [22]. In one study using rhenium-188 [18], 43 of 53 patients with recurrent NMSCs required only one treatment, whereas the remaining patients with thicker lesions needed up to three treatments each. Mean dose decreased from 120 Gy to less than 20 Gy at depths greater than 2 mm, and it is not known why some deeper tumors regressed, or whether this represented true regression or superficial regression with residual deep tumor. A study of 5 patients treated with holmium-166 showed that radiation dosage at depths of 2 mm and deeper was inadequate for treatment of NMSCs [19]. Because of the small number of studies on β-emitting isotopes, their efficacy in the treatment of NMSC remains unclear [1].

Interstitial Brachytherapy

The efficacy of interstitial brachytherapy on NMSC has been evaluated primarily through one randomized controlled trial (RCT), as well as additional prospective and retrospective cohort studies evaluating facial lesions (Table 2). The RCT [27] compared treatment efficacy and cosmetic outcomes between radiotherapy and surgery for the treatment of primary BCC. In this trial, 174 patients were assigned to surgery, and another 173 patients were assigned to radiotherapy. Approximately 55 % of these 173 were assigned to interstitial LDR brachytherapy with 57–76 Gy total dose delivered over a mean of 6.9 days. Four-year recurrence rates were 0.7 % for surgery and 8.8 % for brachytherapy (95 % confidence intervals: 0.1–3.9 % and 4.3–17.1 %, respectively). Good cosmesis was achieved in 87 % of patients treated with surgery and 69 % of patients treated with radiation [27].

In addition, a controlled, retrospective cohort study of 88 BCCs and 9 SCCs of the nose, periorbital area, and ear compared interstitial LDR brachytherapy for patients who were previously untreated to those who had previously received surgery. Total radiation doses were 52–55 Gy over 74–79 h. Five-year disease-free survival was 91 and 80 % in the untreated and previously treated patients, respectively [28]. Another retrospective cohort study of 52 SCCs and 2 BCCs of the lip treated with interstitial LDR brachytherapy at a mean dose of 61.5 Gy over 86.3 h reported a local control rate of 98 % at mean follow-up of 7 years [29]. This local control rate was significantly higher than that previously reported in studies of lip tumors treated with interstitial LDR brachytherapy. Lastly, a prospective cohort study of 19 primary BCCs and 4 primary SCCs of the eyelids treated with interstitial LDR brachytherapy with mean total dose of 40 Gy over 55 h demonstrated local control rate of 91.6 % at mean follow-up of 43 months, with good functional results [30].

Efficacy and Indications

The results of the above studies indicate high local remission rates following both modes of brachytherapy for NMSC at various anatomic locations. Overall, brachytherapy appears to be best suited for the treatment of small, primary NMSCs. Recurrent tumors, tumors of greater depth (>2 mm), and tumors of greater diameter (>2 cm) appear to have a higher failure rate because the inherent dosimetry constraints of brachytherapy result in a steep decline of radiation dose as depth increases [1].

With that said, the primary benefit of brachytherapy compared to other forms of radiation such as external beam radiation therapy is its ability to deliver radiation to the target tissue with less injury to surrounding healthy skin and underlying radiosensitive tissues such as the brain, eye, tendons, and bone. Therefore, brachytherapy may be a preferable radiation modality at certain anatomic sites such as large areas of the scalp, the eyelid, the hand, and very large and irregular skin areas that contain numerous NMSCs.

In addition, historically brachytherapy has been useful for skin cancers in elderly, infirm patients who are unable to tolerate surgery. It is important to note that for these patients a minimal level of functional status is probably necessary before undergoing radiation therapy of any type. However, if the patient is able to provide baseline self-care needs and is able to follow guidelines regarding radiation exposure, brachytherapy may provide a reasonable alternative to surgery.

Notably, although remission rates after brachytherapy are reported to be high, these reported control rates do not necessarily represent cures. Published studies evaluating the treatment of NMSC with brachytherapy have usually followed up patients for less than 2 years [18, 23, 25], while other studies have reported an increased risk of NMSC recurrence for up to 10 years [31]. Therefore, the long-term disease-free survival for brachytherapy remains to be established [1].

Furthermore, data is lacking regarding cure rates for the different subtypes of BCC, and of BCC vs. SCC. Additional research is warranted to clarify the extent to which this modality can effectively treat SCC, BCC, and the subtypes of BCC, as well as the extent to which it can treat large and deep tumors that are not amenable to surgery.

Tolerability, Cosmesis, and Adverse Events

Both forms of brachytherapy have been reported to be well tolerated by patients. Cosmetic and functional results for surface-mold brachytherapy have been evaluated subjectively in various studies by blinded [32] or unblinded observers [25] raters, and objective cosmetic measures have included late radiation effects such as alopecia, telangiectasia, skin atrophy, pigmentation disorders, and scarring (Table 3) [22, 28, 32]. Functional measures such as pain [28] and joint range of motion [32] have also been evaluated. Cosmetic and functional results for interstitial brachytherapy have been evaluated by a single, unblinded examiner in the few studies available, and objective measures have included skin deformity, pigmentation disorders, telangiectasia, and skin atrophy (Table 3). Overall, cosmetic and functional results have been demonstrated to be good for both modes of brachytherapy, based on these potentially biased assessments, with better results generally observed for smaller tumors [22, 28].

However, although brachytherapy has been shown to be associated with good posttreatment cosmesis, patients seeking optimal cosmesis may still elect to undergo surgical excision or Mohs micrographic surgery. It is difficult to make a definitive statement as to the relative cosmetic benefits of these treatment modalities, given the paucity of side-by-side comparisons between brachytherapy and surgical reconstruction. In one study [33], facial BCCs were randomized to surgery or radiotherapy (interstitial brachytherapy, superficial contactherapy involving delivery of low-energy dosages at close proximity to the target site, and conventional radiotherapy). Upon a 4-year follow-up, blinded, observer-rated cosmetic results were statistically superior for lesions treated with surgery for all tumor sites on the face except for the nose. Although notable, this is only a single study, and further investigation is needed.

Table 3 Adverse events reported after brachytherapy

Study	Adverse events—acute	Adverse events—long term
Avril et al. [27]	112/173 Dyspigmentation and telangiectasia	69/173 Scar 9/173 Necrosis 1/173 Cataract 1/173 Lacrimal duct stenosis[a]
Berridge and Morgan [20]	Unknown	10/15 Slight atrophy, pigmentation change, some hair loss 5/15 Patchy atrophy, moderate telangiectasia, total hair loss
Conill et al. [30]	24/24 Erythema, edema	None reported
Conill et al. [29]	54/54 Mucositis	1/54 Achromia and fibrosis
Debois [24]	Dyschromia, telangiectasia	None reported
Guix et al. [22]	136/136 Erythema 14/136 Ulceration	4/136 Radiation necrosis
Lee et al. [19]	5/5 Desquamation, erythema, or ulceration 1/5 Alopecia	None reported
Ozyar and Gurdalli [26]	None reported	None reported
Shields et al. [21]	8/8 Mild postoperative discomfort and tissue edema limits eye movement	None reported
Sedda et al. [18]	53/53 Erythema Bleeding (only large lesions)	None reported
Semrau et al. [34]	1/1 Erythema, ulceration, bleeding	None reported
Somanchi et al. [32]	25/25 Desquamation, crusting, erythema	1/25 Radiation necrosis 17/25 Skin atrophy, telangiectasia, alopecia
Svoboda et al. [23]	26/106 Moist reaction 32/106 Erythema, dry desquamation	6/53 Pigmentation changes, atrophy
Rio et al. [28]	97/97 Inflammatory exudative desquamation	4/34 Epiphora 3/34 Pruritus 1/34 Impairment of eyelid aperture
Rudoltz et al. [25]	1/1 Erythema, moist desquamation	None reported

Adapted from J Am Acad Dermatol, 65(2), Alam M, Nanda S, Mittal BB, Kim NA, Yoo S, The use of brachytherapy in the treatment of nonmelanoma skin cancer: A review, 377–88, Copyright 2011, with permission from Elsevier

[a]Adverse events for this study are for all radiotherapy patients of whom 55 % were brachytherapy patients

Local adverse events have been reported to be mild to moderate. The most common reported acute complications of surface-mold brachytherapy include erythema (77 %), desquamation (65 %), and ulceration (14 %). The most common reported acute complications of interstitial brachytherapy include inflammatory exudative desquamation (80 %), erythema (20 %), and edema (20 %). Sequelae are usually more pronounced for larger tumors, as well as for tumors that received a high total dose, a larger fractionated dose, or a higher dose rate [30].

Conclusion

Brachytherapy has played an important role in the treatment of dermatologic disease for over a century. Although its indications are relatively few in the modern age, it continues to be an effective alternate radiation modality for the treatment of certain NMSCs. Multiple factors must be taken into account when one is deciding which tumors and patients are most likely to benefit from this therapy. Although further investigation is needed in order to clarify the exact role and outcomes that brachytherapy offers in the treatment of dermatologic neoplasms, given recent advancements in the field and bolstered interest worldwide, brachytherapy's presence within the field of dermatology will likely remain for many years to come.

References

1. Alam M, Nanda S, Mittal BB, Kim NA, Yoo S. The use of brachytherapy in the treatment of nonmelanoma skin cancer: a review. J Am Acad Dermatol. 2011;65(2):377–88.
2. Bernier J, Hall EJ, Giaccia A. Radiation oncology: a century of achievements. Nat Rev Cancer. 2004;4(9):737–47.
3. Mould RF. Pierre curie, 1859–1906. Curr Oncol. 2007;14(2):74–82.
4. Kulakowski A. The contribution of Marie Sklodowska-Curie to the development of modern oncology. Anal Bioanal Chem. 2011;400(6):1583–6.
5. Furst CJ, Lundell M, Holm LE. Radiation therapy of hemangiomas, 1909–1959. Acta Oncol. 1987;26(1):33–6.
6. MacKee G. X-ray and radium in the treatment of diseases of the skin. 2nd ed. Philadelphia: Lea & Febiger; 1927.
7. Guadagnolo BA, Ang KK, Ballo MT. The skin. In: Moss WT, Brand WN, Battifora H, editors. Radiation oncology: rationale, technique and results. St. Louis: CV Mosby; 1979. p. 52–82.
8. Belisario JC. Cancer of the skin. London: Butterworth & Co; 1959.
9. Haie-Meder C, Siebert FA, Potter R. Image guided, adaptive, accelerated, high dose brachytherapy as model for advanced small volume radiotherapy. Radiother Oncol. 2011;100(3): 333–43.
10. Phillips TL. 50 years of radiation research: medicine. Radiat Res. 2002;158(4):389–417.
11. Solan MJ, Brady LW. Skin. In: Halperin EC, Perez CA, Brady LW, editors. Perez and Brady's principles and practice of radiation oncology. 5th ed. Philadelphia: Lippincott Williams & Wilkins; 2008. p. 690–701.
12. Ang KK, Weber RS. Cutaneous carcinoma. In: Gunderson LL, Tepper JE, editors. Clinical radiation oncology. 2nd ed. London: Churchill Livingstone; 2006. p. 853–63.
13. Montemaggi P, Guerrieri P, Federico M, Mortellaro G. Clinical applications of brachytherapy: low-dose-rate and pulse-dose-rate. In: Halperin EC, Perez CA, Brady LW, editors. Perez and Brady's principles and practice of radiation oncology. 5th ed. Philadelphia: Lippincott Williams & Wilkins; 2008. p. 476–539.
14. Martinez AA. Brachytherapy. In: Gunderson LL, Tepper JE, editors. Clinical radiation oncology. 2nd ed. London: Churchill Livingstone; 2006. p. 255–82.
15. Devlin PM, editor. Brachytherapy applications and techniques. Philadelphia: Lippincott Williams & Wilkins; 2007.
16. Pathi S, Dorigo O. Radiation therapy for gynecologic cancers. In: DeCherney AH, Nathan L, editors. Current diagnosis and treatment obstetrics and gynecology. 10th ed. New York: McGraw-Hill; 2007.

17. Williamson JF, Brenner DJ. Physics and biology of brachytherapy. In: Halperin EC, Perez CA, Brady LW, Halperin EC, Perez CA, Brady LW, editors. Perez and Brady's principles and practice of radiation oncology. 5th ed. Philadelphia: Lippincott Williams & Wilkins; 2008. p. 423–75.
18. Sedda A, Rossi G, Cipriani C, Carrozzo M, Donati P. Dermatological high-dose-rate brachytherapy for the treatment of basal and squamous cell carcinoma. Clin Exp Dermatol. 2008;33(6):745–9.
19. Lee JD, Park KK, Lee M, Kim E, Rhim KJ, Lee JT, et al. Radionuclide therapy of skin cancers and Bowen's disease using a specially designed skin patch. J Nucl Med. 1997;38(5):697–702.
20. Berridge JK, Morgan DA. A comparison of late cosmetic results following two different radiotherapy techniques for treating basal cell carcinoma. Clin Oncol (R Coll Radiol). 1997;9(6):400–2.
21. Shields JA, Shields CL, Freire JE, Brady LW, Komarnicky L. Plaque radiotherapy for selected orbital malignancies: preliminary observations: the 2002 Montgomery lecture, part 2. Ophthal Plast Reconstr Surg. 2003;19:91–5.
22. Guix B, Finestres F, Tello J, Palma C, Martinez A, Guix J, et al. Treatment of skin carcinomas of the face by high-dose-rate brachytherapy and custom-made surface molds. Int J Radiat Oncol Biol Phys. 2000;47(1):95–102.
23. Svoboda V, Kovarik J, Morris F. High-dose-rate microselectron molds in the treatment of skin tumors. Int J Radiat Oncol Biol Phys. 1995;31(4):967–72.
24. Debois J. Cesium-137 brachytherapy for epithelioma of the skin of the nose: experience with 370 patients. J Belge Radiol. 1994;77(1):1–4.
25. Rudoltz M, Perkins R, Luthmann R, Fracke T, Green T, Eaglstein F, et al. High-dose-rate brachytherapy with a custom-surface mold to treat recurrent squamous cell carcinomas of the skin of the forearm. J Am Acad Dermatol. 1998;38(6 Pt 1):1003–5.
26. Ozyar E, Gurdalli S. Mold brachytherapy can be an optional technique for total scalp irradiation. Int J Radiat Oncol Biol Phys. 2002;54(4):1286.
27. Avril MF, Auperin A, Margulis A, Gerbaulet A, Duvillard P, Benhamou E, et al. Basal cell carcinoma of the face: surgery or radiotherapy? Results of a randomized study. Br J Cancer. 1997;76(1):100–6.
28. Rio E, Bardet E, Ferron C, Peuvrel P, Supiot S, Campion L, et al. Interstitial brachytherapy of periorificial skin carcinomas of the face: a retrospective study of 97 cases. Int J Radiat Oncol Biol Phys. 2005;63(3):753–7.
29. Conill C, Verger E, Marruecos J, Vargas M, Biete A. Low dose rate brachytherapy in lip carcinoma. Clin Transl Oncol. 2007;9:251–4.
30. Conill C, Sanchez-Reyes A, Molla M, Vilalta A. Brachytherapy with ^{192}Ir as treatment of carcinoma of the tarsal structure of the eyelid. Int J Radiat Oncol Biol Phys. 2004;59(5):1326–9.
31. Hadorn DC, Baker D, Hodges JS, Hicks N. Rating the quality of evidence for clinical practice guidelines. J Clin Epidemiol. 1996;49:749–53.
32. Somanchi B, Stanton A, Webb M, Loncaster J, Allan E, Muir L. Hand function after high dose rate brachytherapy for squamous cell carcinoma of the skin of the hand. Clin Oncol (R Coll Radiol). 2008;20(9):691–7.
33. Petit JY, Avril MR, Margulis A, Chassagne D, Gerbaulet A, Duvillard P, et al. Evaluation of cosmetic results of a randomized trial comparing surgery and radiotherapy in the treatment of basal cell carcinoma of the face. Plast Reconstr Surg. 2000;105(7):2544–51.
34. Semrau S, Kunz M, Baggesen K, Vogel H, Buchmann W, Gross G, et al. Successful treatment of field cancerization of the scalp by surface mould brachytherapy. Br J Dermatol. 2008;159:753–5.

Cutaneous Merkel Cell Carcinoma

William M. Mendenhall

Introduction

Cutaneous Merkel cell carcinoma (MCC) is a rare neuroendocrine malignancy [1–3]. The age-adjusted incidence is approximately 0.24–0.44 per 100,000 person years [3]. Risk factors for MCC are sun exposure and immune suppression, including chronic lymphocytic leukemia (CLL), solid organ transplant, and human immunodeficiency virus (HIV) [4–6]. Human polyoma virus (MCPyV) appears to be etiologic in a significant proportion of patients with MCC; the presence of MCPyV DNA in the MCC cells may be associated with an improved prognosis [5]. MCC exhibits a slight male preponderance [2, 7]. The vast majority (over 90–95 %) are Caucasian and approximately 90 % are over 50 years of age [3, 7, 8]. The most common sites include the head and neck and extremities. Andea and colleagues reported on 156 patients and observed the following site distribution: extremity, 42 %; head and neck, 37 %; buttocks, 16 %; and trunk 5 % [3].

The majority of MCCs appear relatively innocuous at diagnosis. Most are 2 cm or less in size and the patients are usually asymptomatic [8]. The most common color is red/pink in over 50 % of patients, followed by blue/violaceous [8]. The lesion is often thought to be benign prior to biopsy [8].

The diagnostic evaluation of the patient includes taking a thorough history, physical examination, chest radiograph, and computed tomography (CT) of the primary site and regional lymphatics. Fluourodeoxyglucose-positron emission tomography (FDG-PET)-CT will likely contribute to altered staging and a change in the treatment plan and should be obtained in most patients [9]. The value of sentinel lymph node biopsy (SLNB) is debatable and depends on treatment philosophy [10]. On the one hand, if patients with a pathologically negative SLNB are to be followed and

W.M. Mendenhall (✉)
Department of Radiation Oncology, College of Medicine, University of Florida,
2000 SW Archer Road, Gainesville, FL 32610, USA
e-mail: mendwm@shands.ufl.edu

A.B. Cognetta and W.M. Mendenhall (eds.), *Radiation Therapy for Skin Cancer*,
DOI 10.1007/978-1-4614-6986-5_14, © Springer Science+Business Media New York 2013

adjuvant nodal RT withheld, then SLNB would be valuable to define this subset of patients. Additionally, one could argue that those with pathologically positive SLNBs could be considered for adjuvant chemotherapy because of the increased risk of distant metastases [11]. However, adjuvant chemotherapy has not been shown to improve outcome in high-risk patients and, because of the high likelihood of subclinical disease in clinically negative regional nodes, it is the author's bias to electively irradiate these regions regardless of SLNB status [11, 12]. Thus, in the latter instance, SLNB does not meaningfully contribute to management decisions.

Several staging systems have been described for MCC [13, 14]. The staging system described by Yiengpruksawan et al. is straightforward and has been widely used: stage I, local disease; stage II, regional disease; and stage III, distant metastasis [13]. The staging system described by the American Joint Committee in Cancer (AJCC) is more complex and is ill-suited to an entity that is relatively rare and where the number of patients included in most single institution outcome studies is relatively small [14]. Mojica et al. reported the following stage distribution in 1,665 patients from the Surveillance Epidemiology and End Results (SEER) database: stage I, 55 %; stage II, 31 %; stage III, 6 %; and no data, 8 % [7].

Surgery and radiotherapy (RT) are the mainstays of treatment for patients with stage I and II MCC [10, 12, 15–20]. Although a subset of patients with stage I disease may be managed with surgery alone, the high likelihood of subclinical disease in the clinically negative regional lymphatics and the modest risk of in-transit metastases suggest that the majority of patients benefit from the addition of RT [7, 20]. Patients with stage II disease have approximately a 75 % local-regional control rate after RT alone or combined with surgery [15, 17]. Although debatable, the addition of surgery to RT probably results in improved local-regional control [15–17, 21].

Radiation Therapy Technique

The RT techniques are the same as those employed for squamous cell carcinoma as are the dose fractionation schedules. Treatment techniques vary with primary site and the location of the first echelon lymph nodes. Dose fractionation schedules vary with the suspected or known amount of disease: elective nodal RT, 50 Gy/25 fractions; negative margins postoperatively, 60 Gy/30 fractions; positive margins postoperatively, 66 Gy/33 fractions; and gross disease, 70 Gy/35 fractions.

Treatment Outcomes

The optimal management of patients with cutaneous MCC is not well-defined in large part due to the relative rarity of the disease. Questions include whether surgery and adjuvant RT improves outcomes compared with surgery alone, the relative

Table 1 Five-year outcomes vs. stage

Outcome	Stage I ($N=24$) (%)	Stage II ($N=16$) (%)	All patients (%)	p-Value
Local control	96	87	92	0.3240
Regional control	87	65	78	0.1587
Local-regional control	87	67	79	0.1607
Distant metastasis-free survival	71	37	57	0.0073
Cause-specific survival	58	27	45	0.0090
Overall survival	48	18	36	0.0037

Source: Reprinted from Am J Otolaryngol, 33(1), Mendenhall WM, Kirwan JM, Morris CG, Amdur RJ, Werning JW, Mendenhall NP, Cutaneous Merkel cell carcinoma, 88–92, Copyright 2012 with permission from Elsevier

efficacy of RT alone compared with surgery and RT, and the efficacy of adjuvant chemotherapy. The following is a discussion of some of these issues.

Mendenhall et al. reported on 40 patients treated with curative intent for de novo MCC with surgery and adjuvant RT (37 patients) or RT alone (3 patients) at the University of Florida between 1984 and 2009 [22]. Adjuvant chemotherapy was administered to 11 patients (28 %). Median follow-up for surviving patients was 4.2 years (range, 2.2–14.2 years). No patients were lost to follow-up. Treatment outcomes are depicted in Table 1. No patients experienced a severe late complication.

Fang et al. reported on 50 patients treated at the University of Washington between 1985 and 2007 for microscopically positive (26 patients) or macroscopically positive (24 patients) nodes [15]. The 2-year regional control rates for 26 patients with microscopically positive SLNBs were 100 % whether the patients were treated with RT alone (19 patients) or neck dissection with or without RT (7 patients). The median follow-up for this subset of patients was 18 months (range, 5–62 months). The 2-year regional control rates for those with macroscopically positive nodes were 78 % after RT alone (9 patients) compared with 73 % after surgery alone or combined with RT (15 patients) ($p=0.8$). The median follow-up was 16 months (range, 5–109 months). The authors concluded that RT alone results in equivalent regional control compared with surgery alone or combined with RT for patients with positive regional nodes. Caveats pertaining to this study are that selection bias could have impacted outcomes, the number of patients is relatively small, and the follow-up is short.

Veness and co-workers reported on an unfavorable series of 43 patients treated at Westmead Hospital (21 patients) and Royal Brisbane/Mater Hospital (22 patients) between 1993 and 2007 with RT alone for medically or technically inoperable MCC [17]. RT was delivered at initial diagnosis in 24 patients (56 %) and for recurrence in the remainder (usually nodal recurrence in a previously untreated nodal basin). The median maximum tumor diameter was 3 cm (range, 0.5–13 cm). The median follow-up was 39 months (range, 4–78 months). The median RT dose to the primary lesion was 51 Gy; the median RT dose to the nodes was 50 Gy. The median dose per fraction was 2 Gy. Recurrence developed in 60 % of patients; 15 (35 %) of 45 patients recurred outside of the RT fields. The in-field control rate was 75 % and the 5-year overall survival rate was 37 %. Interesting points regarding this study are that the in-field control and 5-year survival rates are surprisingly favorable after relatively modest dose RT in an unfavorable series of patients.

Foote et al. reported on 112 patients treated with curative intent RT between 2000 and 2005 at three public radiotherapy treatment centers in Queensland, Australia [18]. Nine patients were treated for recurrent MCC and 103 patients were previously untreated. RT was delivered to the primary site in 88 % of patients for gross (11 %) or subclinical (78 %) disease and to the regional nodes in 89 % of patients, mostly for subclinical disease (71 %). Gross nodal disease was treated with RT in 19 % of patients. The likelihood of failure in the clinically negative regional nodes was 33 % for those who did not receive elective nodal irradiation (ENI), which was significantly higher than for those who did receive ENI. The likelihood of in-field disease control was higher for those who received ≥50 Gy for subclinical disease and ≥55 Gy for gross disease.

Clark and colleagues reported on 110 patients with head and neck MCC treated at Princess Margaret Hospital (Toronto), Westmead Hospital (Sydney), and the Royal Prince Alfred Hospital (Sydney) with either surgery or RT (44 patients) or combined surgery and adjuvant RT (66 patients); survivors had a mean follow-up of 2.3 years [19]. The 5-year local control rate was 84 %; the 5-year regional control rate was 69 %. Surgery and adjuvant RT resulted in improved local control ($p = 0.009$) and regional control ($p = 0.006$) compared with single modality therapy. The 5-year cause-specific and overall survival rates were 62 % and 49 %, respectively. Combined modality treatment resulted in improved disease-free survival ($p = 0.013$) compared with single modality therapy.

Mojica et al. reported on 1,665 patients included in the SEER database from 1973 to 2002; 1,487 patients (89 %) received surgery as a component of their therapy [7]. Adjuvant RT was administered to approximately 40 % of the surgically treated patients and was associated with a significant improvement in median survival compared with surgery alone (63 months vs. 45 months, $p = 0.0002$).

Poulsen and co-workers reported on 40 patients with high-risk MCC who received adjuvant chemotherapy according to the Trans-Tasman Radiation Oncology Group TROG 96:07 study from 1997 to 2001 [11]. Patients had ≥1 of the following high-risk factors: recurrent disease, positive nodes, primary tumor size >1 cm, and gross residual disease after surgery. The primary site and regional nodes received 50 Gy/25 fractions/5 weeks and patients received concomitant carboplatin (AUC 4.5) and etoposide 80 mg/m^2 on days 1–3 of weeks 1, 4, 7, and 10. Patients were compared with a historic group of 62 patients treated between 1988 and 1996 with surgery and RT. Multivariate analyses revealed that the following factors significantly impacted treatment outcomes: (1) overall survival-recurrent disease, age, and presence of residual disease; (2) cause-specific survival-recurrent disease; (3) local-regional control-lower extremity primary site; and (4) distant metastasis-free survival-residual disease. The data suggest that adjuvant chemotherapy had no significant impact in any of the treatment outcomes, including survival.

Conclusion

The likelihood of local-regional control is relatively high after RT alone or combined with surgery. Our treatment philosophy, which does not vary with primary site, is to proceed with surgery if a gross total resection (R0 or R1) can be achieved followed by postoperative RT. An elective node dissection is not indicated because elective nodal RT is likely to be as effective and is employed in all clinically N0 patients. Similarly, SLNB is not required because it does not alter the treatment plan. Our dose fractionation guidelines are similar to those employed for squamous cell carcinoma. Patients with medically or technically unresectable gross disease are treated with RT alone. Although relatively high in-field control rates have been reported with moderate dose RT, our bias is to treat aggressively to 70 Gy in 35 fractions over 7 weeks or to employ altered fractionation, such as 74.4 in 62 twice-daily fractions over 6.5 weeks. Although the dominant failure pattern is distant, there is no convincing evidence that adjuvant chemotherapy improves the likelihood of cure. On the other hand, given the rarity of cutaneous MCC and the existing data, it is not possible to definitively state that adjuvant chemotherapy is ineffective. Patients at particularly high risk for distant relapse, such as those with recurrent disease and/or multiple positive nodes, may be considered for a chemotherapy regimen similar to those used for small cell neuroendocrine carcinoma (i.e., cisplatin and etoposide) given concomitantly with RT.

References

1. Toker C. Trabecular carcinoma of the skin. Arch Dermatol. 1972;105(1):107–10.
2. Asioli S, Righi A, Volante M, Eusebi V, Bussolati G. p63 expression as a new prognostic marker in Merkel cell carcinoma. Cancer. 2007;110(3):640–7.
3. Andea AA, Coit DG, Amin B, Busam KJ. Merkel cell carcinoma: histologic features and prognosis. Cancer. 2008;113(9):2549–58.
4. Koljonen V, Kukko H, Tukiainen E, Bohling T, Sankila R, Joensuu H, et al. Second cancers following the diagnosis of Merkel cell carcinoma: a nationwide cohort study. Cancer Epidemiol. 2010;34(1):62–5.
5. Bhatia K, Goedert JJ, Modali R, Preiss L, Ayers LW. Immunological detection of viral large T antigen identifies a subset of Merkel cell carcinoma tumors with higher viral abundance and better clinical outcome. Int J Cancer. 2010;127(6):1493–6.
6. Samlowski WE, Moon J, Tuthill RJ, Heinrich MC, Balzer-Haas NS, Merl SA, et al. A phase II trial of imatinib mesylate in Merkel cell carcinoma (neuroendocrine carcinoma of the skin): a Southwest Oncology Group study (S0331). Am J Clin Oncol. 2010;33(5):495–9.
7. Mojica P, Smith D, Ellenhorn JD. Adjuvant radiation therapy is associated with improved survival in Merkel cell carcinoma of the skin. J Clin Oncol. 2007;25(9):1043–7.
8. Heath M, Jaimes N, Lemos B, Mostaghimi A, Wang LC, Penas PF, et al. Clinical characteristics of Merkel cell carcinoma at diagnosis in 195 patients: the AEIOU features. J Am Acad Dermatol. 2008;58(3):375–81.
9. Concannon R, Larcos GS, Veness M. The impact of (18)F-FDG PET-CT scanning for staging and management of Merkel cell carcinoma: results from Westmead Hospital, Sydney, Australia. J Am Acad Dermatol. 2010;62(1):76–84.

10. Gupta SG, Wang LC, Penas PF, Gellenthin M, Lee SJ, Nghiem P. Sentinel lymph node biopsy for evaluation and treatment of patients with Merkel cell carcinoma: The Dana-Farber experience and meta-analysis of the literature. Arch Dermatol. 2006;142(6):685–90.
11. Poulsen MG, Rischin D, Porter I, Walpole E, Harvey J, Hamilton C, et al. Does chemotherapy improve survival in high-risk stage I and II Merkel cell carcinoma of the skin? Int J Radiat Oncol Biol Phys. 2006;64(1):114–9.
12. McAfee WJ, Morris CG, Mendenhall CM, Werning JW, Mendenhall NP, Mendenhall WM. Merkel cell carcinoma: treatment and outcomes. Cancer. 2005;104(8):1761–4.
13. Yiengpruksawan A, Coit DG, Thaler HT, Urmacher C, Knapper WK. Merkel cell carcinoma. Prognosis and management. Arch Surg. 1991;126(12):1514–9.
14. American Joint Committee on Cancer, editor. AJCC cancer staging handbook. 7th ed. Chicago: Springer; 2010.
15. Fang LC, Lemos B, Douglas J, Iyer J, Nghiem P. Radiation monotherapy as regional treatment for lymph node-positive Merkel cell carcinoma. Cancer. 2010;116(7):1783–90.
16. Bichakjian CK, Coit DG, Wong SL. Radiation versus resection for Merkel cell carcinoma. Cancer. 2010;116(7):1620–2.
17. Veness M, Foote M, Gebski V, Poulsen M. The role of radiotherapy alone in patients with merkel cell carcinoma: reporting the Australian experience of 43 patients. Int J Radiat Oncol Biol Phys. 2010;78(3):703–9.
18. Foote M, Harvey J, Porceddu S, Dickie G, Hewitt S, Colquist S, et al. Effect of radiotherapy dose and volume on relapse in Merkel cell cancer of the skin. Int J Radiat Oncol Biol Phys. 2010;77(3):677–84.
19. Clark JR, Veness MJ, Gilbert R, O'Brien CJ, Gullane PJ. Merkel cell carcinoma of the head and neck: is adjuvant radiotherapy necessary? Head Neck. 2007;29(3):249–57.
20. Medina-Franco H, Urist MM, Fiveash J, Heslin MJ, Bland KI, Beenken SW. Multimodality treatment of Merkel cell carcinoma: case series and literature review of 1024 cases. Ann Surg Oncol. 2001;8(3):204–8.
21. Kim J, McNiff JM. Nuclear expression of survivin portends a poor prognosis in Merkel cell carcinoma. Mod Pathol. 2008;21(6):764–9.
22. Mendenhall WM, Kirwan JM, Morris CG, Amdur RJ, Werning JW, Mendenhall NP. Cutaneous Merkel cell carcinoma. Am J Otolaryngol. 2012;33(1):88–92.

Radiotherapy for Cutaneous Angiosarcoma

William M. Mendenhall and Nancy P. Mendenhall

Introduction

Cutaneous angiosarcoma (AS) is a rare malignancy of vascular origin that usually arises on the scalp or face of elderly males [1–6]. Soft tissue sarcomas account for less than 1 % of all malignancies and angiosarcomas comprise approximately 2 % of all soft tissue sarcomas [6]. Thus, they are rare. Roughly 60 % of angiosarcomas arise in the skin and superficial soft tissues and approximately 50 % of cutaneous angiosarcomas are found in the head and neck [6, 7]. Angiosarcomas of the breast usually arise in patients who are treated with partial mastectomy and radiotherapy (RT) [8]. Holden et al. reported on 72 patients with AS of the scalp and face; the male to female ratio was 1.57:1 and the age ranged from 56 to 92 years with a peak in the eighth decade [2]. Patients usually present with a lesion that resembles a "spreading bruise" that varies from blue to red in color [1, 2]. A nodular component often develops as the tumor progresses. Although the majority of patients are asymptomatic, some may present with bleeding, edema, and/or ulceration [5]. The median interval between the onset of symptoms and diagnosis reported by Pawlik et al. was 5.1 months (range, 0–12 months) [5].

The primary tumor is often more extensive than is apparent on physical examination. Pawlik et al. reported on 29 patients with AS of the scalp who were treated surgically and observed the following clinical and pathological T-stage: cT1, 62 %; cT2, 38 %; pT1, 25 %; and pT2, 75 % [5]. A significant proportion of patients present with multifocal disease. Pawlik et al. reported that 59 % of patients presented with a single lesion, while the remainder had a multifocal primary tumor or satellite

W.M. Mendenhall (✉)
Department of Radiation Oncology, College of Medicine, University of Florida, 2000 SW Archer Road, Gainesville, FL 32610, USA
e-mail: mendwm@shands.ufl.edu

N.P. Mendenhall
Department of Radiation Oncology, University of Florida Proton Therapy Institute, University of Florida, 2015 North Jefferson Street, Jacksonville, FL 32206, USA

A.B. Cognetta and W.M. Mendenhall (eds.), *Radiation Therapy for Skin Cancer*,
DOI 10.1007/978-1-4614-6986-5_15, © Springer Science+Business Media New York 2013

lesions. Clinically involved regional lymph node metastases are observed in a minority of patients [4]. Hodgkinson et al. observed cervical lymph node metastasis at diagnosis in 3 of 13 patients (23 %) with head and neck cutaneous AS evaluated at the Mayo Clinic; 1 additional patient failed in the regional nodes after treatment [1]. Hematogenous metastases, usually in the lung, at diagnosis are relatively uncommon.

Pathogenesis

AS is thought to arise from the vascular endothelium. A variety of factors may be involved in the pathogenesis and progression of AS [9, 10], including vascular endothelial growth factor (VEGF) and angiopoietin 2 [11, 12].

Diagnostic Evaluation

A history is obtained and a thorough physical examination is performed. Magnetic resonance (MR) imaging may be used to define the extent of the primary tumor [13]. Isoda evaluated 8 patients with AS of the scalp with MR and observed that the tumors enhanced well and exhibited prolonged T_1 and T_2 relaxation times [13]. The lesions were clearly visible on both T_2 weighted and contrast enhanced T_1 weighted MRs with fat saturation. The tumor appeared more extensive on MR compared with physical examination in 4 of 8 patients.

Contrast enhanced computed tomography (CT) may be used to detect involved regional lymph nodes and to evaluate the lungs for distant metastases.

Biopsy is obtained to establish the diagnosis of AS. Although fine needle aspiration may be used to diagnose malignancy in nearly all cases, it is often difficult to diagnose AS, particularly if it is low grade [14].

Histopathology

Well-differentiated AS are composed of well-formed, irregular vascular channels, often lined by flattened endothelial cells. Such tumors are distinguished from hemangiomas by their "collagen dissection pattern" [2], formation of papillae, and anastomosing architecture. Moderately differentiated AS contain more densely packed vessels, and vascular channels are lined by multiple layers of atypical endothelial cells often exhibiting intraluminal proliferation. Poorly differentiated AS are less common in the skin and may closely resemble carcinomas or other soft tissue sarcomas. Some poorly differentiated tumors may contain obvious vasoformative areas, facilitating the diagnosis. Others are composed exclusively of pleomorphic spindled or epithelioid cells with prominent mitotic activity and only subtle vascular lumen formation. Histologic grade is not as accurate in predicting outcome in cutaneous AS as it is with other soft tissue sarcomas.

Staging

There is no staging system for cutaneous AS. Although the American Joint Committee on Cancer (AJCC) staging system may be employed, AS is not included in either the soft tissue sarcoma or skin malignancy sections of the staging manual (Table 1) [15].

Table 1 AJCC staging system for soft tissue sarcomas

Definition of TNM						
Primary tumor (T)						
TX	Primary tumor cannot be assessed					
T0	No evidence of primary tumor					
T1	Tumor 5 cm or less in greatest dimension					
	T1a—superficial tumor					
	T1b—deep tumor					
T2	Tumor more than 5 cm in greatest dimension					
	T2a—superficial tumor					
	T2b—deep tumor					
Note: Superficial tumor is located exclusively above the superficial fascia without invasion of the fascia; deep tumor is located either exclusively beneath the superficial fascia, superficial to the fascia with invasion of or through the fascia, or both superficial yet beneath the fascia. Retroperitoneal, mediastinal, and pelvic sarcomas are classified as deep tumors						
Regional lymph nodes (N)						
NX	Regional lymph nodes cannot be assessed					
N0	No regional lymph node metastasis					
N1[a]	Regional lymph node metastasis					
[a]*Note*: Presence of positive nodes (N1) is considered Stage IV						
Distant metastasis (M)						
MX	Distant metastasis cannot be assessed					
M0	No distant metastasis					
M1	Distant metastasis					
Stage grouping						
Stage I	T1a, 1b, 2a, 2b	N0	M0	G1–2	G1	Low
Stage II	T1a, 1b, 2a	N0	M0	G3–4	G2–3	High
Stage III	T2b	N0	M0	G3–4	G2–3	High
Stage IV	Any T	N1	M0	Any G	Any G	High or low
	Any T	N0	M1	Any G	Any G	High or low

G grade

Used with the permission of the American Joint Committee on Cancer (AJCC), Chicago, Illinois. The original source for this material is the AJCC Cancer Staging Handbook, Seventh Edition (2010) published by Springer Science and Business Media LLC, http://www.springerlink.com

Treatment

The optimal treatment for cutaneous AS is resection of gross disease with wide margins followed by postoperative RT to the primary site and regional lymphatics. Free flap reconstruction of scalp AS should be considered to reduce the risk of a post-RT bone exposure. The main problem with obtaining wide margins is that many lesions are relatively extensive at diagnosis and the majority of cutaneous AS arise on the scalp or face.

RT dose-fractionation schedules are similar to those employed for carcinomas. Patients are treated at 2 Gy per once-daily fraction. The total dose depends on the suspected amount of disease: elective RT for subclinical disease, 50 Gy; postoperative negative margins, 60 Gy; postoperative microscopic positive margins, 66 Gy; and gross disease, 70 Gy. Very wide RT fields are employed to reduce the risk of a marginal miss. Aggressive altered fractionation schedules may be employed for poorly differentiated, rapidly progressing lesions. Scalp AS may be treated with a technique that employs parallel opposed 6 MV photon fields to treat the vertex (the "rind") matched to 6 MeV electron portals to treat the lateral aspects of the scalp, matched to 12 MeV electron fields to treat the parotid and upper neck nodes [16]. Chemotherapy is employed for palliation of patients with incurable disease [7, 17–23]. There is no data to support the use of adjuvant chemotherapy outside of a study setting.

Outcomes

Holden et al. reported on 72 patients treated at St. John's Hospital for AS of the scalp and face; 63 patients had sufficient follow-up to assess outcome [2]. The 5-year survival rate was 12 %; half of the patients died within 15 months of treatment. Survival was significantly influenced by the extent of the primary tumor but not by age, sex, location, or clinical appearance of the primary lesion (bruise-like macule vs. nodule with or without ulceration).

Pawlik et al. reported on 29 patients treated for AS of the scalp at the University of Michigan and had follow-up from 3.2 to 106 months (median, 18.3 months) [5]. Twenty-eight patients underwent wide local excision and postoperative RT; 1 patient with unresectable disease was treated with definitive RT alone. Only 6 of 28 patients (21 %) who underwent resection had negative margins. Twenty-three of 28 patients received postoperative RT that generally consisted of 60 Gy to the whole scalp at 1.8–2 Gy per fraction. The dose to gross disease varied from 60 to 72 Gy. One patient received adjuvant chemotherapy. Twenty-one of 29 patients (72 %) developed a recurrence after treatment: local recurrence, 13 patients; local recurrence and distant metastasis, 4 patients; and distant metastasis alone, 4 patients. Progression-free survival was better for patients with single vs. multifocal lesions ($p=0.02$).

Age, clinical or pathologic T-stage, histologic grade, and margin status did not impact this endpoint. The median overall survival was 28.4 months. Parameters associated with improved overall survival included young age ($p = 0.024$) and less extensive disease at the primary site ($p = 0.013$).

Morrison et al. reported on 14 patients treated with electron beam RT with curative intent at the MD Anderson Cancer Center between 1970 and 1989 for AS of the scalp (11 patients) and face (3 patients) [24]. Three patients were treated with RT alone and 11 patients received RT in addition to chemotherapy (10 patients) and/or surgery (7 patients). Six patients received postoperative RT for subclinical disease to a median dose of 60 Gy (range, 50–66 Gy). Eight patients received RT for gross disease; doses ranged from 55 to 75 Gy. The 5-year local-regional control rate was 40 % for those treated for subclinical disease compared with 24 % for those treated for gross disease ($p = 0.03$). The 5-year "infield" local control rates were 80 % for those treated for subclinical disease and 55 % for those irradiated for gross disease. The 5-year distant metastasis-free and overall survival rates were 37 % and 29 %, respectively. Four of the 6 patients treated for subclinical disease died with cancer and 2 patients were alive and disease-free at 10 years. All 8 patients irradiated for gross disease died with cancer; 7 of 8 died within 2 years and 1 patient died with disease at 130 months.

Scott et al. reported on 41 patients treated with RT for AS at the University of Florida between 1974 and 2009 [16]. Tumor sites included the head and neck (22 patients), breast (14 patients), and other (5 patients). Sixteen AS were RT-induced. Thirty-one patients were treated with surgery and RT (preoperative RT, 12 patients; postoperative RT, 19 patients). RT alone was employed for 10 patients. The median RT dose was 60 Gy (range, 37.5–76 Gy). Once-daily fractionation was employed in 16 patients at 1.8–2.0 Gy/fraction, 7 patients were treated at 1.2–1.5 Gy per twice-daily fraction, and 18 patients were treated 3 times per day at 1.0 Gy per fraction. Median follow-up was 3.7 years. The 5-year local control and overall survival rates were 64 % and 54 %, respectively. Predictors of improved local control were non-scalp primary site, tumor size ≤ 5 cm, RT-induced AS, and combined modality therapy. Predictors of improved survival included non-scalp primary site and tumor size ≤ 5 cm. The best outcomes were for patients with RT-induced breast AS treated with surgery and RT delivered at 1.0 Gy per fractions thrice daily.

Chemotherapy

Fury et al. reported on 125 patients with AS arising from various sites who were treated at the Memorial Sloan Kettering Cancer Center between 1990 and 2003 [7]. Fifty-two of 125 patients received palliative chemotherapy for unresectable disease. The median progression-free survival rates are depicted in Table 2 and range from 1.1 to 5.4 months.

Table 2 Response to palliative chemotherapy—52 patients treated at the Memorial Sloan Kettering Cancer Center, New York

Regimen	No. of administrations[a]	Median line[b]	Median progression-free survival (months)
Doxorubicin	12	2	3.7
Liposomal doxorubicin	11	2	4.2
Ifosfamide	12	2	1.6
Mesna, doxorubicin, ifosfamide	7	1	5.4
Paclitaxel	41	1	4.0
Vinorelbine	6	2.5	3.0
Gemcitabine	11	3	2.2
Other	13	2	1.1

[a]Number of times chemotherapy regimen was initiated
[b]Median line that the drug(s) was used (i.e., first-line, second-line, or third-line)
From Fury MG, Antonescu CR, Van Zee KJ, Brennan MF, Maki RG. A 14-year retrospective review of angiosarcoma: clinical characteristics, prognostic factors, and treatment outcomes with surgery and chemotherapy. Cancer J. 2005 May-Jun;11(3):241–7

Conclusion

Cutaneous AS is a rare, aggressive malignancy that has a high risk of both local-regional and distant relapse after treatment. The optimal therapy is resection of gross disease, preferably with negative margins, followed by wide-field postoperative RT [25]. The risk of regional lymph node metastasis probably varies from 10 to 20 % and our inclination is to treat them electively if they are clinically uninvolved. RT doses are approximately 50 Gy for undissected subclinical disease, 60–66 Gy for dissected subclinical disease, and 70–75 Gy for gross disease. Patients irradiated for gross disease should be considered for altered fractionation. The role of adjuvant chemotherapy remains investigational.

References

1. Hodgkinson DJ, Soule EH, Woods JE. Cutaneous angiosarcoma of the head and neck. Cancer. 1979;44(3):1106–13.
2. Holden CA, Spittle MF, Jones EW. Angiosarcoma of the face and scalp, prognosis and treatment. Cancer. 1987;59(5):1046–57.
3. Sasaki R, Soejima T, Kishi K, Imajo Y, Hirota S, Kamikonya N, et al. Angiosarcoma treated with radiotherapy: impact of tumor type and size on outcome. Int J Radiat Oncol Biol Phys. 2002;52(4):1032–40.
4. Ward JR, Feigenberg SJ, Mendenhall NP, Marcus Jr RB, Mendenhall WM. Radiation therapy for angiosarcoma. Head Neck. 2003;25(10):873–8.
5. Pawlik TM, Paulino AF, McGinn CJ, Baker LH, Cohen DS, Morris JS, et al. Cutaneous angiosarcoma of the scalp: a multidisciplinary approach. Cancer. 2003;98(8):1716–26.
6. Mark RJ, Poen JC, Tran LM, Fu YS, Juillard GF. Angiosarcoma. A report of 67 patients and a review of the literature. Cancer. 1996;77(11):2400–6.

7. Fury MG, Antonescu CR, Van Zee KJ, Brennan MF, Maki RG. A 14-year retrospective review of angiosarcoma: clinical characteristics, prognostic factors, and treatment outcomes with surgery and chemotherapy. Cancer J. 2005;11(3):241–7.
8. Palta M, Morris CG, Grobmyer SR, Copeland III EM, Mendenhall NP. Angiosarcoma after breast-conserving therapy: long-term outcomes with hyperfractionated radiotherapy. Cancer. 2010;116(8):1872–8.
9. Schmid H, Zietz C. Human herpesvirus 8 and angiosarcoma: analysis of 40 cases and review of the literature. Pathology. 2005;37(4):284–7.
10. Zietz C, Rumpler U, Sturzl M, Lohrs U. Inverse relation of Fas-ligand and tumor-infiltrating lymphocytes in angiosarcoma: indications of apoptotic tumor counterattack. Am J Pathol. 2001;159(3):963–70.
11. Amo Y, Masuzawa M, Hamada Y, Katsuoka K. Serum concentrations of vascular endothelial growth factor-D in angiosarcoma patients. Br J Dermatol. 2004;150(1):160–1.
12. Amo Y, Masuzawa M, Hamada Y, Katsuoka K. Observations on angiopoietin 2 in patients with angiosarcoma. Br J Dermatol. 2004;150(5):1028–9.
13. Isoda H, Imai M, Inagawa S, Miura K, Sakahara H. Magnetic resonance imaging findings of angiosarcoma of the scalp. J Comput Assist Tomogr. 2005;29(6):858–62.
14. Klijanienko J, Caillaud JM, Lagace R, Vielh P. Cytohistologic correlations in angiosarcoma including classic and epithelioid variants: Institut Curie's experience. Diagn Cytopathol. 2003;29(3):140–5.
15. American Joint Committee on Cancer, editor. Soft tissue sarcoma. AJCC Cancer Staging Manual. New York, NY: Springer; 2002. p. 193–200.
16. Scott MT, Portnow LH, Morris CG, Marcus RB, Jr., Mendenhall NP, Mendenhall WM, et al. Radiation therapy for angiosarcoma: the 35-year University of Florida experience. Am J Clin Oncol. 2012;36(2):174–80.
17. Isogai R, Kawada A, Aragane Y, Tezuka T. Successful treatment of pulmonary metastasis and local recurrence of angiosarcoma with docetaxel. J Dermatol. 2004;31(4):335–41.
18. Pestoni C, Paredes-Suarez C, Peteiro C, Toribio J. Early detection of cutaneous angiosarcoma of the face and scalp and treatment with placitaxel. J Eur Acad Dermatol Venereol. 2005;19(3):357–9.
19. Wollina U, Fuller J, Graefe T, Kaatz M, Lopatta E. Angiosarcoma of the scalp: treatment with liposomal doxorubicin and radiotherapy. J Cancer Res Clin Oncol. 2001;127(6):396–9.
20. Bong AB, Bonnekoh B, Schon MP, Gollnick H. Treatment of scalp angiosarcoma by controlled perfusion of A. carotis externa with pegylated liposomal doxorubicin and intralesional application of pegylated interferon alfa. J Am Acad Dermatol. 2005;52(2 Suppl 1):20–3.
21. Eiling S, Lischner S, Busch JO, Rothaupt D, Christophers E, Hauschild A. Complete remission of a radio-resistant cutaneous angiosarcoma of the scalp by systemic treatment with liposomal doxorubicin. Br J Dermatol. 2002;147(1):150–3.
22. Skubitz KM, Haddad PA. Paclitaxel and pegylated-liposomal doxorubicin are both active in angiosarcoma. Cancer. 2005;104(2):361–6.
23. Yamada M, Hatta N, Mizuno M, Oishi N, Takehara K. Weekly low-dose docetaxel in the treatment of lung metastases from angiosarcoma of the head. Br J Dermatol. 2005;152(4):811–2.
24. Morrison WH, Byers RM, Garden AS, Evans HL, Ang KK, Peters LJ. Cutaneous angiosarcoma of the head and neck. A therapeutic dilemma. Cancer. 1995;76(2):319–27.
25. Tung SS, Shiu AS, Starkschall G, Morrison WH, Hogstrom KR. Dosimetric evaluation of total scalp irradiation using a lateral electron-photon technique. Int J Radiat Oncol Biol Phys. 1993;27(1):153–60.

Radiotherapy for Dermatofibrosarcoma Protuberans

William M. Mendenhall

Introduction

Dermatofibrosarcoma protuberans (DFSP) is a rare monoclonal cutaneous soft tissue sarcoma [1]. Chang et al. [2] reported on 60 patients treated at the University of Illinois between 1968 and 2001. Approximately 100 patients with soft tissue sarcoma were treated annually so that the proportion of those with DFSP was about 1.8 %. Approximately 85–90 % are low grade; the remainder contain 5 % or more of a high-grade fibrosarcomatous component and are considered to be intermediate grade (DFSP-FS) [3]. DFSPs appear as pink or violet–red plaques; it is usually fixed to the dermis but moves freely over deeper tissues. A nodular growth pattern is not observed until late in the course of the disease. Fixation to deeper structures is usually observed in advanced and/or recurrent tumors [4]. DFSP generally exhibits an indolent growth pattern and are symptom-free for a long time. Lindner et al. [4] reported on a series of 35 patients and observed that the onset of symptoms ranged from 6 months to 30 years (mean, 6.4 years). DFSP usually occurs on the trunk and is more common in men. Enzinger and Weiss [5] reported the following site distribution in a series of 853 patients: trunk, 47 %; lower extremity, 20 %; upper extremity,18 %; and head and neck, 14 %. Rutgers et al. [6] reported a male to female ratio of approximately 3:2 (57 %:43 %) in a series of 264 patients. The tumor usually presents in the fourth decade of life with a wide range [3, 4]. Most tumors are superficial and less than 5 cm in maximum diameter. Bowne et al. [3] reported on the following size distribution in a series of 159 patients treated at the Memorial Sloan Kettering Cancer Center: <5 cm, 134 patients (84 %); 5–10 cm, 21 patients (13 %); and >10 cm, 4 patients (3 %). The tumor was superficial in 121 patients (77 %) and invaded deeper structures in 36 patients (22 %); depth of

W.M. Mendenhall (✉)
Department of Radiation Oncology, College of Medicine, University of Florida,
2000 SW Archer Road, Gainesville, FL 32610, USA
e-mail: mendwm@shands.ufl.edu

A.B. Cognetta and W.M. Mendenhall (eds.), *Radiation Therapy for Skin Cancer*,
DOI 10.1007/978-1-4614-6986-5_16, © Springer Science+Business Media New York 2013

invasion was not reported in 2 patients (1 %). DSFPs rarely exhibit lymphatic or hematogenous dissemination.

DFSP arises from rearrangement of chromosomes 17 and 22 where the collagen type Iα1 gene (COLIα1) is fused to the platelet-derived growth factor (PDGF) β-chain gene that results in deregulated expression of PDGFβ and leads to continuous activation of the PDGF receptor β (PDGFRβ) protein tyrosine kinase that promotes DFSP tumor cell growth [7–9].

Histologically, the tumor is composed of monomorphic, benign-appearing spindle cells in a matted or storiform pattern in which the cells intersect in tight right angles around central vessels [4]. Early in the disease course, there may be a narrow tumor-free zone (grenz zone) between the tumor and the epidermis [4]. Uncommon variants include the Bednar tumor, in which there are melanin-containing dendritic cells, and myxoid DFSP [10, 11]. Approximately 10–15 % of tumors contain a fibrosarcomatous component (DFSP-FS) [3, 12, 13] which may first become apparent if the lesion recurs [14]. Takahira et al. [15] analyzed microsatellite instability (MSI) and p53 mutations in 44 tumors from 36 patients (DFSP, 27 patients; DFSP-FS, 9 patients) treated at the National Kyushu Cancer Center (Fukuoka, Japan) and postulated that MSI and p53 mutations are involved in the progression of DFSP to DFSP-FS and occur as early and late events, respectively [15]. DFSP can be distinguished from solitary fibrous histiocytoma (dermatofibroma) by diffuse CD34 positivity and from plexiform neurofibroma by complete absence of S100 positivity [16].

Sasaki et al. [17] analyzed the MIB-1 labeling index (LI) and p53 overexpression in 16 patients with DFSP and 3 patients with DFSP-FS. Recurrent DFSP had MIB-1 LI that were higher than those seen in previously untreated tumors. The proliferative activity for DFSP-FS was higher than that observed for the DFSP. Overexpression of p53 was observed in 3 of 19 (16 %) with DFSP or DFSP-FS; all 3 tumors also exhibited increased proliferated activity.

Diagnostic Evaluation

Tumor extent and mobility are assessed on physical examination. The regional lymph nodes are assessed by palpation.

Magnetic resonance imaging (MRI) is useful to determine the deep extent of the tumor, particularly for large, recurrent lesions [18]. Computed tomography (CT) is not indicated except in the rare case where underlying bone is thought to be involved. The occasional patient may experience pulmonary metastases, particularly if the lesion is advanced, recurrent, and/or intermediate grade and a chest CT is obtained.

Histologic diagnosis is obtained with a core needle or incisional biopsy; fine needle aspiration (FNA) does not provide enough tissue to render an accurate diagnosis in most previously untreated tumors [19, 20]. In contrast, FNA may be useful to diagnose recurrent disease in previously treated patients where relapse is suspected [20]. DFSP may, at times, be difficult to histologically distinguish from other mesenchymal tumors such as dermatofibroma and benign fibrous histiocytoma and plexiform neurofibroma [21, 22].

Staging

DFSP and DFSP-FS are staged according to the recommendations of the American Musculoskeletal Tumor Society (MSTS) staging system that is based on compartmentalization and tumor grade [23, 24]. A stage IA tumor is low grade and intra-compartmental and could be managed adequately by a wide excision alone (i.e., dissection outside of the reactive zone). A stage IB tumor is low grade and extra-compartmental. Stage II implies high-grade histology and does not apply to DFSP or DFSP-FS. Therefore, the MSTS staging for DFSP and DFSP-FS is as follows: IA, no extension beyond the subcutaneous compartment; and IB, involvement of underlying fascia or muscle [4]. There is no American Joint Committee on Cancer (AJCC) [25] staging system for DFSP or DFSP-FS.

Treatment

The optimal treatment of DFSP and DFSP-FS is resection with wide margins; the likelihood of local recurrence after this procedure is less than 10 % [4]. Experience with Mohs surgery indicates that a high probability of cure is attained as long as the final margins are negative [26–30]. Many Mohs surgeons take an additional layer after frozen section clearance for permanent sections. In contrast, the risk of local recurrence probably exceeds 50 % if the margins are positive [1]. The time interval between treatment and the development of recurrent disease is variable. Chang et al. [2] reported on a series of 60 patients treated surgically at the University of Illinois (Chicago); 10 patients experienced a local recurrence from 1 to 100 months after surgery (mean, 38 months). Three of the ten local recurrences (30 %) were observed more than 5 years after surgery.

Adjuvant radiotherapy (RT) administered either before or after surgery significantly reduces the risk of a local recurrence in patients who have or who are likely to have close or positive margins [1, 31]. The dose-fractionation schedules and treatment techniques are similar to those used for other soft tissue sarcomas [24]. Data pertaining to the efficacy of RT alone for gross disease are scant [1, 31–33].

Outcomes

Bowne et al. [3] reported on 159 patients treated with surgery alone (156 patients) or combined with RT (3 patients) at the Memorial Sloan Kettering Cancer Center between 1950 and 1998 (Table 1). One hundred thirty-four patients (84 %) had DFSP and the remainder had DFSP-FS. Gross total resection was achieved in 157 patients (99 %). Margins were positive in 51 patients (32 %), close (<1 mm) in 15 patients (10 %), and negative in 93 patients (58 %). The 5-year local control rates were as follows: DFSP, 81 %; DFSP-FS, 28 %, and overall, 75 %. Multivariate analysis of local control revealed that close or positive margins ($p<0.001$) and intermediate grade histology

Table 1 Outcomes after surgery alone or combined with adjuvant radiotherapy

Series	Number of patients	Follow-up	Previous treatment (%)	Surgery (%)	Radiotherapy (%)	Local control (interval)	Metastases (%)
MSKCC (3)	159	Median, 4.8 years	30	100	2	75 % (5 years)	1
MDAH (34)	122	Median, 47 months	29	100	16	64 % (5 years)	5
University of Illinois (2)	60	Median, 59 months	–	100	5	76 % (10 years)	–
University of Florida (4)	35	Mean, 58 months	49	100	11	91 %[a]	0
Mayo Clinic (12)	32	–	–	100	16	66 %[a]	6
CGMH (11)	34	Median, 50 months	12	100	29	45 % (7 years)	0
University of California, Davis (26)	24	Median, 4.5 years	54	100	4	100 %[a]	0
University of Heidelberg (28)	22	Mean, 54 months	41	100 (Mohs)	0	100 %[a]	–
University of Michigan (29)	62	Median, 4.4 years	–	100	3	100 %[a]	0
University of Miami, FL/NYU (30)	20	Mean, 56 months	–	100 (Mohs)	0	100 %[a]	–

RT radiotherapy; *Mohs* Mohs surgery; *MSKCC* Memorial Sloan Kettering Cancer Center; *MDAH* M. D. Anderson Hospital; *CGMH* Chang Gung Memorial Hospital; *NYU* New York University

[a]Crude percentage

Source: Mendenhall WM, Zlotecki RA, Scarborough MT. Dermatofibrosarcoma protuberans. Cancer. 2004 Dec 1;101(11):2503–8.

Table 2 Outcomes after radiotherapy alone or combined with surgery

Series	Number of patients	Follow-up	Previous treatment (%)	Surgical margins	Local control (interval)
MGH (1)	18	–	39	Positive/close (83 %) Intralesional (17 %)	88 % (10 years)
MDACC (31)	19	Median, 6 years	–	Negative/positive (95 %) Intralesional (5 %)	95 % (10 years)
CGMH (11)	10	–	–	Positive/close (60 %) Negative (40 %)	80 % (7 years)
University of Florida (33)	10	1.5–15.5 years	50	Negative (40 %) Close (<5 mm) (20 %) Positive (40 %)	90 %[a]
MSKCC (13)	4	–	–	Positive (100 %)	75 %[a]
University of Michigan (29)	2	–	–	Positive (100 %)	100 %[a]

Intralesional, gross disease; *MGH* Massachusetts General Hospital; *MDACC* M. D. Anderson Cancer Center; *CGMH* Chang Gung Memorial Hospital; *MSKCC* Memorial Sloan Kettering Cancer Center

[a]Crude percentage; interval in parentheses

Source: Mendenhall WM, Zlotecki RA, Scarborough MT. Dermatofibrosarcoma protuberans. Cancer. 2004 Dec 1;101(11):2503–8.

($p<0.001$) significantly influenced this endpoint. Two patients with DFSP-FS who underwent resection with positive margins experienced pulmonary metastases.

Cai et al. reported on 260 patients treated for DSFP at Fudan University Shanghai Cancer Center between 1985 and 2006 [32]. Definitive wide excision was performed in 236 patients and 34 patients received postoperative RT. The total RT dose ranged from 33.75 to 73.50 Gy (mean, 57.87 Gy) at 1.8–2.5 Gy per fraction. Follow-up information was available for 31 (91 %) of 34 patients treated with RT. Median follow-up was 79.5 months (range, 24–221 months). Local control was achieved in 28 (90 %) of 31 patients.

Sun et al. [11] reported on 35 patients with DFSP treated at Chang Gung Memorial Hospital (Taiwan) with surgery alone (24 patients) or combined with RT (11 patients) between 1987 and 1998. Follow-up ranged from 11 to 131 months (median, 50 months). The median RT dose was 54 Gy (range, 46–68 Gy) administered at 1.8–2.5 Gy per fraction, 5 days a week. One patient with a $27\times25\times5$ cm tumor who received preoperative RT and incomplete resection experienced local progression. The local control rates for the remaining 34 patients after surgery or surgery and RT were as follows: close or positive margins, 1 of 3 vs. 5 of 6; and negative margins, 14 of 21 (67 %) vs. 4 of 4. The 7-year local control rates were 28 % after surgery and 80 % after surgery and RT. No patient experienced a severe complication.

Ballo et al. [31] reported on 19 patients treated at the M. D. Anderson Cancer Center with RT alone (1 patient) or combined with surgery (18 patients) between 1972 and 1995 (Table 2). Patients had follow-up from 6 months to 23.5 years (median, 6 years). One patient had surgery and experienced a rapid recurrence; RT alone (65 Gy) was used to treat the gross disease and was unsuccessful. The patient subsequently died with disease 21 months after treatment. Two patients received preoperative RT (50 Gy) and surgery and both were locally controlled. Sixteen patients received surgery and postoperative RT (mean, 59 Gy; range, 50–66 Gy); margins were positive in 6 patients and negative in 10 patients. All remained locally controlled. No patient experienced a severe complication.

Dagan et al. reported on 10 patients (DSFP, 9 patients; DSFP-FS, 1 patient) treated at the University of Florida with surgery and postoperative RT and followed from 21 to 185 months [33]. All patients had a gross total resection prior to RT. The external beam RT dose ranged from 59.4 to 65 Gy; one patient received an IR^{192} brachytherapy boost of 22.5 Gy. All 9 patients treated for DSFP have remained disease-free after treatment. The patient with a DFSP-FS experienced a local recurrence and died with disease. No patient experienced a severe complication.

Conclusion

The optimal treatment for patients with DFSP and DFSP-FS is resection with wide margins. The addition of adjuvant RT improves the likelihood of cure in patients with close or positive margins. Although data are scant, RT alone has a reasonable chance of curing the occasional patient with unresectable gross disease. The efficacy of chemotherapy for patients with metastases DFSP is ill defined. There are a few clinical reports indicating that imatinib, a tyrosine kinase inhibitor, can induce regression in patients with recurrent unresectable and/or metastatic DFSP [7].

References

1. Suit H, Spiro I, Mankin HJ, Efird J, Rosenberg AE. Radiation in management of patients with dermatofibrosarcoma protuberans. J Clin Oncol. 1996;14(8):2365–9.
2. Chang CK, Jacobs IA, Salti GI. Outcomes of surgery for dermatofibrosarcoma protuberans. Eur J Surg Oncol. 2004;30(3):341–5.
3. Bowne WB, Antonescu CR, Leung DH, Katz SC, Hawkins WG, Woodruff JM, et al. Dermatofibrosarcoma protuberans: a clinicopathologic analysis of patients treated and followed at a single institution. Cancer. 2000;88(12):2711–20.
4. Lindner NJ, Scarborough MT, Powell GJ, Spanier S, Enneking WF. Revision surgery in dermatofibrosarcoma protuberans of the trunk and extremities. Eur J Surg Oncol. 1999;25(4): 392–7.
5. Enzinger FM, Weiss SW. Fibrohistiocytic tumors of intermediate malignancy. In: Stamatis G, editor. Soft tissue tumors. St. Louis, MO: Mosby; 1988. p. 252–68.
6. Rutgers EJ, Kroon BB, Albus-Lutter CE, Gortzak E. Dermatofibrosarcoma protuberans: treatment and prognosis. Eur J Surg Oncol. 1992;18(3):241–8.
7. McArthur G. Molecularly targeted treatment for dermatofibrosarcoma protuberans. Semin Oncol. 2004;31(2 Suppl 6):30–6.

8. Kiuru-Kuhlefelt S, El-Rifai W, Fanburg-Smith J, Kere J, Miettinen M, Knuutila S. Concomitant DNA copy number amplification at 17q and 22q in dermatofibrosarcoma protuberans. Cytogenet Cell Genet. 2001;92(3–4):192–5.
9. Linn SC, West RB, Pollack JR, Zhu S, Hernandez-Boussard T, Nielsen TO, et al. Gene expression patterns and gene copy number changes in dermatofibrosarcoma protuberans. Am J Pathol. 2003;163(6):2383–95.
10. Sandberg AA, Bridge JA. Updates on the cytogenetics and molecular genetics of bone and soft tissue tumors. Dermatofibrosarcoma protuberans and giant cell fibroblastoma. Cancer Genet Cytogenet. 2003;140(1):1–12.
11. Sun LM, Wang CJ, Huang CC, Leung SW, Chen HC, Fang FM, et al. Dermatofibrosarcoma protuberans: treatment results of 35 cases. Radiother Oncol. 2000;57(2):175–81.
12. Gayner SM, Lewis JE, McCaffrey TV. Effect of resection margins on dermatofibrosarcoma protuberans of the head and neck. Arch Otolaryngol Head Neck Surg. 1997;123(4):430–3.
13. Stojadinovic A, Karpoff HM, Antonescu CR, Shah JP, Singh B, Spiro RH, et al. Dermatofibrosarcoma protuberans of the head and neck. Ann Surg Oncol. 2000;7(9): 696–704.
14. Goldblum JR, Reith JD, Weiss SW. Sarcomas arising in dermatofibrosarcoma protuberans: a reappraisal of biologic behavior in eighteen cases treated by wide local excision with extended clinical follow up. Am J Surg Pathol. 2000;24(8):1125–30.
15. Takahira T, Oda Y, Tamiya S, Yamamoto H, Kawaguchi K, Kobayashi C, et al. Microsatellite instability and p53 mutation associated with tumor progression in dermatofibrosarcoma protuberans. Hum Pathol. 2004;35(2):240–5.
16. Weiss SW, Goldblum JR. Enzinger and Weiss's soft tissue tumors. 4th ed. Philadelphia, PA: Mosby; 2001.
17. Sasaki M, Ishida T, Horiuchi H, MacHinami R. Dermatofibrosarcoma protuberans: an analysis of proliferative activity, DNA flow cytometry and p53 overexpression with emphasis on its progression. Pathol Int. 1999;49(9):799–806.
18. Torreggiani WC, Al-Ismail K, Munk PL, Nicolaou S, O'Connell JX, Knowling MA. Dermatofibrosarcoma protuberans: MR imaging features. AJR Am J Roentgenol. 2002;178(4): 989–93.
19. Domanski HA, Gustafson P. Cytologic features of primary, recurrent, and metastatic dermatofibrosarcoma protuberans. Cancer. 2002;96(6):351–61.
20. Klijanienko J, Caillaud JM, Lagace R. Fine-needle aspiration of primary and recurrent dermatofibrosarcoma protuberans. Diagn Cytopathol. 2004;30(4):261–5.
21. Calikoglu E, Augsburger E, Chavaz P, Saurat JH, Kaya G. CD44 and hyaluronate in the differential diagnosis of dermatofibroma and dermatofibrosarcoma protuberans. J Cutan Pathol. 2003;30(3):185–9.
22. Fanburg-Smith JC, Miettinen M. Low-affinity nerve growth factor receptor (p75) in dermatofibrosarcoma protuberans and other nonneural tumors: a study of 1,150 tumors and fetal and adult normal tissues. Hum Pathol. 2001;32(9):976–83.
23. Enneking WF, Spanier SS, Goodman MA. Current concepts review. The surgical staging of musculoskeletal sarcoma. J Bone Joint Surg Am. 1980;62(6):1027–30.
24. Parsons JT, Zlotecki RA, Reddy KA, Mitchell TP, Marcus RB, Jr, Scarborough MT. The role of radiotherapy and limb-conserving surgery in the management of soft-tissue sarcomas in adults. Hematol Oncol Clin North Am. 2001;15(2):377–88, vii.
25. AJCC. Soft tissue sarcoma. In: Green FL, editor. AJCC cancer staging manual. New York, NY: Springer; 2002. p. 193–200.
26. Khatri VP, Galante JM, Bold RJ, Schneider PD, Ramsamooj R, Goodnight Jr JE. Dermatofibrosarcoma protuberans: reappraisal of wide local excision and impact of inadequate initial treatment. Ann Surg Oncol. 2003;10(9):1118–22.
27. Snow SN, Gordon EM, Larson PO, Bagheri MM, Bentz ML, Sable DB. Dermatofibrosarcoma protuberans: a report on 29 patients treated by Mohs micrographic surgery with long-term follow-up and review of the literature. Cancer. 2004;101(1):28–38.

28. Wacker J, Khan-Durani B, Hartschuh W. Modified Mohs micrographic surgery in the therapy of dermatofibrosarcoma protuberans: analysis of 22 patients. Ann Surg Oncol. 2004;11(4): 438–44.
29. DuBay D, Cimmino V, Lowe L, Johnson TM, Sondak VK. Low recurrence rate after surgery for dermatofibrosarcoma protuberans: a multidisciplinary approach from a single institution. Cancer. 2004;100(5):1008–16.
30. Nouri K, Lodha R, Jimenez G, Robins P. Mohs micrographic surgery for dermatofibrosarcoma protuberans: University of Miami and NYU experience. Dermatol Surg. 2002;28(11):1060–4; discussion 4.
31. Ballo MT, Zagars GK, Pisters P, Pollack A. The role of radiation therapy in the management of dermatofibrosarcoma protuberans. Int J Radiat Oncol Biol Phys. 1998;40(4):823–7.
32. Cai H, Wang Y, Wu J, Shi Y. Dermatofibrosarcoma protuberans: clinical diagnoses and treatment results of 260 cases in China. J Surg Oncol. 2012;105(2):142–8.
33. Dagan R, Morris CG, Zlotecki RA, Scarborough MT, Mendenhall WM. Radiotherapy in the treatment of dermatofibrosarcoma protuberans. Am J Clin Oncol. 2005;28(6):537–9.

Radiation Therapy of Cutaneous Lymphoma

Bradford S. Hoppe and Nancy P. Mendenhall

Introduction

Over 70,000 people are diagnosed with non-Hodgkin lymphoma (NHL) annually in the United States [1]. Ten percent of these patients present with primary cutaneous lymphoma, which is the second most common extranodal site for NHL [2]. Cutaneous lymphoma is divided into primary cutaneous T-cell lymphoma (PCTCL) and primary cutaneous B-cell lymphoma (PCBCL). PCTCL and PCBCL are heterogeneous groups of diseases comprising various histologic subtypes of NHL, each with its own unique clinical features, natural history, prognosis, and treatment strategy.

Diagnosis is based on excisional or incisional biopsy, procuring a sufficient specimen with underlying subcutaneous fat to assess architecture, depth of involvement, and cell morphology and provides tissue for immunophenotyping—using flow cytometry or immunohistochemistry—and genotyping to determine the specific classification.

Work up of a patient with cutaneous lymphoma should include a complete history with an emphasis on B symptoms, and a physical examination with particular attention to the entire skin and lymph node regions. Photographs of the lesions before biopsy can help in treatment planning and response assessment. Laboratory studies should include a complete blood count with differential, a comprehensive chemistry panel, lactate dehydrogenase (LDH), and serum protein electrophoreses (which help exclude a monoclonal gammopathy). In patients with aggressive subtypes, advanced stage, or palpable lymph nodes, imaging should also include computed tomography (CT) scans of the chest, abdomen, pelvis, and neck. Positron emission tomography (PET) scans are appropriate in patients with aggressive subtypes. Bone marrow biopsy should be strongly considered in all cases.

B.S. Hoppe (✉) • N.P. Mendenhall
Department of Radiation Oncology, University of Florida Proton Therapy Institute, University of Florida, 2015 North Jefferson Street, Jacksonville, FL 32206, USA
e-mail: bhoppe@floridaproton.org

A.B. Cognetta and W.M. Mendenhall (eds.), *Radiation Therapy for Skin Cancer*,
DOI 10.1007/978-1-4614-6986-5_17,

The International Society for Cutaneous Lymphoma of the European Organization of Research and Treatment of Cancer (EORTC) developed a tumor-node-metastasis (TNM) classification for cutaneous lymphomas other than mycosis fungoides. The T classification (skin) is composed of T1, solitary skin involvement (T1a <5 cm, T1b >5 cm); T2, regional skin involvement, multiple lesions limited to one body region or two contiguous body regions (T2a, all-disease encompassing <15 cm circular area; T2b, 15–30-cm circular area; T2c, >30-cm diameter circular area); and T3, generalized skin involvement (with T3a, multiple lesions involving two noncontiguous body regions, and T3b, multiple lesions involving ≥3 body regions). The N (nodes) classification includes N0, no lymph node involvement; N1, involvement of 1 peripheral lymph node in a draining area; N2, >1 peripheral lymph node or a single lymph node that does not drain an area of current or prior skin involvement; N3, involvement of central lymph nodes. The M classification (viscera) includes M0, no evidence of extracutaneous non-lymph node disease; and M1, extracutaneous non-lymph node disease present [3].

Treatment is dependent on the specific subtype of cutaneous lymphoma. In general, indolent early-stage lymphoma is often treated with local therapies, such as limited-field RT using electrons, topical chemotherapeutic agents, or steroids. On the other hand, aggressive subtypes or more advanced-stage disease require systemic therapy or total skin electron therapy (TSET), which may or may not be combined with one or more local treatments.

Primary Cutaneous B-Cell Lymphoma

PCBCL comprises approximately 20 % of cutaneous lymphomas with an incidence of approximately one per one million people [4]. It includes primary cutaneous follicle center lymphoma (PCFCL) (50 %), primary cutaneous marginal zone B-cell lymphoma (PCMZL) (30 %), and primary cutaneous large B-cell lymphoma-leg type (PCLBL-LT) (20 %) [4].

Primary Cutaneous Follicular Center Lymphoma

PCFCL predominantly affects elderly patients in the fifth or sixth decades of life with a slight male predominance. It usually appears as solitary or grouped firm erythematous, nonpruritic papules, plaques, or tumors found on the trunk, neck, and head. Lesions are painless and rarely ulcerative, but scaling and surrounding annular erythema can be present [5].

A bone marrow biopsy should be considered in patients with PCFCL, particularly in patients with "B symptoms" and/or elevated LDH.

PCFCL lesions are generally slow growing and only 10 % develop disseminated disease, so aggressive intervention is not warranted. Historic series have demonstrated 10-year cancer-specific survival rates of 95 % and complete response rates (CR) of 99 % with localized RT alone [4]. Relapse rates after RT range from 30–76 %, with larger radiation fields apparently associated with lower rates of recurrence [6, 7]. Excision alone is also associated with approximately 50 % recurrence rates [5]. Other therapies—such as intralesional INF-alpha, intralesional rituximab, systemic rituximab, and systemic chemotherapy—have also been effective in small studies, with complete response rates over 75 %, followed by relapse in half of the patients.

Primary Cutaneous Marginal Zone B-Cell Lymphoma

PCMZL is in the same family as mucosa-associated lymphoid tissue (MALT) lymphoma and is often referred to as "skin-associated lymphoid tissue" (SALT) lymphoma. It develops later in life, typically in the fifth or sixth decade, but cases have occurred in patients as young as 14 years old [5]. Similar to other MALT lymphomas, PCMZL has been linked to bacterial infections, such as *Borrelia burgdorferi*, in Europe, but this relationship has not been observed in the United States or Asia [8, 9]. In areas endemic for *B. burgdorferi*, patients presenting with PCMZL should undergo testing for possible infection. Antibiotic treatment alone has resulted in complete response of the cutaneous lesion in up to 43 % of PCMZL patients with *B. burgdorferi* infection [5]. Cephalosporins are thought to be superior to high-dose tetracyclines in managing patients.

Patients with PCMZL usually present with multifocal red to violaceous papules, plaques, or nodules found on the trunk or upper extremities. Bone marrow biopsies are unnecessary in patients with PCMZL. One study found that only 2 of 82 patients with marginal zone lymphoma had bone marrow involvement [10].

PCMZL is an indolent process that is managed with either limited radiotherapy (RT) or surgical resection, with complete response rates of 85 % or higher and 5-year overall survival rates of 98–100 % [4, 5]. Up to half of patients eventually relapse in another skin site. In an analysis of a series of studies reporting small numbers of patients, a 99 % complete response rate was documented in 132 patients treated with RT to 30–45 Gy with 46 % of patients ultimately relapsing, primarily within the skin [5]. Similarly, 43 % of 75 patients undergoing complete surgical excision also relapsed in the skin [5]. Other case series have also shown some modest responses to intralesional rituximab, interferon alpha, and/or systemic chemotherapy.

Primary Cutaneous Diffuse Large B-Cell Lymphoma-Leg Types

PCLBCL-LTs usually present in the seventh and eighth decades of life with a female predominance of 1:2–3. Formerly classified as a PCFCL, this subtype has been recognized in the last decade as different from PCLBCL-LT in its affliction of older patients, presentation on the lower extremities, and worse prognosis. It accounts for only 5 % of all cutaneous lymphomas and about 20 % of all PCBCL.

A bone marrow biopsy is highly recommended with this diagnosis; 85–90 % of patients present with red or bluish nodules or tumors on the lower legs.

In contrast to the other PCBCLs, PCLBCL-LT requires more aggressive therapy than RT alone. In a collection of studies using RT alone, complete response rates were 88 %, but 60 % of patients relapsed, including 30 % with extracutaneous progression [11]. Multiagent chemotherapy alone has demonstrated similar results with 81 % complete response rates, but relapse rates of approximately 60 % [11]. The poor outcomes with single-modality therapy have led to consensus guidelines for PCLBCL-LT that recommend both RT and aggressive systemic therapy with rituximab and CHOP (cyclophosphamide, doxorubicin, vincristine, and prednisone)-like chemotherapy regimens.

Primary Cutaneous T-Cell Lymphoma

PCTCL accounts for the majority (75–80 %) of cutaneous NHLs and includes mycosis fungoides (MF) [4], adult T-cell leukemia/lymphoma (ATLL), primary cutaneous CD30+ lymphoproliferative disorders, subcutaneous panniculitis-like T-cell lymphoma (SPTL), and primary cutaneous peripheral T-cell lymphoma, unspecified (PTL).

MF accounts for half of all cutaneous lymphomas, predominantly affecting males (2:1 ratio) in the fifth and sixth decades of life [12]. MF is an indolent disease that presents with months to years of pruritus and scaling skin changes, usually distributed along the bathing trunk (buttocks and other sun-protected areas). Lesions may progress into patches, plaques, tumors, generalized erythroderma, poikiloderma, or papules. Erythroderma is associated with significant pruritus, scaling, and adenopathy and may accompany Sézary syndrome. Sézary syndrome is caused by circulating Sézary cells, which are mononuclear cells with a cribriform nucleus. A formal diagnosis requires >1,000 Sézary cells per cubic mm in the peripheral blood.

Skin biopsy (a minimum of a 4 mm punch biopsy is recommended) usually shows small to medium atypical mononuclear cells with cerebriform nuclei infiltrating the upper dermis and epidermal keratinocytes or forming intraepidermal aggregates. Immunophenotyping usually shows mature T-cell markers, including CD3+, CD4+, and CD45RO+ [13]. Loss of chromosome 10q is commonly found.

An algorithm for diagnosis of MF was developed by the International Society for Cutaneous Lymphoma and the European Organization of Research and Treatment of Cancer (ISCL/EORTC) and is a point-based system [14]. A diagnosis is only made when patients have a score of 4 or more points based on clinical, histopathologic, molecular, and immunopathologic criteria (Table 1). In addition to the general work-up of cutaneous lymphoma, a CBC with Sézary cell analysis should be performed. Additionally, all but stage I and IIA patients should undergo a PET-CT scan. A bone marrow biopsy is unnecessary unless visceral disease is identified.

Table 1 International Society for Cutaneous Lymphoma and the European Organization of Research and Treatment of Cancer (ISCL/EORTC) Algorithm for the Diagnosis of Early Mycosis Fungoides

Criteria	Description
Clinical criteria	Patches and plaques plus lesions in a non-sun-exposed location, size/shape variation of lesions, and poikiloderma; 1 point for 1 factor, 2 points for 2 or more factors
Histopathologic criteria	Superficial lymphoid infiltrate present plus epidermotropism without spongiosis and lymphoid atypia (1 point for 1 factor, 2 points for 2 factors)
Molecular-biological criteria	Clonal TCR gene rearrangement is present
Immunopathologic criteria	Fewer than 50 % of the T cells express CD2, CD3, or CD5, <10 % of the T cells express CD7, and there is discordance of epidermal and dermal cells with expression of CD2, CD3, CD5, or CD7 (1 point for any of these present)

Source: Adapted from Olsen E, Vonderheid E, Pimpinelli N, Willemze R, Kim Y, Knobler R, et al. Revisions to the staging and classification of mycosis fungoides and Sézary syndrome: a proposal of the International Society for Cutaneous Lymphomas (ISCL) and the cutaneous lymphoma task force of the European Organization of Research and Treatment of Cancer (EORTC). Blood 2007;110: 1713–22

MF has its own unique staging system (Table 2) [14]. Thirty percent, 35, 20, and 15 % of patients present with T1, T2, T3, or T4 disease, respectively.

Early-stage (IA–IIA) MF has a favorable prognosis with a median survival of 13 years [12] and is generally treated with skin-directed therapies, including topical corticosteroids, topical chemotherapeutic agents (nitrogen mustard and carmustine), topical retinoids (stage IA only), RT (local electron-beam RT for unilesional or total skin electron-beam RT for more extensive and progressive skin disease), and phototherapy using ultraviolet B (UVB) or psoralen + ultraviolet A photochemotherapy (PUVA). No specific treatment is preferred over the others; however, trying a different regimen is recommended on progression after initial treatment. In a study of 103 patients randomized to a combination chemotherapy (cyclophosphamide, doxorubicin, etoposide, and vincristine) and 30 Gy of total skin electron-beam therapy (TSEBT) vs. sequential topical therapy, there was no significant difference in disease-free or overall survival [15]. Because of the morbidity of TSEBT, it is generally reserved for progressive lesions or thicker tumor plaques.

Patients with more advanced MF (stage IIB–IV) have a worse prognosis, with an overall survival rate of 3.5–4 years for stage IIB–III and 1.5 years for stage IV and require more aggressive treatment regimens [12].

Limited stage IIB disease can be treated with a combination of local RT to the tumors with other topical agents applied to adjacent plaques or systemic therapy, while more extensive stage IIB and IIIA disease can be treated with systemic retinoids, interferon, histone deacetylase inhibitors, Denileukin diftitox, systemic

Table 2 Mycosis fungoides TNM classification and staging system for cutaneous T-cell lymphoma

T (skin) classification	
T1	Limited patch or plaque on <10 % of the skin surface
T2	Generalized patch or plaque on >10 % of the skin surface involved
T3	Tumorous skin involvement
T4	Erythroderma
N (lymph nodes) classification	
N0	No clinically abnormal lymph nodes
N1	Clinically abnormal lymph nodes with histopathology Dutch grade 1 or NCI LN0-2
N2	Histopathology Dutch grade 2 or NCI LN3
N3	Histopathology Dutch grades 3–4 or NCI LN4
M (visceral organs) classification	
M0	No visceral involvement
M1	Visceral involvement
B (blood) classification	
B0	No significant blood involvement with ≤5 % Sézary cells
B1	Low blood tumor burden
B2	High blood tumor burden with positive clone plus one of the following: ≥1,000/μL Sézary cells, CD4/CD8 ≥ 10, CD4+CD7− cells ≥40 %, or CD4+CD26− cells ≥30 %
Clinical stage	
IA	T1N0M0B0-1
IB	T2N0M0B0-1
IIA	T1-2N1-N2B0-1
IIB	T3N0-2M0B0-1
IIIA	T4N0-2M0B0
IIIB	T4N0-2M0B1
IVA1	T1-4N0-2M0B2
IVA2	T1-4N3M0B0-2
IVB	T1-4N0-3M1B0-2

LN0 no atypical lymphocytes; *LN3* aggregates of atypical lymphocytes; nodal architecture Preserved; *LN4* partial/complete effacement of nodal architecture by atypical lymphocytes or frankly neoplastic cells

Source: Adapted from Olsen E, Vonderheid E, Pimpinelli N, Willemze R, Kim Y, Knobler R, et al. Revisions to the staging and classification of mycosis fungoides and Sézary syndrome: a proposal of the International Society for Cutaneous Lymphomas (ISCL) and the cutaneous lymphoma task force of the European Organization of Research and Treatment of Cancer (EORTC). Blood 2007;110: 1713–22

chemotherapy, and TSEBT. Generally TSEBT is only used in stage IIB disease, because patients with more advanced disease may suffer severe desquamation after doses as low as 4 Gy.

Stage IIIB and IV requires systemic therapy to target malignant cells in the blood and may include extracorporeal photochemotherapy, systemic retinoids, interferon, histone deacetylase inhibitors, Denileukin diftitox, methotrexate, or allogeneic stem cell transplantation. These systemic agents can be combined with skin-directed therapies.

Table 3 Acronyms

NHL	non-hodgkin lymphoma
PCTCL	primary cutaneous T-cell lymphoma
PCBCL	primary cutaneous B-cell lymphoma
LDH	lactate dehydrogenase
CT	computed tomography
PET	Positron emission tomography
EORTC	European Organization of Research and Treatment of Cancer
TNM	tumor-node-metastasis
TSET	total skin electron therapy
PCMZL	primary cutaneous marginal zone B-cell lymphoma
PCLBL-LT	primary cutaneous large B-cell lymphoma-leg type
CR	complete response
MALT	mucosa-associated lymphoid tissue
SALT	skin-associated lymphoid tissue
RT	radiotherapy
MF	mycosis fungoides
ATLL	adult T-cell leukemia/lymphoma
SPTL	subcutaneous panniculitis-like T-cell lymphoma
PTL	peripheral T-cell lymphoma, unspecified
ISCL	International Society for Cutaneous Lymphoma
UVB	ultraviolet B
PUVA	psoralen + ultraviolet A
TSEBT	total skin electron-beam therapy
C-ALCL	cutaneous-anaplastic large-cell lymphoma
LyP	lymphomatoid papulosis
HTLV-1	human T-cell leukemia virus-1
SPTL-AB	subdivided into an alpha/beta
SPTL-GD	subdivided into an gamma/delta

Total Skin Electron Beam Treatment

TSEBT is one of the most complex and labor-intensive radiation therapy applications and, as such, requires experienced radiation oncologists, a robust physics and dosimetry team, and equipment not usually available in the community setting. TSEBT delivers a total prescription dose of 30–36 Gy over 9–10 weeks. Typically, a 6-field technique is used, which includes anterior, posterior, and four opposed oblique fields. Three fields are treated each day (usually the anterior with two posterior oblique fields on one day followed by the posterior with two anterior oblique fields on the second day). A total skin dose of 1.5–2 Gy is delivered over each 2-day cycle [16]. Additional small boost fields are generally required to augment the dose to the top of the scalp, perineum, and the soles of the feet. Acute toxicity from TSEBT includes erythema, desquamation, alopecia, fingernail and toenail loss, and loss of sweat glands for the first 6–12 months following treatment. Long-term toxicities include scattered telangiectasias and cutaneous malignancies.

Non-MF CTCL

Primary cutaneous CD30+ lymphoproliferative disorders are made up of several different subtypes, including primary cutaneous-anaplastic large-cell lymphoma (C-ALCL), lymphomatoid papulosis (LyP), and other borderline cases. C-ALCL presents with solitary lesions in up to 75 % of patients, with multiple lesions in about 25 % [17]. It generally has a favorable prognosis with a 5-year disease-specific survival rate of greater than 90 % [18, 19]. Treatment generally involves RT or surgical excision, while systemic therapy is reserved for patients with multiple lesions or extracutaneous disease. LyP typically presents as chronic, recurrent, self-healing papulonecronic or papulondular skin disease. No therapy with curative potential has been identified; >90 % of relapses are in the skin. Methotrexate may be effective in delaying future skin lesions. Despite high relapse rates, overall survival at 5 and 10 years has been reported at 100 and 92 %, respectively [17].

ATLL that is limited to the skin is a slowly progressive lymphoma compared with the usual variant, which is widely disseminated. The skin variant presents with lesions similar to MF, but can be distinguished by the clonally integrated human T-cell leukemia virus-1 (HTLV-1) genes found in all cases and can be helpful in distinguishing it from MF [20]. Skin-directed therapies, similar to MF, are effective in managing this indolent version of ATLL.

SPTL primarily affects the legs and has been subdivided into an alpha/beta (SPTL-AB) or gamma/delta (SPTL-GD) component [21]. Due to the poor outcomes with SPTL-GD (5 years DSS-11 %), however, SPTL-GD has been reclassified as a PTL, unspecified. Although 5-year disease-specific survival rate is approximately 85 % for SPTL-AB, hemophagocytic syndrome occurs in 17 % of patients and results in a 5 years DSS as low as 46 % compared with 91 % in those without hemophagocytic syndrome [4]. Management of SPTL-AB is with systemic chemotherapy or corticosteroids [21].

PTL, unspecified, is a heterogeneous group of different rare lymphoma types. They generally have a more aggressive clinical course with 5-year disease-specific survival rate of 10–30 % and require treatment with systemic chemotherapy.

References

1. Siegel R, Naishadham D, Jemal A. Cancer statistics, 2012. CA Cancer J Clin. 2012;62:10–29.
2. Burg G, Kerl H, Przybilla B, Braun-Falco O. Some statistical data, diagnosis, and staging of cutaneous B-cell lymphomas. J Dermatol Surg Oncol. 1984;10:256–62.
3. Kim YH, Willemze R, Pimpinelli N, Whittaker S, Olsen EA, Ranki A, et al. TNM classification system for primary cutaneous lymphomas other than mycosis fungoides and Sezary syndrome: a proposal of the International Society for Cutaneous Lymphomas (ISCL) and the Cutaneous Lymphoma Task Force of the European Organization of Research and Treatment of Cancer (EORTC). Blood. 2007;110:479–84.
4. Willemze R, Jaffe ES, Burg G, Cerroni L, Berti E, Swerdlow SH, et al. WHO-EORTC classification for cutaneous lymphomas. Blood. 2005;105:3768–85.

5. Senff NJ, Hoefnagel JJ, Jansen PM, Vermeer MH, van Baarlen J, Blokx WA, et al. Reclassification of 300 primary cutaneous B-cell lymphomas according to the new WHO-EORTC classification for cutaneous lymphomas: comparison with previous classifications and identification of prognostic markers. J Clin Oncol. 2007;25:1581–7.
6. Eich HT, Eich D, Micke O, Suttzer H, Casper C, Krieg T, et al. Long-term efficacy, curative potential, and prognostic factors of radiotherapy in primary cutaneous B-cell lymphoma. Int J Radiat Oncol Biol Phys. 2003;55:899–906.
7. Piccinno R, Caccialanza M, Berti E. Dermatologic radiotherapy of primary cutaneous follicle center cell lymphoma. Eur J Dermatol. 2003;13:49–52.
8. Takino H, Li C, Hu S, Kuo TT, Geissinger E, Muller-Hermelink HK, et al. Primary cutaneous marginal zone B-cell lymphoma: a molecular and clinicopathological study of cases from Asia, Germany, and the United States. Mod Pathol. 2008;21:1517–26.
9. Goodlad JR, Davidson MM, Hollowood K, Ling C, MacKenzie C, Christie I, et al. Primary cutaneous B-cell lymphoma and Borrelia burgdorferi infection in patients from the Highlands of Scotland. Am J Surg Pathol. 2000;24:1279–85.
10. Senff NJ, Kluin-Nelemans HC, Willemze R. Results of bone marrow examination in 275 patients with histological features that suggest an indolent type of cutaneous B-cell lymphoma. Br J Haematol. 2008;142:52–6.
11. Senff NJ, Noordijk EM, Kim YH, Bagot M, Berti E, Cerroni L, et al. European Organization for Research and Treatment of Cancer and International Society for Cutaneous Lymphoma consensus recommendations for the management of cutaneous B-cell lymphomas. Blood. 2008;112:1600–9.
12. Kim YH, Liu HL, Mraz-Gernhard S, Varghese A, Hoppe RT. Long-term outcome of 525 patients with mycosis fungoides and Sezary syndrome: clinical prognostic factors and risk for disease progression. Arch Dermatol. 2003;139:857–66.
13. Oshtory S, Apisarnthanarax N, Gilliam AC, Cooper KD, Meyerson HJ. Usefulness of flow cytometry in the diagnosis of mycosis fungoides. J Am Acad Dermatol. 2007;57:454–62.
14. Olsen E, Vonderheid E, Pimpinelli N, Willemze R, Kim Y, Knobler R, et al. Revisions to the staging and classification of mycosis fungoides and Sezary syndrome: a proposal of the International Society for Cutaneous Lymphomas (ISCL) and the cutaneous lymphoma task force of the European Organization of Research and Treatment of Cancer (EORTC). Blood. 2007;110:1713–22.
15. Kaye FJ, Bunn Jr PA, Steinberg SM, Stocker JL, Ihde DC, Fischmann AB, et al. A randomized trial comparing combination electron-beam radiation and chemotherapy with topical therapy in the initial treatment of mycosis fungoides. N Engl J Med. 1989;321:1784–90.
16. Hoppe RT, Fuks Z, Bagshaw MA. Radiation therapy in the management of cutaneous T-cell lymphomas. Cancer Treat Rep. 1979;63:625–32.
17. Liu HL, Hoppe RT, Kohler S, Harvell JD, Reddy S, Kim YH. CD30+ cutaneous lymphoproliferative disorders: the Stanford experience in lymphomatoid papulosis and primary cutaneous anaplastic large cell lymphoma. J Am Acad Dermatol. 2003;49:1049–58.
18. Bekkenk MW, Geelen FA, van Voorst Vader PC, Heule F, Geerts ML, van Vloten WA, et al. Primary and secondary cutaneous CD30(+) lymphoproliferative disorders: a report from the Dutch Cutaneous Lymphoma Group on the long-term follow-up data of 219 patients and guidelines for diagnosis and treatment. Blood. 2000;95:3653–61.
19. Vergier B, Beylot-Barry M, Pulford K, Michel P, Bosq J, de Muret A, et al. Statistical evaluation of diagnostic and prognostic features of CD30+ cutaneous lymphoproliferative disorders: a clinicopathologic study of 65 cases. Am J Surg Pathol. 1998;22:1192–202.
20. Ohshima K, Suzumiya J, Sato K, Kanda M, Sugihara M, Haraoka S, et al. Nodal T-cell lymphoma in an HTLV-I-endemic area: proviral HTLV-I DNA, histological classification and clinical evaluation. Br J Haematol. 1998;101:703–11.
21. Willemze R, Jansen PM, Cerroni L, Berti E, Santucci M, Assaf C, et al. Subcutaneous panniculitis-like T-cell lymphoma: definition, classification, and prognostic factors: an EORTC Cutaneous Lymphoma Group Study of 83 cases. Blood. 2008;111:838–45.

Squamous and Basal Cell Carcinomas with Perineural Invasion

William M. Mendenhall and Jeffrey Bennett

Introduction

The majority of skin carcinomas are basal cell carcinomas (BCCs) and squamous cell carcinomas (SCCs) and are treated successfully with surgery or radiotherapy (RT) [1, 2]. Perineural invasion (PNI) occurs in 2–6 % of skin cancers and is associated with a poorer prognosis [3–19]. The frequency of PNI varies according to different factors, such as the number of histologic sections examined, the stains used, and the diligence of the pathologist or Mohs surgeon. PNI is of particular concern when it is associated with skin cancers arising in the head and neck because of proximity to cranial nerves (CNs) and the increased difficulty obtaining wide margins depending on the primary site. The risk of PNI is increased with mid-face location, male gender, increasing tumor size, recurrence after prior treatment, and poor histologic differentiation [18–22]. The nerves most commonly involved are the second division of CN V and CN VII [21].

Patients with tumors with PNI may be asymptomatic (incidental) or may present with CN deficits (clinical) because of tumor invasion [23, 24]. Patients with clinical PNI are symptomatic and/or have radiographic evidence of PNI; radiographic evidence of PNI is rare in an asymptomatic patient. The initial symptoms of PNI are often subtle such as a feeling of ants crawling underneath the skin (formication) [21]. The symptoms may slowly progress to pain, numbness, and/or facial weakness over 6 months to 2 years before the diagnosis is made. The patient may be incorrectly diagnosed as having Bell's palsy or trigeminal neuralgia and undergo

W.M. Mendenhall (✉)
Department of Radiation Oncology, College of Medicine, University of Florida,
2000 SW Archer Road, Gainesville, FL 32610, USA
e-mail: mendwm@shands.ufl.edu

J. Bennett
Department of Radiology, University of Florida, 2000 SW Archer Road,
Gainesville, FL 32608, USA

A.B. Cognetta and W.M. Mendenhall (eds.), *Radiation Therapy for Skin Cancer*,
DOI 10.1007/978-1-4614-6986-5_18, © Springer Science+Business Media New York 2013

one or more non-diagnostic magnetic resonance imaging (MRI) scans before the presence of PNI is appreciated.

The aim of this chapter is to discuss the management and outcomes of patients with PNI, in particular those arising on the head and neck.

Diagnosis

Most of the time, PNI is identified on histologic examination of a relatively asymptomatic skin cancer following excision. Histologically, the tumor cells usually surround the nerve and extend along the nerve; skip lesions are common. Intraneural extension is usually not appreciated, particularly for patients with incidental PNI. Although proximal spread towards the central nervous system (CNS) is the usual mode of invasion, distal spread may also occur [10, 21].

PNI may be difficult to appreciate histologically. Peritumoral fibrosis, which is the presence of concentric layers of fibrous tissue that surround or are surrounded by tumor, may mimic PNI [17, 25]. The addition of the $p75^{NGFR}$ (nerve growth factor receptor) immunostain to the hematoxylin and eosin (H & E) stain with or without the S-100 immunostain may enhance the detection of PNI [25].

MRI is the most sensitive radiographic study to detect and define the extent of PNI [23]. Expansion of neural foramina and canals such as the inferior alveolar canal, infraorbital foramen, foramen rotundum, or facial canal may be apparent on computed tomography (CT) scan. The use of high-field 3T MRI may increase the sensitivity in detecting PNI [26]. Radiographic evidence of PNI includes enlargement or abnormal enhancement of the nerve, obliteration of the fat plane surrounding the nerve with loss of the distinction between the nerve and the perineural vascular plexus, and/or erosion or enlargement of the related foramen (Fig. 1) [23].

Patients with PNI have an increased risk of metastases to the regional lymph nodes [4, 9, 27] which can also be assessed on MRI but preferably with contrast-enhanced CT. Sentinel lymph node biopsy (SLNB) may also be considered to assess the regional nodes [28].

Treatment

Patients with microscopic PNI have almost always undergone excision of the primary lesion prior to the diagnosis. Whether or not to routinely add postoperative RT following complete excision is controversial. A survey of approximately 25 % of the membership of the American College of Mohs Surgery revealed that most respondents considered in-transit metastases and PNI as the major factors leading to consideration of radiographic staging, SLNB, and adjuvant RT for patients with high-risk SCC [15]. In 2009, Jambusaria-Pahlajani et al. [29] reported on a literature review of reports on high-risk SCC with PNI treated with either surgery alone

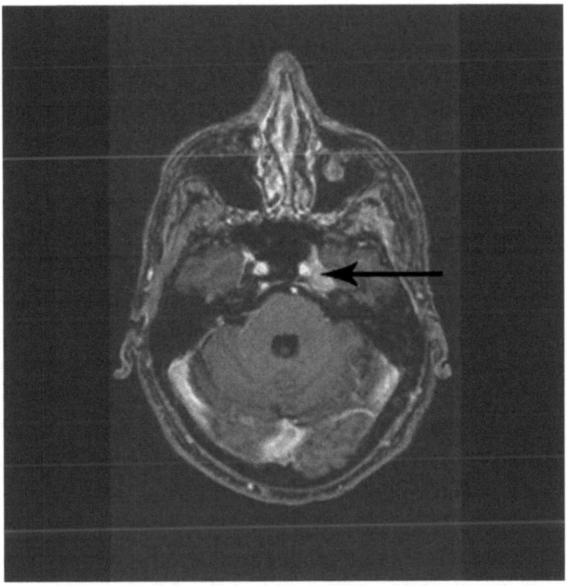

Fig. 1 Patient with squamous cell carcinoma of the skin with clinical perineural invasion of the second division of the trigeminal nerve and the facial nerve. Gross tumor extends through the skull base and invades the left cavernous sinus (*arrow*)

or surgery and adjuvant RT. They observed that, for 74 patients with PNI, the outcomes after surgery alone and surgery plus RT were similar and concluded that, in the presence of clear surgical margins, the benefit of adjuvant RT was unclear. The disadvantage of retrospective literature reviews is that the patients at higher risk for recurrence are probably more likely to receive adjuvant RT, thus biasing the comparison. In relation to the surgical technique, Mohs micrographic surgery (MMS) is likely superior in terms of local control to standard surgical resection in SCC with PNI.

In 2009, Ross et al. [12] reported that the diameter of the nerve involved with PNI may be useful to predict outcome with PNI. They reported on 48 patients with SCC and PNI treated at the University of Pennsylvania between 1996 and 2005 with surgery (46 patients), RT alone (1 patient), and desiccation and curettage (1 patient) [12]. Surgery was combined with adjuvant RT in 25 patients. The median diameter of involved nerves was 0.09 mm (range, 0.02–0.6 mm). Overall, 17 % of patients died from recurrent SCC. PNI of nerves less than 0.1 mm was associated with a cause-specific death rate of 0 % compared with 32 % for those PNI of larger caliber nerves. Other parameters significantly associated with diminished survival included recurrent or poorly differentiated SCC, tumor diameter ≥2 cm, and/or depth of invasion of ≥1 cm. Thus the diameter of the involved nerve may be useful to select patients for treatment with surgery alone.

The indications for postoperative RT in patients with incidental PNI are not well-defined. A subset of patients with focal incidental PNI with negative margins is likely to be cured with surgery alone, particularly a BCC that is not adjacent to a major CN. Alternatively, those with multifocal PNI should be considered for post-operative RT, particularly patients with recurrent cancers, SCCs, and mid-face locations in proximity to CNs V and VII. Patients with extensive microscopic PNI associated with BCC have a high risk of recurrence with extension to the skull base after surgery alone and should be considered for postoperative RT. Patients who are immunocompromised due to solid organ transplant and/or chronic lymphocytic leukemia tend to have more aggressive cancers and should be strongly considered for postoperative RT.

In practice, the majority of patients with SCC and microscopic PNI undergo postoperative RT to reduce the risk of locoregional recurrence. RT fields usually encompass the primary site with a surrounding margin. With extensive PNI with positive margins, the involved nerve is included in the RT treatment volume to the skull base. The latter patients experience more treatment-related toxicity because of the increased volume of tissue irradiated and have a worse prognosis due to selection bias [23]. The risk of lymph node metastases is approximately 15–20 % in patients with SCC and microscopic PNI, hence clinically negative regional nodes should be electively treated [23, 24]. Although SLNB may be considered, our practice is to forego the procedure.

Patients with clinical PNI have a worse prognosis and their management is less controversial. If the gross disease appears to be completely resectable, they are treated with resection and postoperative RT. A significant subset of patients with tumor that extends proximally to the skull base has unresectable disease. Aggressive subtotal resection of such tumors, such as those that involve the cavernous sinus, results in multiple CN deficits and significant residual disease without meaningfully enhancing the probability of cure. Thus, such patients are better treated with definitive RT. Treatment volumes are individualized based on the location and extent of the tumor. The volume is initially generous because the extent of subclinical disease is often difficult to define. The clinician must be aware that the tumor involving CN V may involve CN VII via the auriculotemporal nerve, or vice versa [30]. Patients are treated with hyperfractionation at 1.2 Gy per fraction twice daily to doses in the range of 64.8–74.4 Gy postoperatively (depending on the margins) and 74.4 Gy for definitive RT. Hyperfractionation is preferred to once-daily fractionation to reduce the risk of radiation retinopathy and/or optic neuropathy in cases where the retina, optic nerve(s), and/or chiasm is included in the RT volume to high dose [31]. There are no data to support the use of adjuvant chemotherapy in patients with skin cancer and PNI; nevertheless, local failure is the dominant mode of recurrence in patients who are treated for clinical PNI. It may well be reasonable to extrapolate data from patients treated for mucosal head and neck SCCs and consider adding concomitant chemotherapy, such as weekly cisplatin 30 mg/m^2, to improve the likelihood of local control [32].

Outcomes

In 2009, Jackson et al. [14] reported on 118 patients with cutaneous BCC or SCC and incidental (97 patients) or clinical (21 patients) PNI treated with RT between 1992 and 2000. RT was definitive in 4 patients and administered postoperatively in

Table 1 Five-year outcomes

Five-year outcomes	Incidental PNI (*N*=107) (%)	Clinical PNI (*N*=109; %)	*p* Value
Overall survival	55	54	0.8252
Cause-specific survival	73	64	0.0856
Local control	80	54	0.0038
Local-regional control	70	51	0.0648
Freedom from distant metastases	90	94	0.1918

PNI perineural invasion

Source: Balamucki CJ, DeJesus R, Galloway TJ, Mancuso AA, Amdur RJ, Morris CG, Kirwan JM, Mendenhall WM. Impact of radiographic findings on prognosis skin cancer with perineural invasion. Amer J Clin Oncol. 2013; In press

114 patients. Median follow-up was 84 months (range, 4–201 months). The 5-year outcomes after treatment for incidental vs. clinical PNI were: local control, 90 and 57 % ($p<0.0001$); relapse-free survival, 76 and 46 % ($p=0.003$); cause-specific survival, 90 and 76 % ($p=0.002$); and overall survival, 69 and 57 % ($p=0.03$), respectively. Patients with microscopic PNI and BCC had improved local control compared with those who had incidental PNI and SCC, 97 % vs. 84 % ($p=0.02$).

In 2011, Balamucki et al. [33] reported on 216 patients treated with curative intent at the University of Florida between 1965 and 2007 for skin carcinomas with incidental (107 patients) or clinical (109 patients) PNI. Median follow-up for living patients was 6.6 years (range, 0.6–23 years); 14 patients were lost to follow-up at a median of 35 months (range, 7.8–168.1 months). One hundred and five patients (78 %) had SCCs; the remainder had BCCs or metatypical BCCs. One hundred and thirty-three patients (62 %) had cancers that were recurrent after prior surgery.

Treatment for the 107 patients with microscopic PNI included surgery and postoperative RT (99 patients), preoperative RT and surgery (4 patients), and RT alone (4 patients) [33]. Twenty six of 107 patients (24 %) presented with clinically positive nodes. Margins were positive in 41 (40 %) of 103 patients treated surgically. The 5-year outcomes are depicted in Table 1 [33]. Seventeen of 107 patients (16 %) experienced 24 RT-severe related complications; 10 patients (9 %) required surgical interventions (Table 2). There were no fatal treatment complications.

Treatment of the 109 patients with clinical PNI included surgery and postoperative RT (58 patients), preoperative RT and surgery (2 patients), and definitive RT (49 patients) [33]. Nineteen patients received adjuvant chemotherapy including 6 patients who received postoperative RT and 13 patients who received definitive RT. Fifteen of 109 patients (14 %) presented with clinically positive neck nodes. The outcomes 5 years after treatment are shown in Table 1. Ninety percent of recurrences were observed within 5 years of treatment. Most failures were local. Multivariate analysis of local control revealed that none of the variables tested, including whether the patient was treated with surgery and RT vs. RT alone, significantly improved this endpoint. Cranial neuropathies improved in 14 of 62 patients (23 %) who experienced continuous local control after treatment. Fifty-four severe complications were observed in 39 of 109 patients (36 %); 13 patients (12 %) required surgical intervention. There were no fatal treatment complications.

Table 2 Complications (grade ≥3)

Complication	Incidental PNI (%) $N=107$	Clinical PNI (%) $N=109$
Soft-tissue necrosis	5 (5 %)	6 (6 %)
Bone exposure	7 (7 %)	12 (11 %)
Osteoradionecrosis	3 (3 %)	3 (3 %)
Fistula formation	0	5 (5 %)
Wound infection	3 (3 %)	6 (6 %)
Dehiscence	1 (1 %)	1 (1 %)
Blindness[a]	0	12 (11 %)
Other	5 (5 %)	9 (8 %)
Total events	24	54

PNI perineural invasion
Source: Balamucki CJ, DeJesus R, Galloway TJ, Mancuso AA, Amdur RJ, Morris CG, Kirwan JM, Mendenhall WM. Impact of radiographic findings on prognosis skin cancer with perineural invasion. Amer J Clin Oncol. 2013; In press
[a]Blindness: ipsilateral (9), contralateral (1), and bilateral (2)

Table 3 Clinical perineural invasion—5-year outcomes vs. pretreatment radiographic findings (45 patients)

	Radiographic findings			
5-Year outcome	Imaging negative ($n=10$; %)	Minimal or moderate peripheral PNI ($n=14$; %)	Central and/or macroscopic PNI ($n=21$; %)	p Value
Local control	76	57	25	0.2027
Cause-specific survival	100	56	61	0.0206
Overall survival	90	50	58	0.0817

PNI perineural invasion
Source: Balamucki CJ, DeJesus R, Galloway TJ, Mancuso AA, Amdur RJ, Morris CG, Kirwan JM, Mendenhall WM. Impact of radiographic findings on prognosis skin cancer with perineural invasion. Amer J Clin Oncol. 2013; In press

Galloway et al. [23] correlated the pretreatment radiographic findings on MRI and/or CT with outcome in 45 patients with PNI who were treated with surgery and adjuvant RT (24 patients) or definitive RT (21 patients) at the University of Florida between 1986 and 2002. Four patients received concomitant chemotherapy. Minimum follow-up on living patients was 2 years. Forty-four patients had clinical PNI, and 1 patient had only radiographic evidence of PNI. Patients defined as having minimal or moderate peripheral disease were those with abnormal nerve enhancement without enlargement or nerve enlargement 2–3 times the size of the normal nerve. Central and/or macroscopic disease was defined as enlargement more than 3 times the size of the normal nerve and/or involvement of the nerve between the skull base and the brainstem. Ten patients (22 %) had no radiographic evidence of PNI, 14 patients (31 %) had minimal or moderate peripheral disease, and 21 patients (47 %) had central and/or macroscopic disease. The 5-year local control and survival rates are depicted in Table 3 [23]. Local control was inversely related to radiographic evidence of proximal PNI. The survival rates in the two groups with radiographic evidence of PNI may be similar, in part, due to the relatively slow rate of disease progression after local recurrence in some cases.

Conclusion

BCCs and SCCs with PNI are relatively uncommon and have a worse prognosis compared with patients without evidence of this mode of spread. The optimal treatment is likely resection and postoperative RT for patients with apparently resectable disease [34]. Those with unresectable cancers are treated with definitive RT. Patients with clinically negative nodes but who have a high risk of spread to regional nodes should have the nodes treated electively. Because most recurrences are local, strategies to improve local control (including altered fractionation and concomitant chemotherapy) should be considered. Emerging technologies, such as intensity modulated radiation therapy (IMRT) or proton beam RT, may be employed to produce a more conformal dose distribution to dose escalate and/or reduce the dose to adjacent normal tissues (such as the optic chiasm or brainstem) and further improve the therapeutic ratio [35].

References

1. Mendenhall WM, Amdur RJ, Hinerman RW, Cognetta AB, Mendenhall NP. Radiotherapy for cutaneous squamous and basal cell carcinomas of the head and neck. Laryngoscope. 2009;119(10):1994–9.
2. Mourouzis C, Boynton A, Grant J, Umar T, Wilson A, Macpheson D, et al. Cutaneous head and neck SCCs and risk of nodal metastasis—UK experience. J Craniomaxillofac Surg. 2009;37(8):443–7.
3. Clayman GL, Lee JJ, Holsinger FC, Zhou X, Duvic M, El-Naggar AK, et al. Mortality risk from squamous cell skin cancer. J Clin Oncol. 2005;23(4):759–65.
4. Moore BA, Weber RS, Prieto V, El-Naggar A, Holsinger FC, Zhou X, et al. Lymph node metastases from cutaneous squamous cell carcinoma of the head and neck. Laryngoscope. 2005;115(9):1561–7.
5. Cassarino DS, Derienzo DP, Barr RJ. Cutaneous squamous cell carcinoma: a comprehensive clinicopathologic classification. Part one. J Cutan Pathol. 2006;33(3):191–206.
6. Cassarino DS, Derienzo DP, Barr RJ. Cutaneous squamous cell carcinoma: a comprehensive clinicopathologic classification–part two. J Cutan Pathol. 2006;33(4):261–79.
7. Backous DD, DeMonte F, El-Naggar A, Wolf P, Weber RS. Craniofacial resection for nonmelanoma skin cancer of the head and neck. Laryngoscope. 2005;115(6):931–7.
8. Faustina M, Diba R, Ahmadi MA, Esmaeli B. Patterns of regional and distant metastasis in patients with eyelid and periocular squamous cell carcinoma. Ophthalmology. 2004;111(10): 1930–2.
9. Cherpelis BS, Marcusen C, Lang PG. Prognostic factors for metastasis in squamous cell carcinoma of the skin. Dermatol Surg. 2002;28(3):268–73.
10. Ballantyne AJ, McCarten AB, Ibanez ML. The extension of cancer of the head and neck through peripheral nerves. Am J Surg. 1963;106:651–67.

11. Begemann M, Rosenblum MK, Loh J, Kraus D, Raizer JJ. Leptomeningeal metastases from recurrent squamous cell cancer of the skin. J Neurooncol. 2003;63(3):295–8.
12. Ross AS, Whalen FM, Elenitsas R, Xu X, Troxel AB, Schmults CD. Diameter of involved nerves predicts outcomes in cutaneous squamous cell carcinoma with perineural invasion: an investigator-blinded retrospective cohort study. Dermatol Surg. 2009;35(12):1859–66.
13. Mendenhall WM, Amdur RJ, Hinerman RW, Werning JW, Malyapa RS, Villaret DB, et al. Skin cancer of the head and neck with perineural invasion. Am J Clin Oncol. 2007;30(1): 93–6.
14. Jackson JE, Dickie GJ, Wiltshire KL, Keller J, Tripcony L, Poulsen MG, et al. Radiotherapy for perineural invasion in cutaneous head and neck carcinomas: toward a risk-adapted treatment approach. Head Neck. 2009;31(5):604–10.
15. Jambusaria-Pahlajani A, Hess SD, Katz KA, Berg D, Schmults CD. Uncertainty in the perioperative management of high-risk cutaneous squamous cell carcinoma among Mohs surgeons. Arch Dermatol. 2010;146(11):1225–31.
16. DeAmbrosis K, De'Ambrosis B. Nonmelanoma skin cancer with perineural invasion: report of outcomes of a case series. Dermatol Surg. 2010;36(1):133–8.
17. Leibovitch I, Huilgol SC, Selva D, Hill D, Richards S, Paver R. Cutaneous squamous cell carcinoma treated with Mohs micrographic surgery in Australia II Perineural invasion. J Am Acad Dermatol. 2005;53(2):261–6.
18. Leibovitch I, Huilgol SC, Selva D, Richards S, Paver R. Basal cell carcinoma treated with Mohs surgery in Australia III Perineural invasion. J Am Acad Dermatol. 2005;53(3):458–63.
19. Goepfert H, Dichtel WJ, Medina JE, Lindberg RD, Luna MD. Perineural invasion in squamous cell skin carcinoma of the head and neck. Am J Surg. 1984;148(4):542–7.
20. Mendenhall WM, Parsons JT, Mendenhall NP, Brant TA, Stringer SP, Cassisi NJ, et al. Carcinoma of the skin of the head and neck with perineural invasion. Head Neck. 1989; 11(4):301–8.
21. Mendenhall WM, Amdur RJ, Williams LS, Mancuso AA, Stringer SP, Price MN. Carcinoma of the skin of the head and neck with perineural invasion. Head Neck. 2002;24(1):78–83.
22. Salmon PJ, Hussain W, Geisse JK, Grekin RC, Mortimer NJ. Sclerosing squamous cell carcinoma of the skin, an underemphasized locally aggressive variant: a 20-year experience. Dermatol Surg. 2011;37(5):664–70.
23. Galloway TJ, Morris CG, Mancuso AA, Amdur RJ, Mendenhall WM. Impact of radiographic findings on prognosis for skin carcinoma with clinical perineural invasion. Cancer. 2005;103(6):1254–7.
24. Farasat S, Yu SS, Neel VA, Nehal KS, Lardaro T, Mihm MC, et al. A new American Joint Committee on Cancer staging system for cutaneous squamous cell carcinoma: creation and rationale for inclusion of tumor (T) characteristics. J Am Acad Dermatol. 2011;64(6):1051–9.
25. Lewis Kelso R, Colome-Grimmer MI, Uchida T, Wang HQ, Wagner Jr RF. p75(NGFR) immunostaining for the detection of perineural invasion by cutaneous squamous cell carcinoma. Dermatol Surg. 2006;32(2):177–83.
26. Penn R, Abemayor E, Nabili V, Bhuta S, Kirsch C. Perineural invasion detected by high-field 3.0-T magnetic resonance imaging. Am J Otolaryngol. 2010;31(6):482–4.
27. Fagan JJ, Collins B, Barnes L, D'Amico F, Myers EN, Johnson JT. Perineural invasion in squamous cell carcinoma of the head and neck. Arch Otolaryngol Head Neck Surg. 1998;124(6):637–40.
28. Wagner JD, Evdokimow DZ, Weisberger E, Moore D, Chuang TY, Wenck S, et al. Sentinel node biopsy for high-risk nonmelanoma cutaneous malignancy. Arch Dermatol. 2004; 140(1):75–9.
29. Jambusaria-Pahlajani A, Miller CJ, Quon H, Smith N, Klein RQ, Schmults CD. Surgical monotherapy versus surgery plus adjuvant radiotherapy in high-risk cutaneous squamous cell carcinoma: a systematic review of outcomes. Dermatol Surg. 2009;35(4):574–85.
30. Gluck I, Ibrahim M, Popovtzer A, Teknos TN, Chepeha DB, Prince ME, et al. Skin cancer of the head and neck with perineural invasion: defining the clinical target volumes based on the pattern of failure. Int J Radiat Oncol Biol Phys. 2009;74(1):38–46.

31. Bhandare N, Monroe AT, Morris CG, Bhatti MT, Mendenhall WM. Does altered fractionation influence the risk of radiation-induced optic neuropathy? Int J Radiat Oncol Biol Phys. 2005;62(4):1070–7.
32. Mendenhall WM, Riggs CE, Vaysberg M, Amdur RJ, Werning JW. Altered fractionation and adjuvant chemotherapy for head and neck squamous cell carcinoma. Head Neck. 2010;32(7):939–45.
33. Balamucki CJ, Mancuso AA, Amdur RJ, Kirwan JM, Morris CG, Flowers FP, et al. Skin carcinoma of the head and neck with perineural invasion. Am J Otolaryngol. 2011;33(4): 447–54.
34. Kropp L, Balamucki CJ, Morris CG, Kirwan J, Cognetta AB, Stoer CB, et al. Mohs resection and postoperative radiotherapy for head and neck cancers with incidental perineural invasion. Am J Otolaryngol. 2013; In press.
35. Mendenhall WM, Amdur RJ, Palta JR. Intensity-modulated radiotherapy in the standard management of head and neck cancer: promises and pitfalls. J Clin Oncol. 2006;24(17):2618–23.

Adjuvant Radiotherapy for Cutaneous Melanoma

William M. Mendenhall

Introduction

The dominant pattern of failure is distant in patients with locally advanced melanoma, but the likelihood of a local-regional recurrence is also high and may cause significant morbidity [1–16]. Patients are staged according to the TNM classifications of the seventh edition of the American Joint Committee on Cancer Staging Handbook [17]. Melanoma has long been thought to be relatively radio-resistant and, thus, the mainstay of treatment has been surgery [18, 19]. While systemic biologic therapy, such as interferon, may enhance disease-free survival, it likely does not impact locoregional control and probably has little, if any, impact on overall survival [20–24]. Radiotherapy (RT) has a relatively low likelihood of achieving long-term control in patients with gross residual disease; however, it has been increasingly employed postoperatively to improve local-regional control in patients at high risk for residual subclinical disease after surgery [18, 19, 24–33].

The purpose of this chapter is to review the factors that are associated with a high risk of residual subclinical local-regional disease after surgery and to discuss the role of adjuvant postoperative RT. Throughout the discussion, local recurrence refers to failure at the primary site, regional recurrence indicates failure in the at-risk nodal basin, and in-transit metastases refers to recurrence in the dermal lymphatics. RT probably is relatively ineffective at controlling in-transit disease because the dermal lymphatics have no valves and the likelihood of recurrence outside of the RT fields is high.

W.M. Mendenhall (✉)
Department of Radiation Oncology, College of Medicine, University of Florida,
2000 SW Archer Road, Gainesville, FL 32610, USA
e-mail: mendwm@shands.ufl.edu

A.B. Cognetta and W.M. Mendenhall (eds.), *Radiation Therapy for Skin Cancer*,
DOI 10.1007/978-1-4614-6986-5_19, © Springer Science+Business Media New York 2013

Factors Associated with Local-Regional Recurrence after Surgery

Local-regional recurrence may occur as a failure at the primary site, in-transit metastases in the dermal lymphatics adjacent to the primary site, and/or a recurrence in the regional lymph nodes.

Local Recurrence

The likelihood of local recurrence is related to the extent of the primary tumor and its location, which may determine the ability to obtain wide surgical margins with an acceptable cosmetic and functional outcome.

O'Brien and co-workers reported on 629 patients who received their entire treatment for head and neck melanomas at the Sydney Melanoma Unit between 1960 and 1990 [34]. The rates of local recurrence versus tumor thickness were: <0.76 mm, 2 %; 0.76–1.49 mm, 5 %; 1.5–3.99 mm, 15 %; and ≥4 mm, 20 %. Shen and colleagues reported on 197 patients with positive nodes treated surgically at the John Wayne Cancer Center between 1971 and 1998 [35]. The incidence of dermal relapse at the primary site was 24 %.

Incidence of Positive Sentinel Lymph Node Biopsy

Joseph and co-workers reported on 600 patients without regional or distant metastases who underwent SLNB at the H. Lee Moffitt Cancer Center (Tampa, FL) for melanomas arising in the head and neck (110 patients), trunk (246 patients), and extremities (244 patients). Sentinel lymph nodes were identified via technetium 99 (Tc99) lymphoscintography and blue dye [4]. The rates of positive SLNB vs. primary tumor thickness were: <0.76 mm, 0 of 15 patients (0 %); 0.76 to <1 mm, 5 of 83 patients (6 %); 1.0 to <1.5 mm, 12 of 169 patients (7 %); 1.5 to <4 mm, 48 of 267 patients (18 %); and ≥4 mm, 19 of 62 patients (30 %). McMasters and associates reported on SLNB in 961 patients with melanomas 1.0 mm or more in thickness who were enrolled in a multi-institutional study [6]. Sentinel lymph nodes were successfully identified in 99.7 % of patients and were then serial-sectioned and underwent immunohistochemical staining for S-100. Two hundred eight (21 %) of 961 patients had a positive SLNB. Multivariate analysis revealed that SLNB was more likely to be positive with increasing Breslow thickness ($p=0.0005$), ulceration ($p=0.0003$), Clark's level of 4 or more ($p=0.008$), and age ≤60 years ($p=0.008$). The rates of SLNB positivity vs. Breslow thickness are depicted in Table 1 for several selected series. Patients with a Breslow thickness of 1.5 mm or greater have a relatively high risk of positive sentinel lymph nodes.

Table 1 Primary depth of invasion versus sentinel lymph node biopsy (SLNB) positivity

		Depth of invasion (No. of patients)			
Series	Primary site	≤1 mm	1.01–2.00 mm	2.01–4.00 mm	>4.00 mm
Rousseau et al. [39], M.D. Anderson Hospital	Various	4 % (388)	12 % (522)	28 % (314)	44 % (151)
Emery et al. [40], University of Oregon	Various	2 % (41)	13 % (85)	20 % (35)	27 % (11)
Paek et al. [41], University of Michigan	Various	–	19 % (490)	32 % (301)	45 % (119)
Kruper et al. [42], University of Pennsylvania	Various	5 % (251)	10 % (228)	20 % (140)	38 % (63)
Leong et al. [43], Multicenter	Head and neck	3 % (134)	7 % (230)	21 % (160)	13 % (63)
Berk et al. [44], Stanford University	Various	0 % (45)	18 % (115)	19 % (64)	16 % (32)

Adapted from Mendenhall WM, Amdur RJ, Grobmyer SR, George TJ Jr, Werning JW, Hochwald SN, Mendenhall NP. Adjuvant radiotherapy for cutaneous melanoma. Cancer. 2008 Mar 15;112(6):1189–96

Table 2 Pathologically positive residual nodes in completion node dissection after positive sentinel lymph node biopsy (SLNB)

Series	No. of patients	Site	Percent positive residual nodes
Sabel et al. [45], University of Michigan	132	Inguinal	17
Pearlman et al. [37], University of Colorado	80	Various	21
Vuylsteke et al. [36], Vrije Universiteit	38	Various	24
Wagner et al. [9], Indiana University	53	Various	28

Adapted from Mendenhall WM, Amdur RJ, Grobmyer SR, George TJ Jr, Werning JW, Hochwald SN, Mendenhall NP. Adjuvant radiotherapy for cutaneous melanoma. Cancer. 2008 Mar 15;112(6):1189–96

The likelihood of nodal recurrence in a negative SLNB basin is relatively low. Vuylsteke and colleagues reported on 209 patients with stage I and II melanomas who underwent SLNB at the Vrije Universiteit between 1993 and 1996 [36]. SLNB was successful in 208 of 209 patients (99 %) and survivors were followed for 5 years. Four of 168 patients (2 %) with a negative SLNB recurred in the nodal basin and 11 patients (7 %) developed a local-regional dermal recurrence.

Incidence of Residual Positive Nodes in a Completion Node Dissection After a Positive SLNB

The likelihood of positive residual nodes after a positive SLNB probably ranges from 20 to 30 % (Table 2). Additionally, the likelihood of positive residual nodes may be related to the tumor burden detected in the sentinel lymph nodes. Pearlman and co-workers reported on 504 patients who underwent SLNB at the University of

Colorado (Denver) between 1996 and 2005 [37]. Ninety patients (18 %) had a positive SLNB and 80 of 90 patients underwent a completion node dissection; the remaining 10 patients declined further surgery. Additional positive nodes were detected in the completed dissection in 3 of 49 patients (6 %) with SLNB tumor deposits of ≤2 mm vs. 14 of 31 patients (45 %) with SLNB metastases >2 mm and/or extracapsular extension ($p<0.0001$).

Recent data suggest that patients who undergo an immediate completion node dissection after a positive SLNB may have improved survival compared with those who are observed. Morton and colleagues reported on 1,269 patients enrolled in the Multicenter Selective Lymphadenectomy Trial (MSLT-I) between 1994 and 2002 and followed for a median of 5 years [7]. Patients had either Clark's level III and Breslow thickness of 1 mm or more or Clark's level IV or V and any Breslow thickness. Patients underwent a wide local excision and were randomized to SLNB or observation; those with a positive SLNB were to undergo a completion node dissection. One hundred twenty two (16 %) of 764 patients randomized to SLNB had positive sentinel nodes. Patients with a positive SLNB who declined completion node dissection and were observed had a 52 % 5-year survival rate compared with 72 % in those who underwent the completion node dissection.

Incidence of Regional Recurrence in Patients with Positive Lymph Nodes

The likelihood of a regional recurrence in patients with positive nodes depends on the number of involved nodes, extracapsular extension, location of the metastases, whether the node dissection was therapeutic or elective, and length of follow-up [22, 23, 35]. The rates of regional recurrence after surgery for patients with positive nodes are depicted in Tables 3 and 4. Patients were generally treated with surgery alone; few, if any, received postoperative RT. The overall risk of a regional recurrence in the nodal basin is probably at least 20 % and increases with multiple positive nodes and/or extracapsular extension.

Adjuvant Radiotherapy

Bonnen and co-workers reported on 157 clinically N0 patients with head and neck melanomas who received resection of the primary lesion followed by postoperative elective neck irradiation (157 patients) alone or combined with RT to the primary site (154 patients) between 1983 and 1998 at the M.D. Anderson Cancer Center [33]. One hundred fifty-five of 157 patients had a primary tumor with a Breslow thickness of ≥1.5 mm or ≥Clark's level IV. Postoperative RT consisted of 30 Gy in 5 fractions over 2.5 weeks. The 10-year outcomes were: local control, 94 %; regional control, 89 %; local-regional control, 86 %; distant metastases-free survival, 49 %;

Table 3 Regional recurrence after node dissection for positive regional nodes

Series	Site	No. of patients	Follow-up	Regional recurrence (follow-up)
Pathak et al. [46], SWHSC	Head and neck	31	Mean, 45 months (range, 1–108 months)	31 % (5 years)
Meyer et al. [20], University of Erlangen	Various	140	Median, 20 months (range, 4–237 months)	34 %[a,b]
Hughes et al. [47], Royal Marsden Hospital	Inguinal	132	Median, 43 months[c] (range, 2–154 months)	Groin: 19 %[b] Pelvis: 6 %[b]
Kretschmer et al. [21], Martin Luther University	Inguinal	104	68 months[c] (range, 28–141 months)[c]	34 %[b]
Shen et al. [35], John Wayne Cancer Center	Head and neck	196	Median 20 months Median 32 months[c]	17 % (5 years)
Lee et al. [22], Roswell Park Memorial Institute	Various	338	Mean, 54 months (range, 12–306 months)	30 % (10 years)
O'Brien et al. [34], Sydney Melanoma Unit	Head and neck	386	NS	19 %[b]

Adapted from Mendenhall WM, Amdur RJ, Grobmyer SR, George TJ Jr, Werning JW, Hochwald SN, Mendenhall NP. Adjuvant radiotherapy for cutaneous melanoma. Cancer. 2008 Mar 15;112(6):1189–96

SWHSC Sunnybrook and Women's Health Sciences Center; *NS* not stated

[a]First site of recurrence

[b]Crude recurrence rate

[c]Follow-up on surviving patients

Table 4 Regional recurrence after node dissection for positive nodes

Series	No. of patients	Follow-up	Parameters	Regional recurrence (interval)	*p*-Value
Calabro et al. [23], M.D. Anderson Hospital	1,001	Minimum, 10 years[a]	*No. of positive nodes*		
			1	9 %[b]	
			2–4	15 %[b]	
			5–10	17 %[b]	≤0.05
			>10	33 %[b]	
			Matted	29 %[b]	
			Extracapsular extension		
			Absent	15 %[b]	
			Present	28 %[b]	<0.001
Lee et al. [22], Roswell Park Memorial Institute	338	Mean, 54 months (range, 12–306 months)	*No. of positive nodes*		
			1–3	25 %[b]	
			4–10	46 %[b]	0.0001
			>10	63 %[b]	
			Extracapsular extension		
			Absent	23 %[b]	
			Present	63 %[b]	<0.0001
			Site		
			Cervical	43 %[b]	
			Axillary	28 %[b]	0.0008
			Inguinal	23 %[b]	

Adapted from Mendenhall WM, Amdur RJ, Grobmyer SR, George TJ Jr, Werning JW, Hochwald SN, Mendenhall NP. Adjuvant radiotherapy for cutaneous melanoma. Cancer. 2008 Mar 15;112(6):1189–96

[a]Follow-up on surviving patients

[b]Crude recurrence rates

overall survival, 22 %; and cause-specific survival, 58 %. One patient sustained a severe complication which was a temporal lobe necrosis.

Ballo and colleagues reported on 36 patients with head and neck melanomas who presented synchronous (20 patients) or metachronous (16 patients) positive cervical nodes between 1983 and 2003 at the M.D. Anderson Cancer Center [30]. Patients underwent limited excision of the clinically positive node(s) followed by postoperative RT (30 Gy/5 fractions/2.5 weeks). Patients had 1–3 positive nodes (median, 1); the size of the involved nodes ranged from 0.6 to 6 cm (median, 2 cm). Nine patients (25 %) had extracapsular extension. Postoperative RT consisted of 30 Gy/5 fractions/2.5 weeks: follow-up on survivors ranged from 2.9 to 243 months (median, 63 months). The 5-year outcomes were: regional control, 93 %; distant metastases-free survival 59 %; disease-free survival, 59 %; and cause-specific survival, 69 %. One patient developed a severe complication which was a mandibular osteoradionecrosis after a dental extraction that necessitated hyperbaric oxygen treatments.

Stevens and co-workers reported on 174 patients with stage I-III melanoma treated with surgery and postoperative RT to the primary site (35 patients) or positive regional nodes (139 patients) at the Royal Prince Alfred Hospital between 1989 and 1998 [32]. Indications for RT to the primary site included close or positive margins, neurotropic desmoplastic melanoma, recurrence with perineural invasion, tumor satellites, and/or early or multiple recurrences. Postoperative RT consisted of 30–36 Gy in 5–7 fractions over 2.5 weeks. Infield local control was obtained in 154 patients (89 %) and the 5-year survival rate was 41 %. O'Brien and colleagues reported on 143 patients with melanoma metastases to the parotid and/or cervical nodes who were treated with surgery alone (107 patients) or combined with postoperative RT (36 patients) at the Royal Prince Alfred Hospital between 1987 and 1995 [31]. Patients treated with postoperative RT tended to have more advanced lesions (≥2 positive nodes, 65 %; extracapsular extension, 48 %) compared with surgery alone (≥2 positive nodes, 40 %; extracapsular extension, 19 %). Regional control was achieved in 94 % after surgery and postoperative RT compared with 81 % after surgery alone ($p=0.005$). Multivariate analysis revealed that postoperative RT was associated with a trend towards improved regional control ($p=0.065$) but not survival.

Burmeister and colleagues reported on two prospective trials conducted by the Trans-Tasman Radiation Oncology Group (TROG) that included 234 node-positive melanoma patients who underwent node dissection and postoperative RT [27]. Sites included the head and neck, 77 patients; axilla, 109 patients; and ilioinguinal, 48 patients. RT consisted of approximately 48 Gy in 20 fractions. One hundred seventy-six patients (75 %) had extracapsular extension and 164 patients (70 %) had 2 or more positive nodes. Median follow-up was 58 months (range, 21–158 months); 2 patients were lost to follow-up. The 5-year outcomes were: regional control, 91 %; progression-free survival, 27 %; and overall survival, 36 %. The most significant late complication was grade 3 lymphedema which was not observed in any head and neck patients, 9 of 109 (8 %) axillary patients, and 19 of 48 (40 %) ilioinguinal patients.

Chang and co-workers reported on 56 patients who were at high risk for a local-regional recurrence who were treated with surgery and postoperative RT at the University of Florida between 1980 and 2004 [19]. High risk was determined by

Table 5 Outcomes after surgery and postoperative radiotherapy at the M.D. Anderson Cancer Center for node positive melanoma patients

Series	No. of patients	Site	Follow-up[a]	RC[b]	DMFS[b]	Survival[b]
Ballo et al. [29], 2003	160	Cervical	Median, 78 months (range, 6–224 months)	94 % (10 years)	43 % (10 years)	CSS = 48 % (10 years)
Ballo et al. [30], 2002	89	Axilla	Median, 58 months (range, 7–159 months)	87 % (5 years)	49 % (5 years)	OS = 50 % (5 years)
Ballo et al. [28], 2004	40	Ilioinguinal	Median, 23 months (range, 4–107 months)	74 % (3 years)	35 % (3 years)	OS = 38 % (3 years)

Adapted from Mendenhall WM, Amdur RJ, Grobmyer SR, George TJ Jr, Werning JW, Hochwald SN, Mendenhall NP. Adjuvant radiotherapy for cutaneous melanoma. Cancer. 2008 Mar 15;112(6):1189–96
RC regional control; *DMFS* distant metastasis-free survival; *CSS* cause-specific survival; *OS* overall survival
[a]Follow-up for surviving patients
[b]Outcome (interval)

gross residual disease, close or positive margins, disease recurrence, in-transit metastases, and/or regional node metastases. Sites included the head and neck, 49 patients; axilla, 3 patients; upper torso, 2 patients; inguinal, 1 patient; and upper extremity, 1 patient. Forty one patients were treated with hypofractionation (30 Gy/5 fractions/2.5 weeks) and 15 patients with conventional fractionation. Fourteen patients were treated once daily to a median dose of 60 Gy (range, 50–70 Gy) at a median 2 Gy per fraction. One patient was treated twice daily to 74.4 Gy in 62 fractions. Median follow-up on survivors was 4.4 years (range, 0.6–14.4 years). Five-year outcomes were: infield local-regional control, 87 %; freedom from distant metastases, 43 %; cause-specific survival, 57 %; and overall survival, 46 %. Fractionation schedule did not significantly impact infield local-regional control. Two patients (4 %) experienced severe late complications that included temporal bone osteoradionecrosis and a partial brachial plexopathy; both were treated with hypofractionated RT.

Some of the largest published series of postoperative RT for node-positive melanoma patients are from the M.D. Anderson Cancer Center (Table 5). RT consisted of a hypofractionated regimen consisting of 30 Gy in 5 fractions over 2.5 weeks. The highest regional control rates are for patients irradiated for head and neck melanomas whereas the lowest are for those irradiated for ilioinguinal disease. The main late complication was lymphedema, which was observed more often in patients treated for ilioinguinal or axillary disease compared with those who receive head and neck RT. The 5-year rates of arm edema in 89 patients who received axillary RT were: grade 2 (requiring medical intervention), 19 %; and grade 3 (requiring surgical intervention), 1 % [38]. Although 15 of 40 (38 %) patients had lymphedema after ilioinguinal RT, 7 of 15 patients had lymphedema prior to irradiation [28]. In contrast, only 9 of 160 patients (6 %) treated for head and neck melanomas had a grade 2 complication and no patients had a severe (grade 3) complication [29].

Conclusion

Postoperative RT likely improves local-regional control in patients at high risk for relapse after surgery. This includes patients with close ($\leq$1 cm) or positive margins at the primary site who are not suitable for reexcision as well as those with locally recurrent disease at the primary site. In addition, it includes patients with multiple positive nodes or extracapsular extension following node dissection. Wider margins are likely necessary for desmoplastic neurotropic melanoma; it is unclear whether postoperative RT should be routinely administered for this histology. Adjuvant RT is associated with good regional nodal control, particularly in the head and neck, and may be considered in patients with clinically negative nodes in lieu of an elective node dissection. It is unlikely that postoperative RT significantly improves survival. The vast majority of the reported experiences with adjuvant RT has been with hypofractionated treatment schedules, such as those employed at the M.D. Anderson Cancer Center and the Royal Prince Alfred Hospital. These appear to be safe and effective, requiring little time to deliver relative to adjuvant immunotherapy. Hypofractionation schedules are particularly attractive for patients who are at high risk for hematogenous dissemination and may be candidates for adjuvant systemic therapy after completion of local-regional treatment. Patients who require adjuvant RT to sites where cosmesis may be an issue as well as those who require a large volume of tissue to be irradiated may benefit from conventionally fractionated RT.

References

1. Monsour PD, Sause WT, Avent JM, Noyes RD. Local control following therapeutic nodal dissection for melanoma. J Surg Oncol. 1993;54:18–22.
2. Carlson GW, Murray DR, Greenlee R, Alazraki N, Fry-Spray C, Poole R, et al. Management of malignant melanoma of the head and neck using dynamic lymphoscintigraphy and gamma probe-guided sentinel lymph node biopsy. Arch Otolaryngol Head Neck Surg. 2000;126:433–7.
3. Krag DN, Meijer SJ, Weaver DL, Loggie BW, Harlow SP, Tanabe KK, et al. Minimal-access surgery for staging of malignant melanoma. Arch Surg. 1995;130:654–8.
4. Joseph E, Brobeil A, Glass F, Glss J, Messina J, DeConti R, et al. Results of complete lymph node dissection in 83 melanoma patients with positive sentinel nodes. Ann Surg Oncol. 1998;5:119–25.
5. Statius Muller MG, Borgstein PJ, Pijpers R, van Leeuwen PA, van Diest PJ, Gupta A, et al. Reliability of the sentinel node procedure in melanoma patients: analysis of failures after long-term follow-up. Ann SurgOncol. 2000;7:461–8.
6. McMasters KM, Wong SL, Edwards MJ, Ross MI, Chao C, Noyes RD, et al. Factors that predict the presence of sentinel lymph node metastasis in patients with melanoma. Surgery. 2001;130:151–6.
7. Morton DL, Thompson JF, Cochran AJ, Mozzillo N, Elashoff R, Essner R, et al. Sentinel-node biopsy or nodal observation in melanoma. N Engl J Med. 2006;355:1307–17.
8. Wagner JD, Park HM, Coleman III JJ, Love C, Hayes JT. Cervical sentinel lymph node biopsy for melanomas of the head and neck and upper thorax. Arch Otolaryngol Head Neck Surg. 2000;126:313–21.

9. Wagner JD, Gordon MS, Chuang TY, Coleman III JJ, Hayes JT, Jung SH, et al. Predicting sentinel and residual lymph node basin disease after sentinel lymph node biopsy for melanoma. Cancer. 2000;89:453–62.
10. Kane M, McClay E, Bellet RE. Frequency of occult residual melanoma after excision of a clinically positive regional lymph node. Ann Surg. 1987;205:88–9.
11. O'Brien CJ, McNeil EB, McMahon JD, Pathak I, Lauer CS. Incidence of cervical node involvement in metastatic cutaneous malignancy involving the parotid gland. Head Neck. 2001;23:744–8.
12. Karakousis CP, Rizos S, Driscoll DL. Residual nodal disease after excisional biopsy of a palpable, positive node in melanoma. Am J Surg. 1994;168:69–70.
13. Anderson TD, Weber RS, Guerry D, Elder D, Schuchter L, Loevner LA, et al. Desmoplastic neurotropic melanoma of the head and neck: the role of radiation therapy. Head Neck. 2002;24:1068–71.
14. Bastiaannet E, Beukema JC, Hoekstra HJ. Radiation therapy following lymph node dissection in melanoma patients: treatment, outcome and complications. Cancer Treat Rev. 2005; 31:18–26.
15. Kavanagh D, Hill AD, Djikstra B, Kennelly R, McDermott EM, O'Higgins NJ. Adjuvant therapies in the treatment of stage II and III malignant melanoma. Surgeon. 2005;3:245–56.
16. Fuhrmann D, Lippold A, Borrosch F, Ellwanger U, Garbe C, Suter L. Should adjuvant radiotherapy be recommended following resection of regional lymph node metastases of malignant melanomas? Br J Dermatol. 2001;144:66–70.
17. American Joint Committee on Cancer. Melanoma of the skin. In: Edge SB, Byrd DR, Compton CC, Fritz P, Greene FL, Trotti A, editors. AJCC cancer staging handbook. New York: Springer; 2010. p. 387–415.
18. Mendenhall WM, Amdur RJ, Hinerman RW, Werning JW, Villaret DB, Mendenhall NP. Head and neck mucosal melanoma. Am J Clin Oncol. 2005;28:626–30.
19. Chang DT, Amdur RJ, Morris CG, Mendenhall WM. Adjuvant radiotherapy for cutaneous melanoma: comparing hypofractionation to conventional fractionation. Int J Radiat Oncol Biol Phys. 2006;66:1051–5.
20. Meyer T, Merkel S, Gohl J, Hohenberger W. Lymph node dissection for clinically evident lymph node metastases of malignant melanoma. Eur J Surg Oncol. 2002;28:424–30.
21. Kretschmer L, Neumann C, Preusser KP, Marsch WC. Superficial inguinal and radical ilioinguinal lymph node dissection in patients with palpable melanoma metastases to the groin–an analysis of survival and local recurrence. Acta Oncol. 2001;40:72–8.
22. Lee RJ, Gibbs JF, Proulx GM, Kollmorgen DR, Jia C, Kraybill WG. Nodal basin recurrence following lymph node dissection for melanoma: implications for adjuvant radiotherapy. Int J Radiat Oncol Biol Phys. 2000;46:467–74.
23. Calabro A, Singletary SE, Balch CM. Patterns of relapse in 1001 consecutive patients with melanoma nodal metastases. Arch Surg. 1989;124:1051–5.
24. Gyorki DE, Ainslie J, Joon ML, Henderson MA, Millward M, McArthur GA. Concurrent adjuvant radiotherapy and interferon-alpha2b for resected high risk stage III melanoma—a retrospective single centre study. Melanoma Res. 2004;14:223–30.
25. Vongtama R, Safa A, Gallardo D, Calcaterra T, Juillard G. Efficacy of radiation therapy in the local control of desmoplastic malignant melanoma. Head Neck. 2003;25:423–8.
26. Bron LP, Traynor SJ, McNeil EB, O'Brien CJ. Primary and metastatic cancer of the parotid: comparison of clinical behavior in 232 cases. Laryngoscope. 2003;113:1070–5.
27. Burmeister BH, Mark SB, Burmeister E, Baumann K, Davis S, Krawitz H, et al. A prospective phase II study of adjuvant postoperative radiation therapy following nodal surgery in malignant melanoma-Trans Tasman Radiation Oncology Group (TROG) Study 96.06. Radiother Oncol. 2006;81:136–42.
28. Ballo MT, Zagars GK, Gershenwald JE, Lee JE, Mansfield PF, Kim KB, et al. A critical assessment of adjuvant radiotherapy for inguinal lymph node metastases from melanoma. Ann SurgOncol. 2004;11:1079–84.

29. Ballo MT, Bonnen MD, Garden AS, Myers JN, Gershenwald JE, Zagars GK, et al. Adjuvant irradiation for cervical lymph node metastases from melanoma. Cancer. 2003;97:1789–96.
30. Ballo MT, Garden AS, Myers JN, Lee JE, Diaz Jr EM, Sturgis EM, et al. Melanoma metastatic to cervical lymph nodes: can radiotherapy replace formal dissection after local excision of nodal disease? Head Neck. 2005;27:718–21.
31. O'Brien CJ, Petersen-Schaefer K, Stevens GN, Bass PC, Tew P, Gebski VJ, et al. Adjuvant radiotherapy following neck dissection and parotidectomy for metastatic malignant melanoma. Head Neck. 1997;19:589–94.
32. Stevens G, Thompson JF, Firth I, O'Brien CJ, McCarthy WH, Quinn MJ. Locally advanced melanoma: results of postoperative hypofractionated radiation therapy. Cancer. 2000;88: 88–94.
33. Bonnen MD, Ballo MT, Myers JN, Garden AS, Diaz Jr EM, Gershenwald JE, et al. Elective radiotherapy provides regional control for patients with cutaneous melanoma of the head and neck. Cancer. 2004;100:383–9.
34. O'Brien CJ, Coates AS, Petersen-Schaefer K, Shannon K, Thompson JF, Milton GW, et al. Experience with 998 cutaneous melanomas of the head and neck over 30 years. Am J Surg. 1991;162:310–4.
35. Shen P, Wanek LA, Morton DL. Is adjuvant radiotherapy necessary after positive lymph node dissection in head and neck melanomas? Ann SurgOncol. 2000;7:554–9.
36. Vuylsteke RJ, van Leeuwen PA, Statius Muller MG, Gietema HA, Kragt DR, Meijer S. Clinical outcome of stage I/II melanoma patients after selective sentinel lymph node dissection: long-term follow-up results. J Clin Oncol. 2003;21:1057–65.
37. Pearlman NW, McCarter MD, Frank M, Hurtubis C, Merkow RP, Franklin WA, et al. Size of sentinel node metastases predicts other nodal disease and survival in malignant melanoma. Am J Surg. 2006;192:878–81.
38. Ballo MT, Strom EA, Zagars GK, Bedikian AY, Prieto VG, Mansfield PF, et al. Adjuvant irradiation for axillary metastases from malignant melanoma. Int J Radiat Oncol Biol Phys. 2002;52:964–72.
39. Rousseau Jr DL, Ross MI, Johnson MM, Prieto VG, Lee JE, Mansfield PF, et al. Revised American Joint Committee on Cancer staging criteria accurately predict sentinel lymph node positivity in clinically node-negative melanoma patients. Ann SurgOncol. 2003;10:569–74.
40. Emery RE, Stevens JS, Nance RW, Corless CL, Vetto JT. Sentinel node staging of primary melanoma by the "10% rule": pathology and clinical outcomes. Am J Surg. 2007;193: 618–22.
41. Paek SC, Griffith KA, Johnson TM, Sondak VK, Wong SL, Chang AE, et al. The impact of factors beyond Breslow depth on predicting sentinel lymph node positivity in melanoma. Cancer. 2007;109:100–8.
42. Kruper LL, Spitz FR, Czerniecki BJ, Fraker DL, Blackwood-Chirchir A, Ming ME, et al. Predicting sentinel node status in AJCC stage I/II primary cutaneous melanoma. Cancer. 2006;107:2436–45.
43. Leong SP, Accortt NA, Essner R, Ross M, Gershenwald JE, Pockaj B, et al. Impact of sentinel node status and other risk factors on the clinical outcome of head and neck melanoma patients. Archives of Otolaryngology–Head and Neck. Surgery. 2006;132:370–3.
44. Berk DR, Johnson DL, Uzieblo A, Kiernan M, Swetter SM. Sentinel lymph node biopsy for cutaneous melanoma: the Stanford experience, 1997–2004. Arch Dermatol. 2005;141:1016–22.
45. Sabel MS, Griffith KA, Arora A, Shargorodsky J, Blazer III DG, Rees R, et al. Inguinal node dissection for melanoma in the era of sentinel lymph node biopsy. Surgery. 2007;141: 728–35.
46. Pathak I, Gilbert R, Yoo J, Hilton M. Outcome of neck dissection for node-positive melanoma. J Otolaryngol. 2002;31:147–9.
47. Hughes TM, A'Hern RP, Thomas JM. Prognosis and surgical management of patients with palpable inguinal lymph node metastases from melanoma. Br J Surg. 2000;87:892–901.

Getting Started in Superficial Radiation for the Dermatology Practice

David E. Kent

Introduction

Management of nonmelanoma skin cancer (NMSC) is routinely performed by dermatologist and nondermatologist's practices in both an office setting and outpatient surgery centers. Traditional treatment options include surgical (excision with and without frozen section evaluation, Mohs surgery, curettage, and electrodesiccation) and nonsurgical options (topical therapies and radiation therapy).

Many patients that present for management of NMSC are candidates for nonsurgical treatment with radiation. Up to this point, radiation centers using linear accelerators with electrons delivered in a concrete bunker have been the primary option. Those patients with poor health who may be elderly and frail, or who want to avoid potential scarring are prime candidates for superficial X-ray therapy. As noted, dermatologists were at the forefront of utilizing ionizing radiation for NMSC with superficial X-ray machines. They have been involved with delivering superficial X-ray treatments for over one century. Until recently, there have been few if any options for purchasing new updated equipment for providing this service in an office setting safely and efficiently. Superficial X-ray therapy for NMSC in dermatology offices was limited to machines that were dated and at times temperamental.

Now with the availability of updated new superficial X-ray machines, the supply issue is solved. Making the decision to provide superficial X-ray for treatment of NMSC rests on the dermatologist's ability to critically examine their practice's suitability for this service. The following discussion is aimed to assist the dermatologists at examining their practice for suitability in adding this modality for managing NMSC. It is important to note from the onset that the patients who will receive superficial X-ray will comprise a minority of NMSC patients. Patient selection is

D.E. Kent (✉)
Dermatologic Surgery Specialists, PC, 308 Coliseum Drive #200, Macon, GA 31217, USA
e-mail: dekent@dsspc.com

A.B. Cognetta and W.M. Mendenhall (eds.), *Radiation Therapy for Skin Cancer*,
DOI 10.1007/978-1-4614-6986-5_20, © Springer Science+Business Media New York 2013

key just as it is in all fields of medicine. Our discussion will transit the physician through the stages necessary for considering "getting started" with superficial X-ray. The main steps involved in this process include: planning, purchase, implementation, regulatory issues including potential outside negative forces, staff and physician training, and all supporting educational information and documentation forms.

Planning

In the planning stage of assessing a medical practice's suitability for adding superficial X-ray, the physician or practice administrator must critically look at several key questions:

1. Does the practice have a volume of skin cancer patients who will fit the profile of the "ideal candidate" for superficial X-ray?
2. What lesional criteria are necessary in order to be considered for superficial X-ray? What will we treat and what will we not treat?
3. Does the physician and practice currently specialize in managing a wide range of NMSC? Or, is the practice geared toward managing only a narrow patient profile for NMSC or more focused on other aspects of dermatological care including cosmetic services?
4. Does the practice have sufficient space that is appropriately located and accessible?
5. Is the practice committed to adding the personnel required?
6. Is the physician willing to commit to becoming expert in all phases of superficial X-ray therapy for their patients? This will require training or retraining in areas that include radiation biology and physics. Many of us have had didactic training in our residency or through the AAD annual meeting. Some of us have been "exposed" to radiation by our older colleagues or while in training.
7. Does your practice have access to capital for purchase or lease and will it be a financial burden that could choke off cash flow that all businesses rely on for stability and health?
8. Does it make economic sense to add this service; what would be a realistic return on investment (ROI)?
9. Will this service be dependent on a single physician being present each and every day or additional physicians and providers to evaluate patients who present assessment for their daily treatment in case a question or other issue arises?
10. Are there any regulatory issues in one's state that would be difficult to satisfy such as a Certificate of Need (CON)? Can one anticipate any resistance to your practice providing this service?
11. What options for superficial X-ray are currently available in your community?
12. Can the treatments be delivered efficiently without having the patients wait?

Let us examine the above questions individually.

1 and 2. The ideal candidate should satisfy the following criteria:

- Age—greater than 65 unless special circumstances are present. Patients younger than 65 that have a longer life expectancy and will have more time to potentially develop chronic radiation changes to the treatment site. For example, we have treated a patient less than age 60; however, they had a profoundly serious constellation of medical problems including severe cardiovascular disease, CHF, ICD, diabetes, on three different blood thinners, and had several lesions present. These multiple facial lesions could be treated concurrently.
- Lesion diagnosis—basal cell and squamous cell carcinomas should not have aggressive histology. Sclerosing, metatypical, or infiltrative BCC lesions should not be selected for superficial X-ray therapy. Infiltrative, aggressive growth SCCs should be avoided. Lesions with perineural involvement should be avoided. Only primary lesions should be selected for treatment. If a patient is not a surgical candidate and has an aggressive histologic lesion, then they should be considered for treatment in a linear accelerator with electrons.
- Location—primarily the head and neck with extreme care for lesions on the lids and external ear. Ideal locations include the cheeks, forehead, temples, nose, and neck.

3. *Practice mix*. Those practices that have multiple providers, specialize in managing NMSC, have multiple office locations, see a wide range of patients, or serve as a regional referral center for skin managing NMSC such as a multispecialty group or a large single specialty practice are well suited to provide superficial X-ray. Alternatively, a smaller practice with fewer patients, or a practice geared toward medical dermatology or focused on cosmetics may lack sufficient patient volume to choose the proper candidates for this service.
4. *Appropriate space*. Specific criteria are necessary:

- Size—a treatment room must be large enough to have a power treatment table and X-ray machine as well as the necessary cabinetry for fashioning shielding supplies, etc.
- Leaded glass window for direct observation of the patient while treatment is being delivered.
- Audio intercom to directly communicate with the patient at all times.
- Positioning of the treatment room—ideally should be close to or adjacent to the pod of rooms the physician responsible for supervising treatments is located. This will reduce unnecessary steps and delays for all parties and improve office efficiency.
- Perimeter room on outside wall is preferable away from high patient traffic flow.
- A trained physicist can scrutinize the room selected for necessary shielding with lead.

5. *Personnel.* Required placements include:
   - Treatment technician. Radiology technicians are well suited as they have received basic training in radiation biology and physics. This individual is a key hire and should possess solid communication skills, have a commitment to excellence, have an eye for precise detail, and be extremely dependable. Sources for these positions are regional technical colleges, schools, or university medical centers with training programs. Frequently these educational institutions have placement services. Be sure to carefully screen the top candidates of the class.
   - Nontechnical operational support in the business office to ensure proper coding and keeping up to date with other issues such as regulatory issues, safety badges, etc. These duties do not require a full time equivalent employee just for this job.
6. *Physician commitment to becoming expert in superficial X-ray treatments.* Most training programs have lectures in radiation biology that deal with superficial X-ray. In many cases, the physician may have to review and relearn the details necessary to provide these services. After all, the physician under the learned intermediary doctrine is ultimately responsible for each phase of treatment including patient selection; dosimetry, treatment safety, and patient followup. This database is manageable and should not pose as a hurdle that cannot be mastered. The treatment team including the treatment technologist who will be generating the initial treatment plans for your review must receive adequate expert training. These training centers are few in number currently. A direct observational visit to one of these centers for physician and treating technologist is mandatory.
7. *Access to capital.* The business side of adding a service that is capital intensive when you take in all aspects of adding superficial X-ray. These include purchase cost, room preparation, personnel required, and regulatory inspections. This can easily top $200,000. Therefore, consideration of purchase or lease should be reviewed with the practice business advisor, CPA, and be absolutely sure it fits with the business model of the practice and it "makes sense." Larger single specialty practices and multispecialty practices are more likely to be able to absorb the up front capital costs and generate enough patients for appropriate use to become cash flow positive as soon as possible. The provider must remember that this service is suitable for a specific, defined patient profile, and most likely not the majority of patients that present for treatment of NMSC.
8. *Return on investment.* Again, larger practices will see a more brisk population of the appropriate patients that will bring that practice to a cash flow positive position much sooner than smaller practices.
9. *Physician oversight.* A physician or practitioner or qualified technician should see each patient each time a treatment is delivered. This can be a brief encounter to quickly assess the patient's response to treatment. Practices with multiple physicians and providers will be better equipped to share the supervisory duties and responsibilities day to day than practices with few providers that cannot satisfy this requirement. If a physician works less than a full week, it may reduce the flexibility of dosing schedules that can be offered patients. We as physicians must always remember: we can delegate duties but we cannot delegate responsibilities.

10. *Regulatory issues*. Strict regulations are in place in each state for delivering superficial X-ray services whether they be diagnostic or in our case therapeutic. These regulations are for the most part very straightforward and can be satisfied with due diligence. The secretary of state's office will provide you with a list of regulatory requirements. Fortunately, the manufacturer of this equipment along with independent professional physicists can successfully assist the practice to satisfy each and every requirement.
11. *Available services for radiation treatment for NMSC in your community*. One must carefully evaluate the options for treatment currently available. It is possible to receive resistance to your delivering this service in your community. It is unlikely to come from other dermatologists rather from more traditional centers of radiation therapy. While the coexistence of both radiation centers and dermatologists who provide superficial X-ray treatments seems logical, it is possible for some centers to feel some degree of threat or competition. Attempts to quash a dermatologist providing this service could come in the form of attempted regulatory hurdles typically reserved for linear accelerators in traditional radiation centers. These circumstances can prove taxing and require legal representation and the aid of dermatologists who are expert in the field of delivering superficial X-ray treatments. After all, the radiation delivered is very similar to a dental X-ray. Our practice had such an experience. Fortunately, we were able to prevail with a common sense approach with expert documentation and assistance from our dermatology colleagues.
12. *Successful delivery of superficial services in a timely, efficient manner*. To ensure that this service is provided in a manner that is safe, effective, and efficient, it will be necessary to develop appropriate supporting paperwork for documentation at each phase of the process. This includes: patient education materials; consultation flow sheets to be sure complete informed consent is discussed; details of each phase of treatment; a schedule of appointments; photos of patients who have completed treatment; and reassurance that if a patient needs assistance after hours they will have definite access.

Implementation

Once appropriate planning and due diligence have been performed as outlined above and you have purchased your treatment machine, staff has been hired and all are trained, regulatory issues have been satisfied, and all paperwork has been generated, you are ready to implement actual treatments. Prior to scheduling the first patient for treatment, you must carefully introduce this modality to the entire office and practice group. This will most likely require a series of sessions explaining the how, why, where, and who you want to treat. Safety concerns, especially women of childbearing age or pregnant employees, must be addressed and plans for them put in place. Careful statistics in the form of a treatment log detailing all patients treated should be carefully updated in real time. Routine followup for identification of any adverse event, signs of recurrence, and patient satisfaction should be documented.

Patient simulations and actual trial patient treatments should be performed until the entire team is comfortable with providing the services. Once you have successfully implemented this service into your practice, you will be ready to let potential referral sources know about your center. To this point, marketing pieces geared toward education can be prepared and personally distributed to area dermatologists and nondermatologists alike.

I would like to at this time recognize my friend and mentor in superficial X-ray therapy for NMSC: Dr. Armand Cognetta in Tallahassee, Florida. It is because of his extreme generosity, teaching, commitment to excellence, ethics, and patience that we are able to provide superficial X-ray therapy for our patients.

Index

A.B. Cognetta and W. Mendenhall (eds.), *Radiation Therapy for Skin Cancer*, DOI 10.1007/978-1-4614-6986-5,

MIX
Papier aus verantwortungsvollen Quellen
Paper from responsible sources
FSC® C105338

If you have any concerns about our products,
you can contact us on
ProductSafety@springernature.com

In case Publisher is established outside the EU,
the EU authorized representative is:
Springer Nature Customer Service Center GmbH
Europaplatz 3, 69115 Heidelberg, Germany

Printed by Libri Plureos GmbH
in Hamburg, Germany